W0112657

MEDICINAL PLANTS

MEDICINAL PLANTS

Mr. E. Edwin Jarald

M.Pharm, IDCRCT (Ph.D)
Reader, Department of Pharmacognosy
B.R.Nahata College of Pharmacy &
BRNSS Contract research Center
Mandsaur-458001 (M.P)

Mrs. Sheeja Edwin Jarald

M.Pharm, IDCRCT (Ph.D)
Principal (Diploma) & Sr. Lecturer
B.R.Nahata College of Pharmacy &
BRNSS Contract research Center
Mandsaur-458001 (M.P)

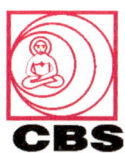

CBS

CBS PUBLISHERS & DISTRIBUTORS PVT. LTD.

New Delhi • Bengaluru • Pune • Kochi • Chennai

Dedicated
To Our
Loving Parents and God

ISBN : 81-239-1360-5

First Edition : 2006
Reprint : 2012

Copyright © Authors & Publisher

All rights reserved. No part of this book may be reproduced or transmitted in any form or by any means, electronic or mechanical, including photocopying, recording, or any information storage and retrieval system without permission, in writing, from the publisher.

Published by Satish Kumar Jain and produced by V.K. Jain for
CBS Publishers & Distributors Pvt. Ltd.,
CBS Plaza, 4819/XI Prahlad Street, 24 Ansari Road, Daryaganj,
New Delhi - 110002, India.   • Website: www.cbspd.com
e-mail: delhi@cbspd.com, cbspubs@airtelmail.in
Ph.: 23289259, 23266861, 23266867   • Fax: 011-23243014

Branches:
• *Bengaluru:* Seema House, 2975, 17th Cross, K.R. Road,
  Bansankari 2nd Stage, Bengaluru - 560070   Ph.: +91-80-26771678/79
  • E-mail: cbsbng@gmail.com, bangalore@cbspd.com
• *Pune:* Bhuruk Prestige, Sr. No. 52/12/2+1+3/2,
  Narhe, Haveli (Near Katraj-Dehu Road By-pass), Pune - 411051
  Ph.: +91-20-64704058/59, 32342277   • E-mail: pune@cbspd.com
• *Kochi:* 36/14, Kalluvilakam, Lissie Hospital Road,
  Kochi - 682018, Kerala • Ph.: +91-484-4059061-65
  Fax: +91-484-4059065   • E-mail: cochin@cbspd.com
• *Chennai:* 20, West Park Road, Shenoy Nagar, Chennai - 600030
  Ph.: +91-44-26260666, 26208620   E-mail: chennai@cbspd.com

Printed at : Dynamic Print Grafix, Delhi

Foreword

It gives me immense pleasure to write a foreword to the "Medicinal Plants" authored by Mr. E. Edwin Jarald and Mrs. Sheeja Edwin Jarald. This book provides collective information for more than 130 plants widely occurring in our country. This book is an outcome of a vast practical study and experience by the authors from different part of the country.

Among the entire flora, 35,000 to 70,000 species have been used for medicinal purposes. Herbs have proved its medicinal value, since the existence of medicine and mankind. Among the important plant derived drugs used in one or more countries, 77% were regarded as having been discovered as a result of plants from traditional medicine. Our country has a collection of a vast variety of plants and the proper identification of these plants is very vital tool towards the development of a new drug in today's competitive field of medicine.

The book provides information regarding the vernacular names, botanical name, family, constituents, uses, botanical classification and photos of plants, which would be very useful for the researchers, teachers and students of several field related to plant sciences and even to traditional medical practitioners.

The authors Mr. E. Edwin Jarald and Mrs. Sheeja Edwin Jarald deserve appreciation and I congratulate them for bringing out such an extremely interesting and useful book at an early stage of their career.

Dr. V.B. Gupta
Director,
B.R. Nahata College of Pharmacy &
BRNSS Contract Research Center
Mandsaur 458001, M.P.

Date : 20/1-/05

Place: Mandsaur

Preface

Natural products from the medicinal plant source are the main cast of modern drug in clinical use. Herbs are used by man from the beginning of human culture as a source of medicine. For the maintenance of good health majority of the population of the world are turning towards natural products. WHO estimates that more than 80 % of the world's population relies on plants as the primary medicinal source for the treatment of common illness. People not only use herbs as medicines but also as food and cosmetics.

Though most of the people whose studies are related to plant sciences have knowledge regarding medicinal plants, they lack in identifying the plants and they easily get confused regarding the different species of a same genus or else to identify a well-known plant by its botanical name. This book not only serves for the students, faculties of technical courses but also for vaidyas and hakims who could make use of this book by its photographs in communicating their ideas.

We have attempted to bring together many herbs along with their photos and botanical classification that could be a useful tool for the students and researchers in several disciplines of sciences.

E. EDWIN JARALD
SHEEJA EDWIN JARALD

Acknowledgement

We are delighted to acknowledge some of the organizations and individuals for their support in completing this work.

First and foremost we would like to thank Mr. Rahul Nahata who had sown the idea of writing a book in our minds. Our heartfelt thanks to the management for the encouragement rendered to us from the beginning of this work and for providing all the needful facilities to carry out this work.

We gratefully acknowledge the Director of our college, Dr. V. B. Gupta, the head and staff of KNK College of Horticulture, Mandsaur for extending their cooperation. We thank Dr. A. Amal Raj for being an inspiration.

Special thanks to our students Mr Vaibhav Tiwari and Mr Emmanual Toppo for helping us during this period. We also extend our acknowledgement to our colleagues especially Ms Smita Gupta and the other faculties for their encouragement and help provided by them.

Not the least, we would like to thank our father Dr. G. Elias, (Siddha Medical practitioner) without whom this work could never be completed.

Before closing the ritual of acknowledgement we earnestly invite your valuable suggestions for the book, so that we could come with another better edition later on.

Contents

NOTE

Abrus precatorius Linn

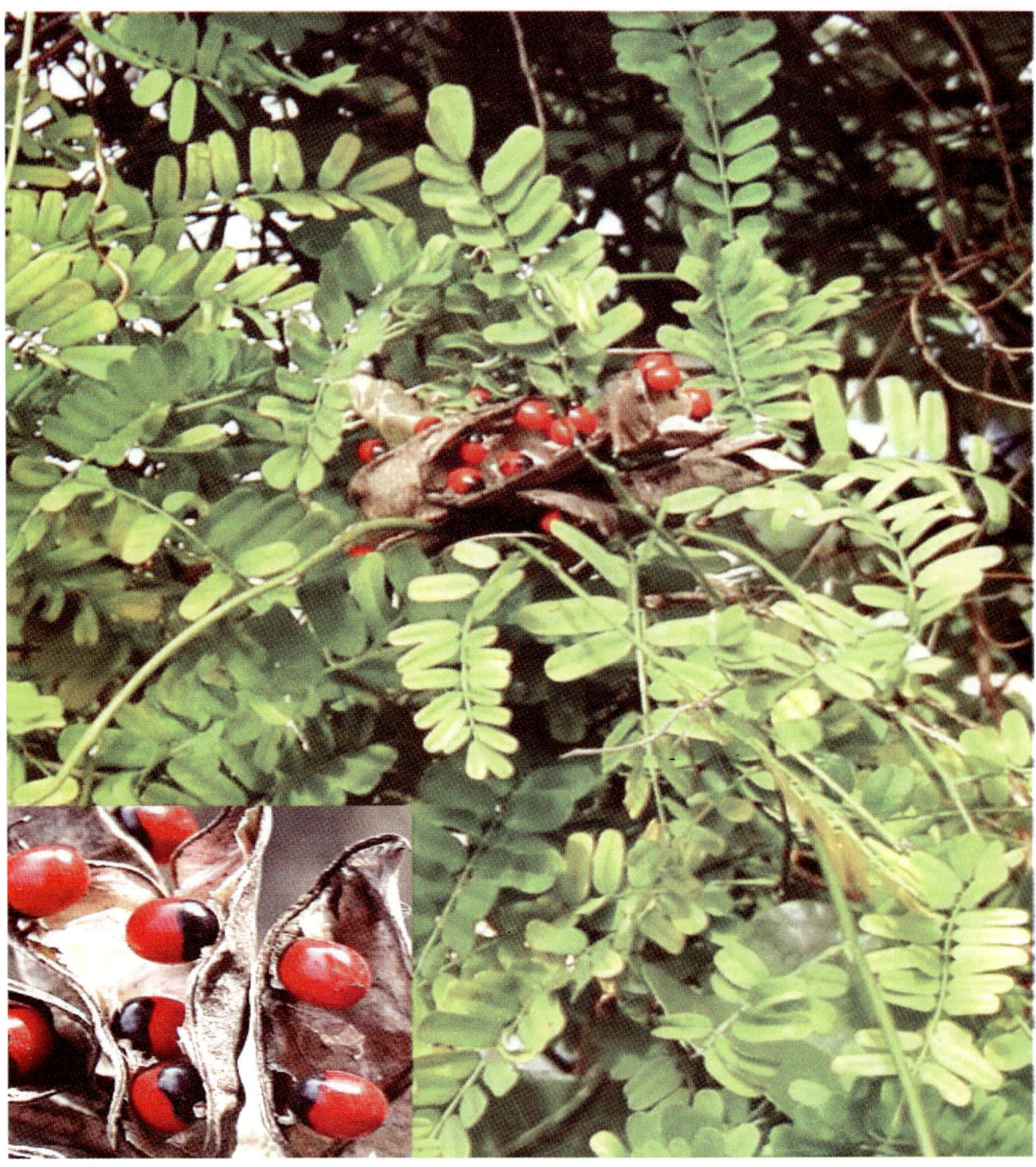

PLATE
1

Abrus precatorius Linn

PAPILIONACEAE

Common Names

Eng   :   Rosary pea.
Hind   :   Rati
Sans   :   Gunja
Ben   :   Kunch
Tam   :   Gundumani
Mal   :   Kunni, Gundumani

Parts Used

Roots, seeds, leaves

Constituents

The methanolic extract of leaves have highly sweet triterpenoid glycosides known as abrusoside A, B, C, and D along with other constituents like abrusgenic acid, abruslactone A. Seeds contain poisonous protein, a flat-splitting enzyme, glucose, abrussic acid, haemagglutinn and albuminous substance called abrin.

Uses

Seeds are purgative, emetic, anti phlogistic, anti-fertility, anti-ophthalmic, aphrodisiac. The methanolic extract of the seeds inhibits the motility of human spermatozoa. Agglutinins isolated from seeds are used in the treatment of AIDS and hepatitis. Leaves are applied on painful swelling. Root syrup is given frequently in cough.

Classification	
Kingdom	Plantae – Plants
Subkingdom	Tracheobionta – Vascular plants
Superdivision	Spermatophyta – Seed plants
Division	Magnoliophyta – Flowering plants
Class	Magnoliopsida – Dicotyledons
Subclass	Rosidae –
Order	Fabales –
Family	Fabaceae – Pea family
Genus	Abrus Adans. – abrus

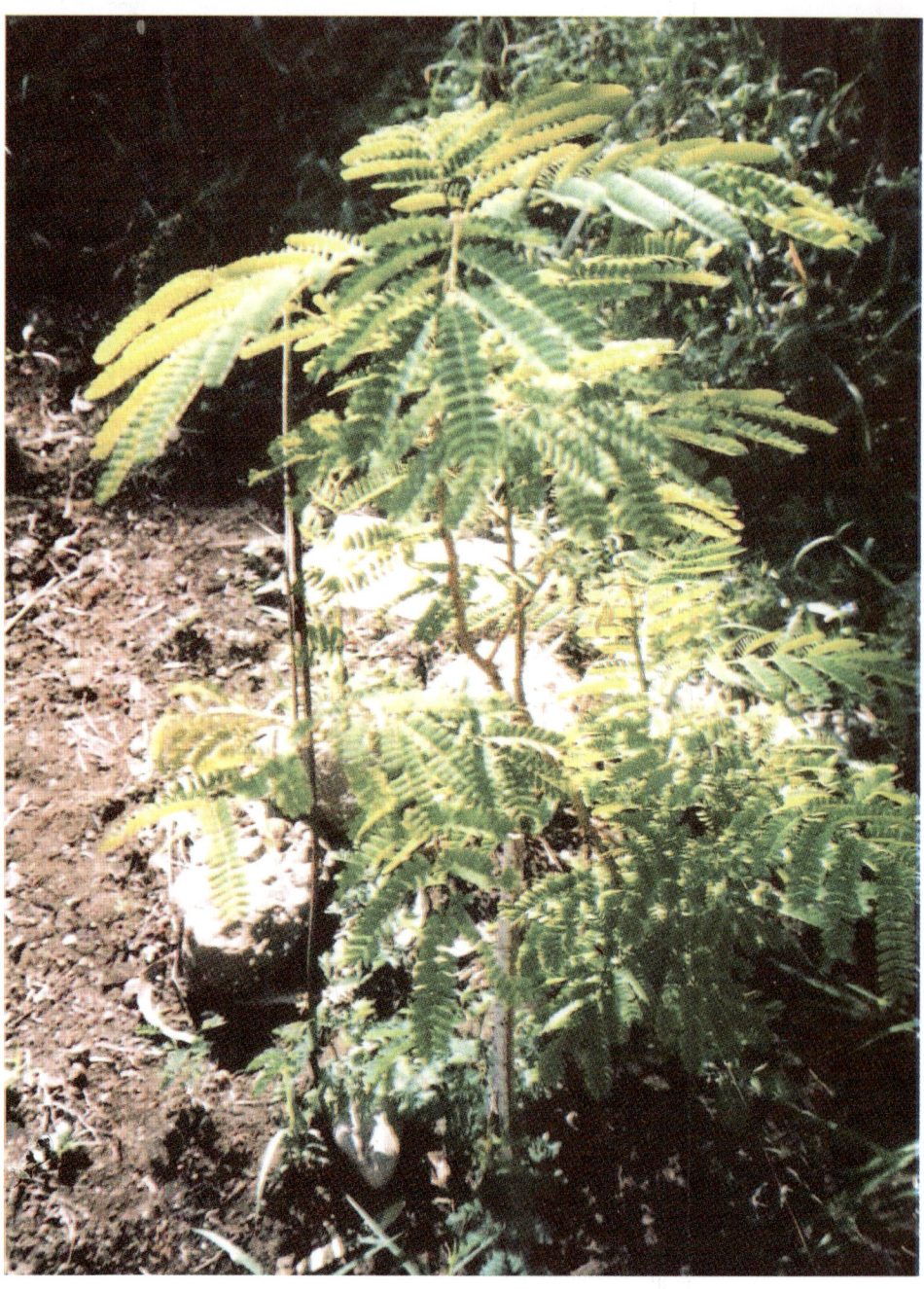

PLATE

2

Acacia concinna Dc

MIMOSACEAE

Common Names

Eng	:	Sompoy
Hind	:	Shikakai
Sans	:	Saptala
Ben	:	Banritha
Tel	:	Cheekaya
Tam	:	Sheeyakai
Mal	:	Cheeyakayi

Parts Used

Pods and leaves.

Constituents

Alkaloids, saponins, gums, coloring matters.

Uses

Promotes growth of hair and removes dandruff, also used as mild laxative, in malarious fever and in jaundice.

Classification	
Kingdom	Plantae – Plants
Subkingdom	Tracheobionta – Vascular plants
Superdivision	Spermatophyta – Seed plants
Division	Magnoliophyta – Flowering plants
Class	Magnoliopsida – Dicotyledons
Subclass	Rosidae –
Order	Fabales –
Family	Fabaceae – Pea family
Genus	Acacia Dc. – acacia

Acalypha indica Linn

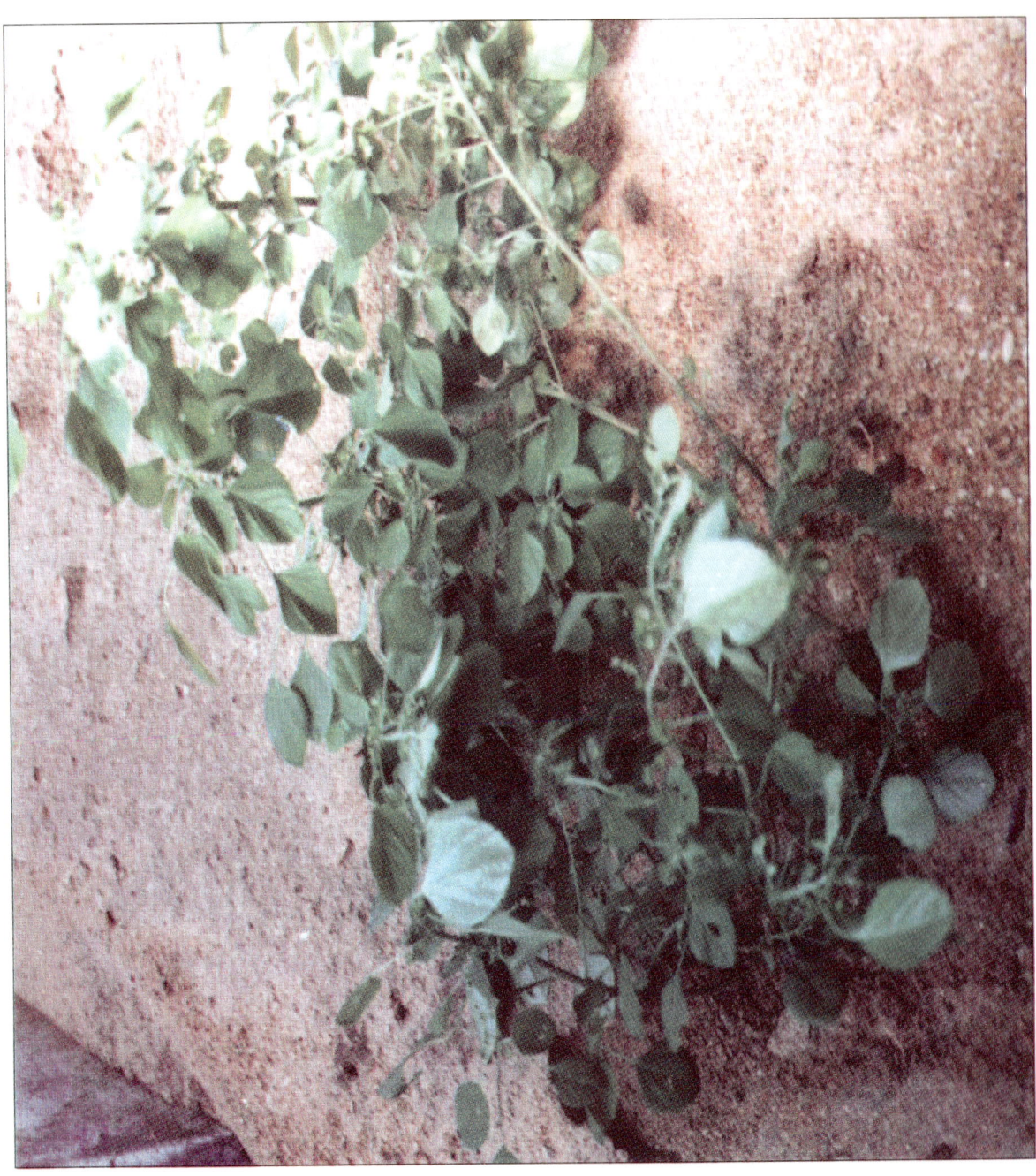

PLATE

3

Acalypha indica Linn

EUPHORBIACEAE

Common Names

Eng	:	Indian acalpyha
Hind	:	Kuppu
Sans	:	Arittamanjarie
Tam	:	Kuppaimeni
Mal	:	Kuppamani

Parts Used

Leaves, roots, flowers

Constituents

Alkaloids – acalphus, acalphine.

Uses

Cathartic, anthelmintic, expectorant, emetic, anodyne, hypnotic and antimicrobial. The juice of fresh leaves is given in painful rheumatism.

Classification	
Kingdom	Plantae – Plants
Subkingdom	Tracheobionta – Vascular plants
Superdivision	Spermatophyta – Seed plants
Division	Magnoliophyta – Flowering plants
Class	Magnoliopsida – Dicotyledons
Subclass	Rosidae –
Order	Euphorbiales –
Family	Euphorbiaceae – Spurge family
Genus	Acalypha L. – copperleaf

Achyranthes aspera Linn

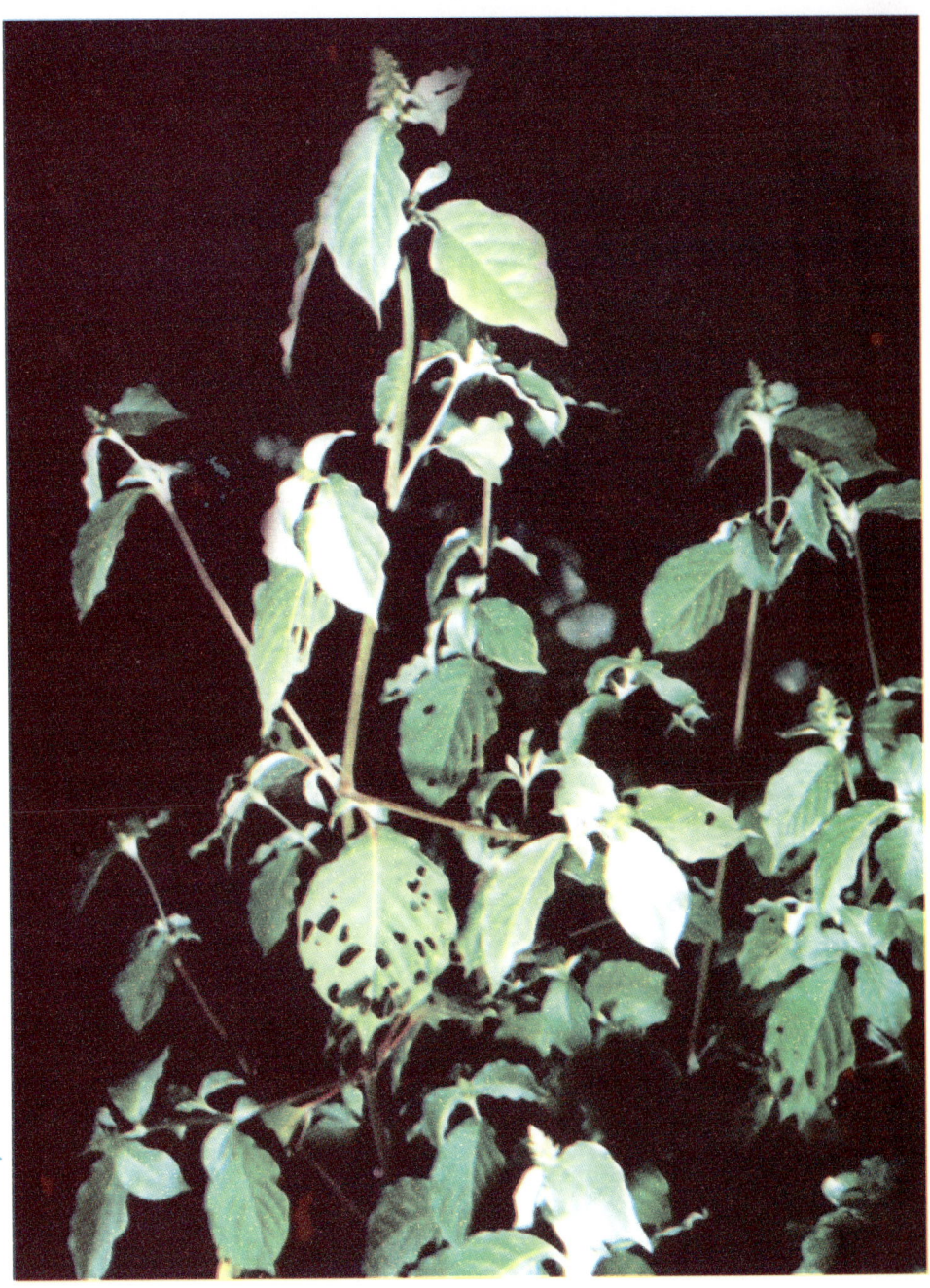

PLATE
4

Achyranthes aspera Linn

AMARANTHACEAE

Common Names

Eng	:	Rough Chaff Tree
Hind	:	Latjira, Chirchira
Sans	:	Apamarga
Ben	:	Apang
Tam	:	Nayuruvi
Mal	:	Kadaladi, Katalati

Parts Used

Roots, seeds, leaves

Constituents

Shoot contains glycosides, tannins, essential oil, 36, 47- dihydroxyhenpentacontan -4- one, tritriacontanol, 27- cyclohexylheptacosan 7-ol. Betaine and ecdysterone from root are also reported.

Uses

Eye and liver complications, rheumatism, scabies. It is used as tranquillizing agent and expectorant. It is also used in veterinary medicine to expel placenta. It also shows abortificiant activity, anti periodic, mild astringent.

Classification	
Kingdom	Plantae – Plants
Subkingdom	Tracheobionta – Vascular plants
Superdivision	Spermatophyta – Seed plants
Division	Magnoliophyta – Flowering plants
Class	Magnoliopsida – Dicotyledons
Subclass	Caryophyllidae –
Order	Caryophyllales –
Family	Amaranthaceae – Amaranth family
Genus	Achyranthes L. – chaff flower

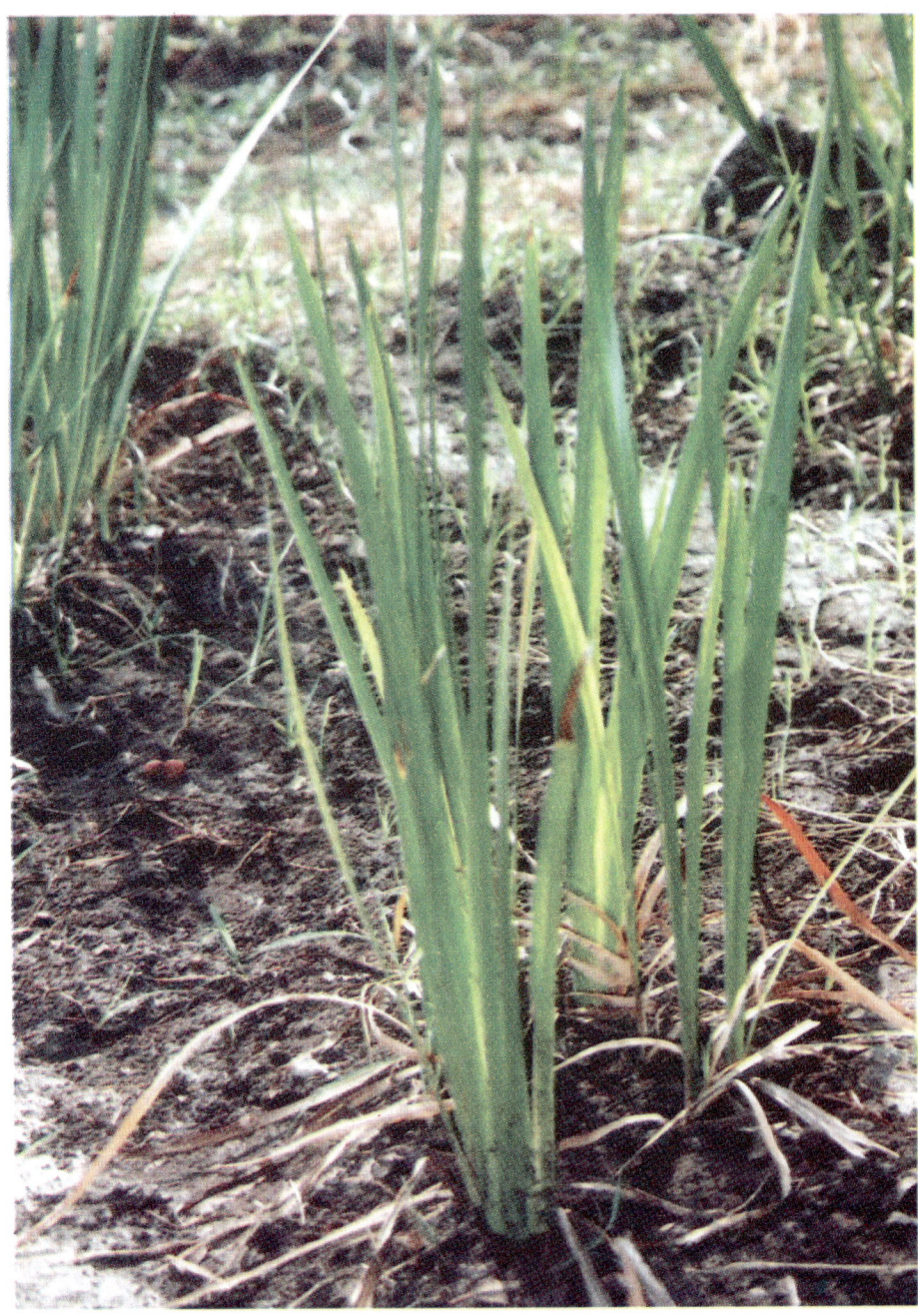

PLATE

5

Acorus calamus Linn

ACORACEAE

Common Name

Eng	:	Sweetflag
Hind	:	Bach, Gora-bach
Sans	:	Vacha, Shadgranthalolomi
Ban	:	Bach, Gora-bach
Tam	:	Vashambu
Mal	:	Vayambhu

Parts Used

Rhizome

Constituents

Rhizomes contain β-cis asarone, asaraldehyde, acoradin, phenylindane and phenyl propane derivatives. Essential oil, acorin, bitter principle acoretin, calamine, starch, mucilage, tannins, palmitic acid, eugenol.

Uses

Rhizomes are potent tranquilizer with neuroleptic, anti-inflammatory and anti anxity property, it is also used in loss of memory. The fresh rhizomes are chewed to prevent intoxication from alcohol and also they are stimulant, emetic, stomachic, aromatic, expectorant, carminative, antispasmodic.

Classification	
Kingdom	Plantae – Plants
Subkingdom	Tracheobionta – Vascular plants
Superdivision	Spermatophyta – Seed plants
Division	Magnoliophyta – Flowering plants
Class	Liliopsida – Monocotyledons
Subclass	Arecidae –
Order	Arales –
Family	Acoraceae – Calamus family
Genus	Acorus L. – sweetflag

Adhatoda vasica Linn

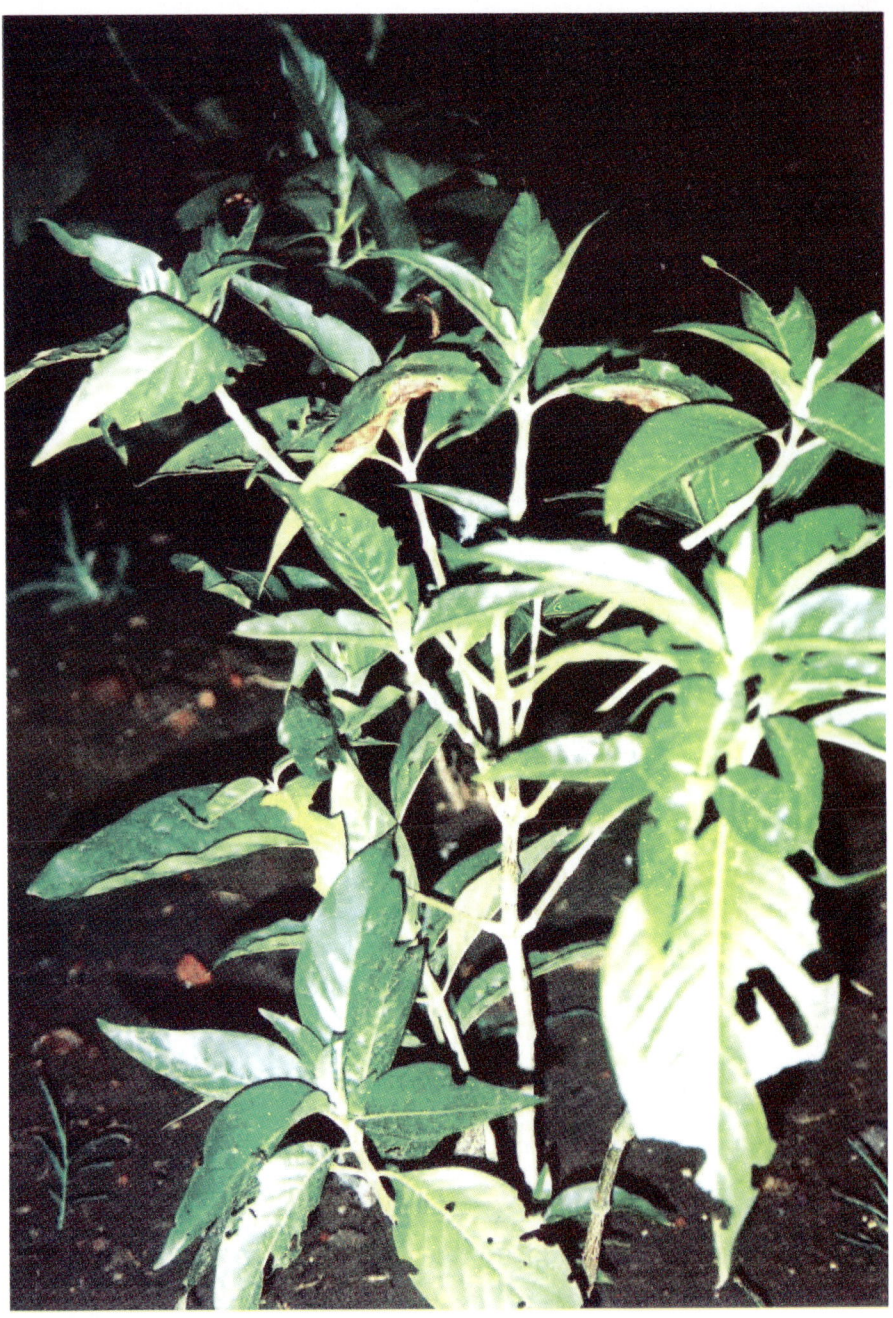

PLATE
6

Adhatoda vasica Linn

ACANTHACEAE

Common Names

Eng	:	Malabar Nut
Hind	:	Arusha
Sans	:	Sinhaparni, Vasaka
Ben	:	Basak, Vasaka
Tam	:	Adhotodai
Mal	:	Ataloetakam

Parts Used

Roots, leaves, flowers & bark

Constituents

Vasicine, a nonvolatile alkaloid, organic acid known as adhatodic acid, β-sitasterol, vasicinol and anisotine.

Uses

Expectorant, diuretic, antispasmodic, spasm of bronchioles.

Classification	
Kingdom	Plantae – Plants
Subkingdom	Tracheobionta – Vascular plants
Superdivision	Spermatophyta – Seed plants
Division	Magnoliophyta – Flowering plants
Class	Magnoliopsida – Dicotyledons
Subclass	Asteridae –
Order	Scrophulariales –
Family	Acanthaceae – Acanthus family
Genus	Adhatoda L – water-willow

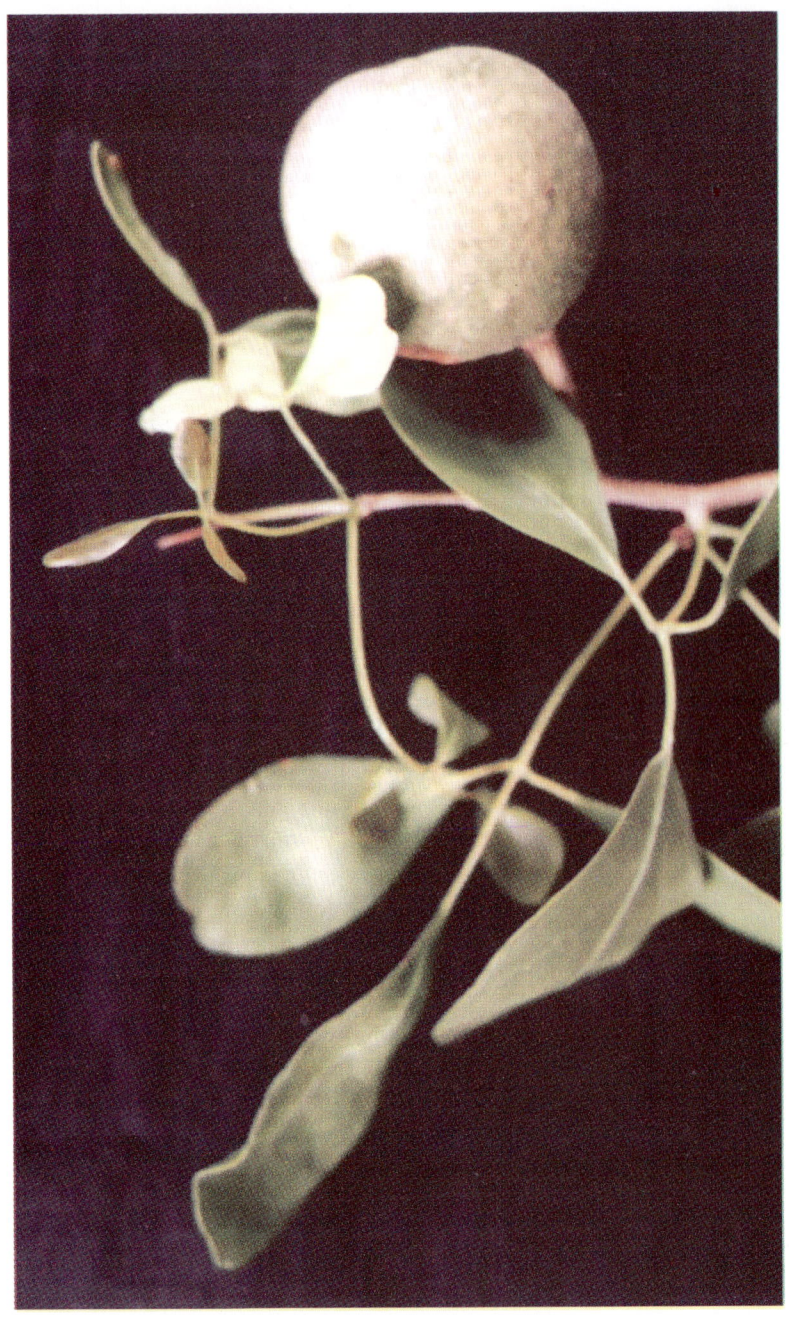

PLATE

7

Aegle marmelos Corr

RUTACEAE

Common Names

Eng	:	Bael, Bengal quince
Hind	:	Bel, Bael sripal
Sans	:	Bilvam
Ben	:	Bela
Tam	:	Vilvam
Mal	:	Kooralam

Parts Used

Roots, fruit, leaves, stem

Constituents

The stem contains Lignan- glucoside, Lyoniresinol 2 alpha –O-beta – D-glucopyranoside, coumarin, marmin, umbelliferone, skimmianine, marmin, tannin, phlobotannis aegeline, flavon -3 Old, leuconthocyanins, ordinol, and ethyl cinnamamide.

Uses

Leaves are used in jaundice, coumarin and marmin isolated from roots show anti-inflammatory activity, the tree is tolerant to pollution, it also exhibit laxative, diuretic activity and the unripe fruits are stomachic, digestive, diarrhoeal agents.

Classification	
Kingdom	Plantae – Plants
Subkingdom	Tracheobionta – Vascular plants
Superdivision	Spermatophyta – Seed plants
Division	Magnoliophyta – Flowering plants
Class	Magnoliopsida – Dicotyledons
Subclass	Rosidae –
Order	Sapindales –
Family	Rutaceae – Rue family
Genus	Aegle Corr. – aegle

Allium cepa Linn

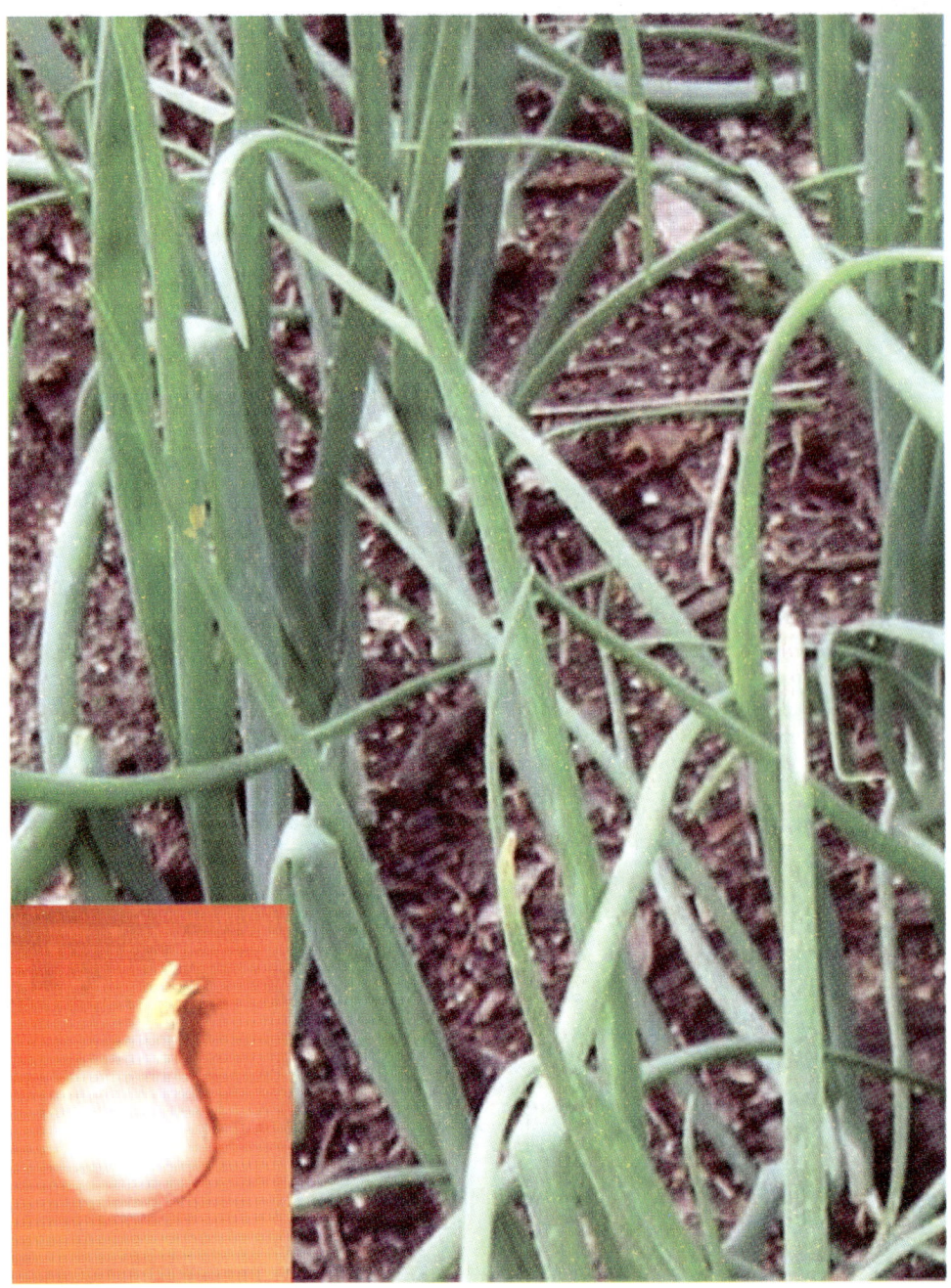

PLATE

8

Allium cepa Linn

LILIACEAE

Common Names

Eng	:	Onion
Hind	:	Piyaz
Sans	:	Palandu
Ben	:	Piyaj
Tam	:	Vengayam
Mal	:	Eerulli

Parts Used

Bulbs

Constituents

Several thiosulfonates and á sulfinyl disulfides were isolated and identified in the extract of the bulbs. Volalile oil that is allyl-propyl disulphide, cycloallin an amino acid, propyl sulfenic acid etc. are also present.

Uses

All the compounds indicates potent inhibitory effect on collagen- induced aggregation of human platelets, it has high fungitoxic activity and antimicrobial activity. Onion Juice is aphrodisiac, hypoglycemic, Stimulant, diuretic and expectorant.

Classification	
Kingdom	Plantae – Plants
Subkingdom	Tracheobionta – Vascular plants
Superdivision	Spermatophyta – Seed plants
Division	Magnoliophyta – Flowering plants
Class	Liliopsida – Monocotyledons
Subclass	Liliidae –
Order	Liliales –
Family	Liliaceae – Lily family
Genus	Allium L. – onion

Allium sativum Linn

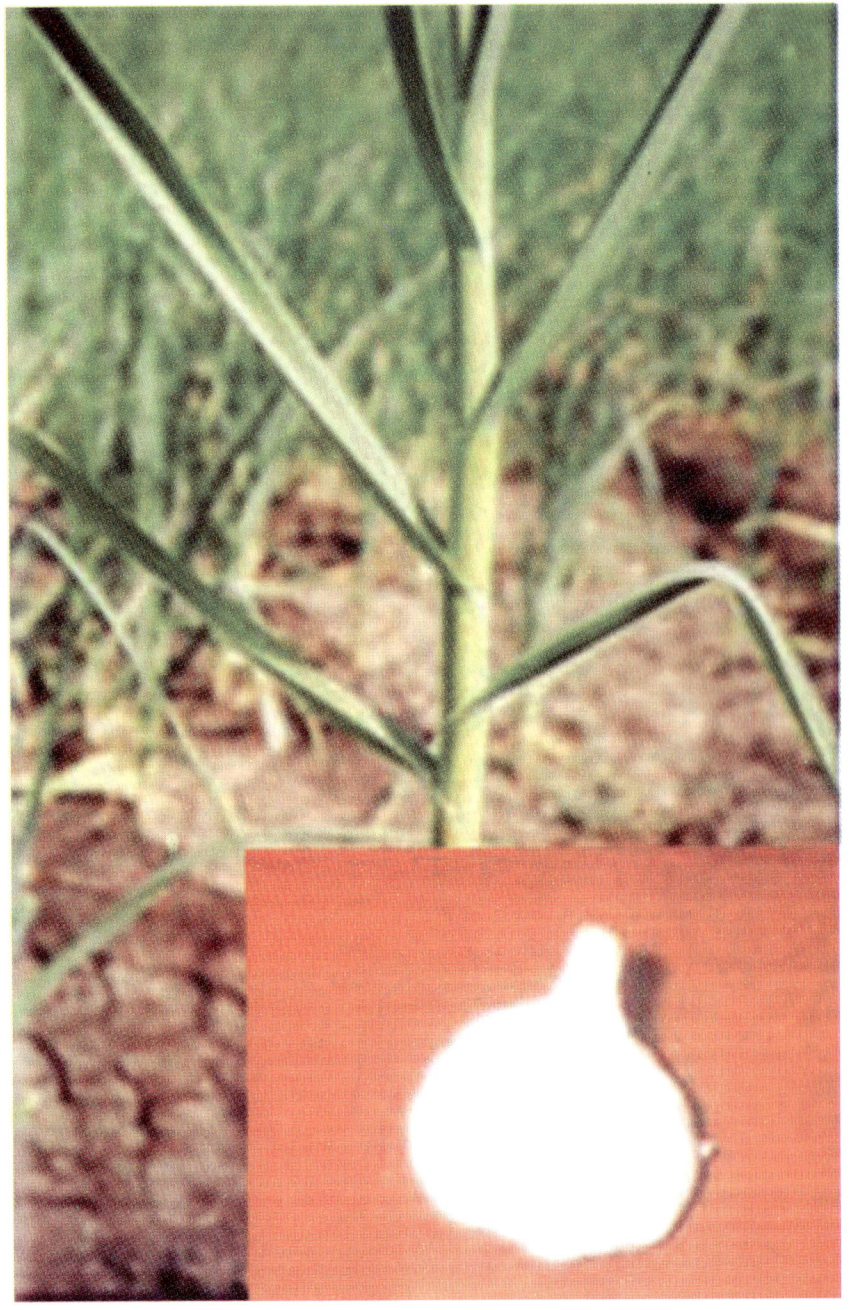

PLATE

9

Allium sativum Linn

LILIACEAE

Common Names

Eng	:	Garlic
Hind	:	Lasan
Sans	:	Lasuna
Ben	:	Rasum
Tam	:	Vellapundu
Mal	:	Vellulli

Parts Used

Bulbs

Constituents

Oil obtained from the bulb contains diallyl mono, di, tri, tetra, hexa and heptasulfides, vinyldithiins and ajoenes. Fifteen sulfides are isolated. Allyl, propyl disulphide and other organic sulphide or sulphur compounds diallyl disulphide the oclourous compound scordinin A, allicin, allinase are also reported.

Uses

Garlic oil shows anti tubercular activity. The volatile oil and its components are reported to possess hepatoprotective activity. It prevented free radical formation and lipidperoxidation. The garlic extract is also used as antiarthritis, anti-inflammatory, stimulant, carminative, emmenagogue, anthelmintic, dyspepsia, antiseptic, antispasmodic, asthma and whooping cough.

Classification	
Kingdom	Plantae – Plants
Subkingdom	Tracheobionta – Vascular plants
Superdivision	Spermatophyta – Seed plants
Division	Magnoliophyta – Flowering plants
Class	Liliopsida – Monocotyledons
Subclass	Liliidae –
Order	Liliales –
Family	Liliaceae – Lily family
Genus	Allium L. – onion

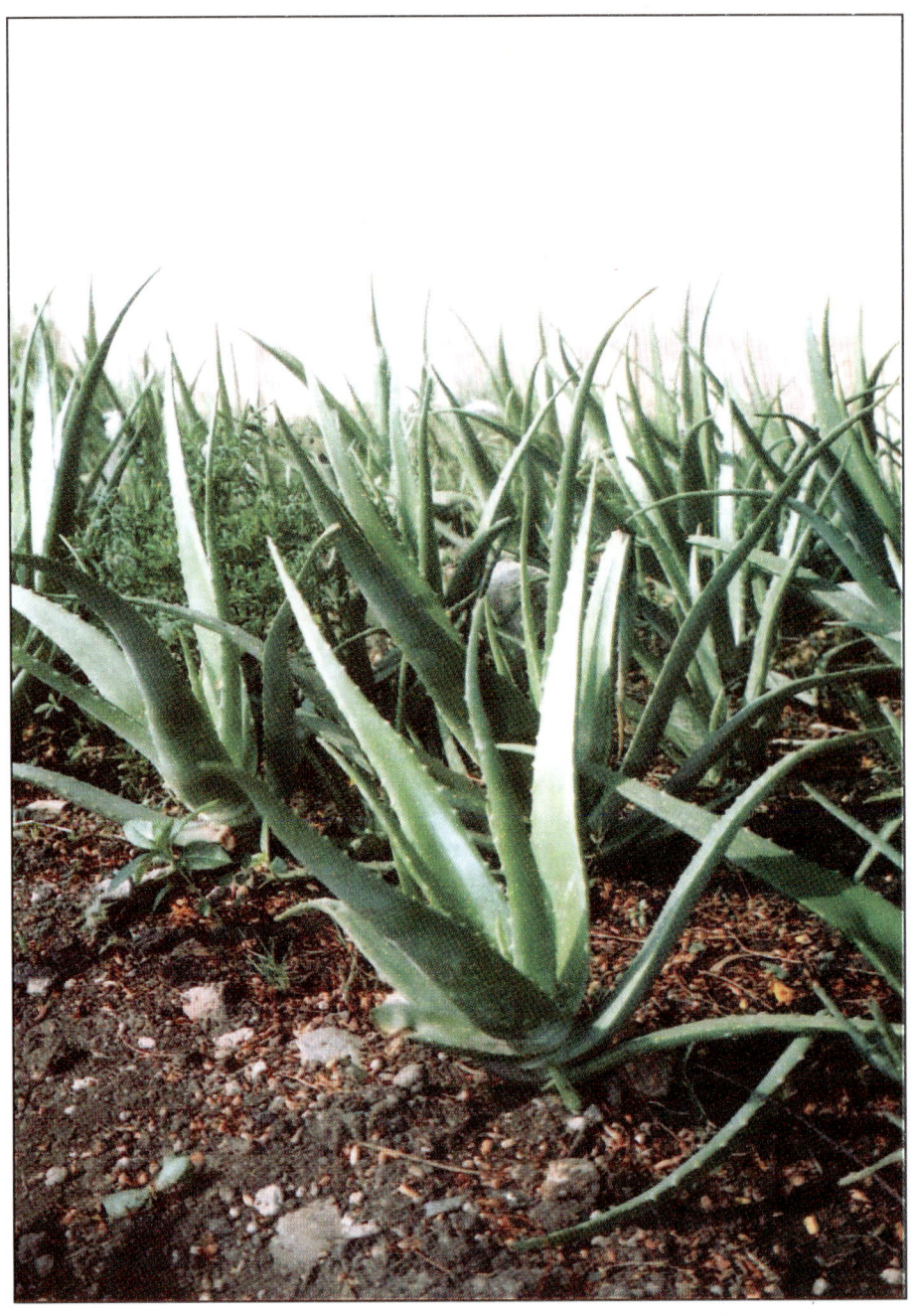

PLATE 10

Aloe vera (L.) Burm. F.

LILIACEAE

Common Names

Eng	:	Indian aloe
Hind	:	ghikanvar, kumari
Sans	:	Ghrita-kumari
Ben	:	Ghrita-kumari
Tam	:	Kattalai
Mal	:	Kattavala

Parts Used

Dried Juice of leaves and pulp

Constituents

Aloin, isobarbaloin, emodin, aloe- emodin, β-barbaloin

Uses

Cathartic, hypoglycemic, remedy for the intestinal worms in children, pulp with honey and turmeric is given in cough, Lutins isolated from aloe gel are strong haemagglutinating and mitogenic agents. Extracts from the parenchymatous leaf gel showed glutathione peroxidase activity.

Classification	
Kingdom	Plantae – Plants
Subkingdom	Tracheobionta – Vascular plants
Superdivision	Spermatophyta – Seed plants
Division	Magnoliophyta – Flowering plants
Class	Liliopsida – Monocotyledons
Subclass	Liliidae –
Order	Liliales –
Family	Aloeaceae – Aloe family
Genus	Aloe L. – aloe

Andrographis paniculata (Burm. F.) Wall. Ex Nees

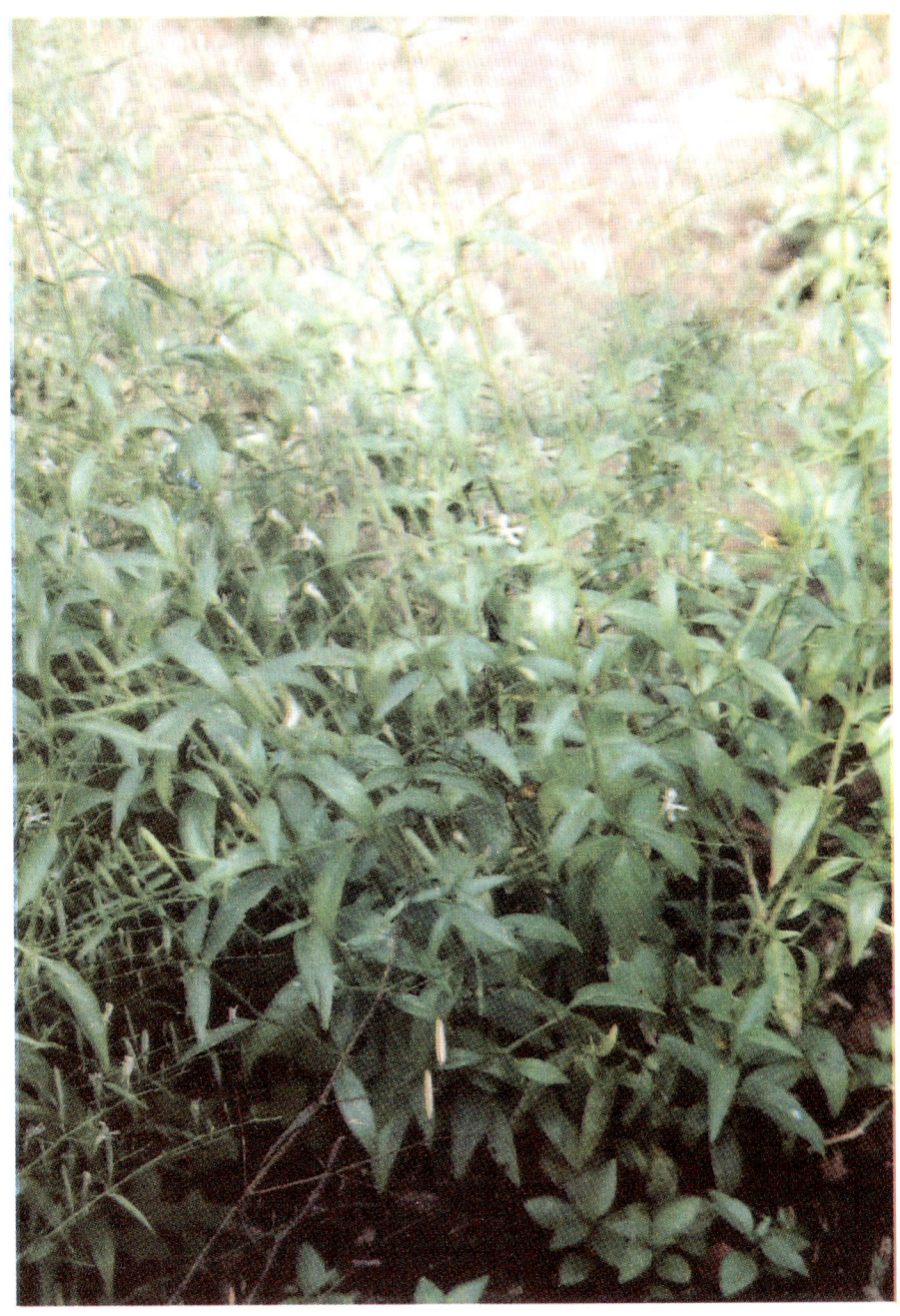

PLATE 11

Andrographis paniculata (Burm. F.) Wall. Ex Nees

ACANTHACEAE

Common Names

Eng	:	King of bitters
Hind	:	Kiryat, kalmegh
Sans	:	Bhunimba, Mahatikta
Ben	:	Kalmegh
Tam	:	Nilavembu
Mal	:	Nilavepu, Kiriyat

Parts Used

Whole herb

Constituents

It contains irridoid glucoside, procumbide along with 14- deoxyandrographolide-19-β-D-glucoside, andrographolide-19-β-D-glucoside, 5-hydroxy-2', 5-dihydroxy-7, diterpenoids and neo andrographolide. Andragrapholide, andrographin, panicolin, apigenin di-methyl ether, and diacaffeylquinic acid are also present.

Uses

Plant suppresses the parasitaemia level, antipyretic and antihepatotoxic activities are attributed to the presence of andrographolide, diterpenoids and neo andrographolide present in the plant. It is also used as antimalarial, stomachic, anthelmintic, remedy in griping loss of appetite, flatulence, diarrhoea in children, febrifuge, bittes tonic, etc.

Classification	
Division	Angiosperms
Class	Dicotyledonae
Subclass	Gamopetalae
Series	Bicarpellatae
Order	Personales
Tribe	Justicieae
Family	Acanthaceae
Genus	Andrographis

Anethum graveolens Linn

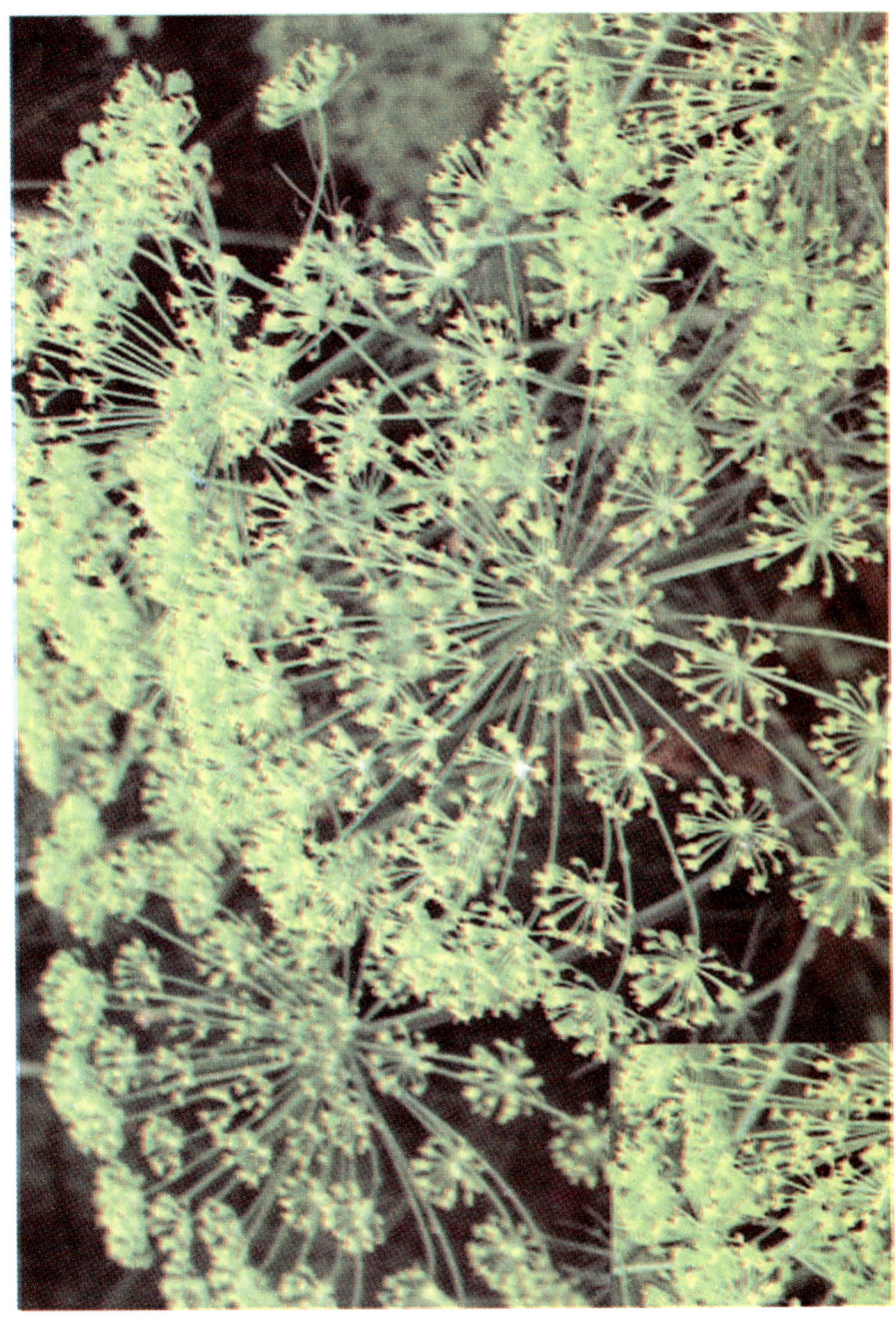

Medicinal Plants

PLATE

12

Anethum graveolens Linn

UMBELLIFERAE

Common Names

Eng	:	Dill
Hind	:	Sowa
Sans	:	Misroya
Ben	:	Soolpha
Tam	:	Shatakupivirai
Mal	:	Chatukuppa

Parts Used

Fruit

Constituents

Monogalactosyl and digalactosyl are the main constituents of glycolipid. Phosphatidylglycerol is predominant in leaves where as phosphatidylcholine is predominant in stem. The major fatty acids present are linolenic acid, and palmitic acid. Carvene, protein, dihydrocarvene, D-limonene, phellandrene, terpenes are also reported.

Uses

Dill oil is powerful pesticide, aromatic, stimulant, and carminative property is also reported.

Classification	
Kingdom	Plantae – Plants
Subkingdom	Tracheobionta – Vascular plants
Superdivision	Spermatophyta – Seed plants
Division	Magnoliophyta – Flowering plants
Class	Magnoliopsida – Dicotyledons
Subclass	Rosidae –
Order	Apiales –
Family	Apiaceae – Carrot family
Genus	Anethum L. – dill

Annona squamosa Linn

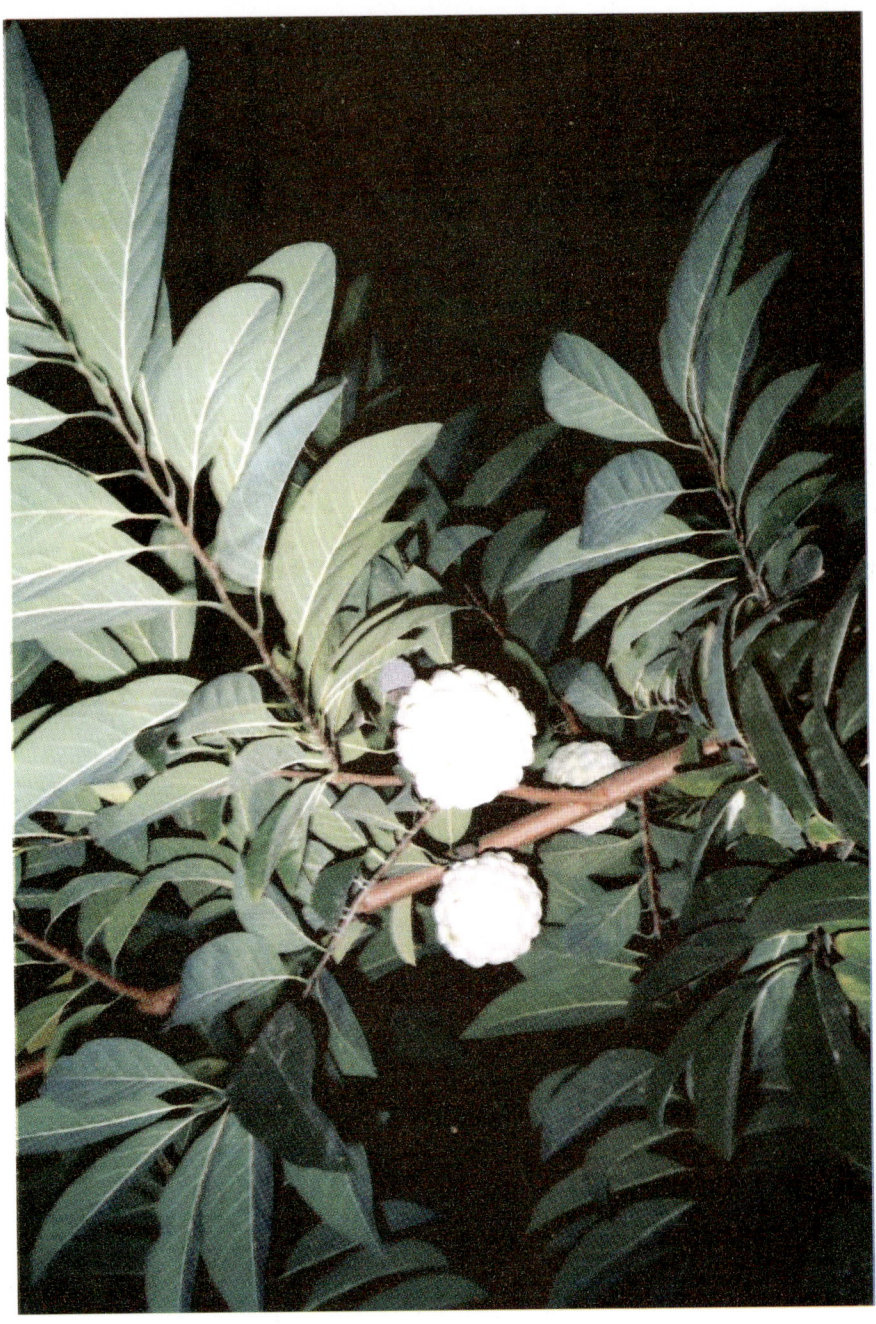

PLATE

13

Annona squamosa Linn

ANNONACEAE

Common Names

Eng   :   Custard apple
Hind   :   Sitaphal
Sans   :   Shuba
Ben   :   Ata
Tam   :   Sitapalam
Mal   :   Sirpha

Parts Used

Leaves, barks, seeds, roots and fruit

Constituents

Alkaloids, resins, sugars.

Uses

Vermicide, insecticide, anthelmintic, astringent, tonic, diarrhoea, dysentery, etc.

Classification	
Kingdom	Plantae – Plants
Subkingdom	Tracheobionta – Vascular plants
Superdivision	Spermatophyta – Seed plants
Division	Magnoliophyta – Flowering plants
Class	Magnoliopsida – Dicotyledons
Subclass	Magnoliidae –
Order	Magnoliales –
Family	Annonaceae – Custard-apple family
Genus	Annona L. – annona

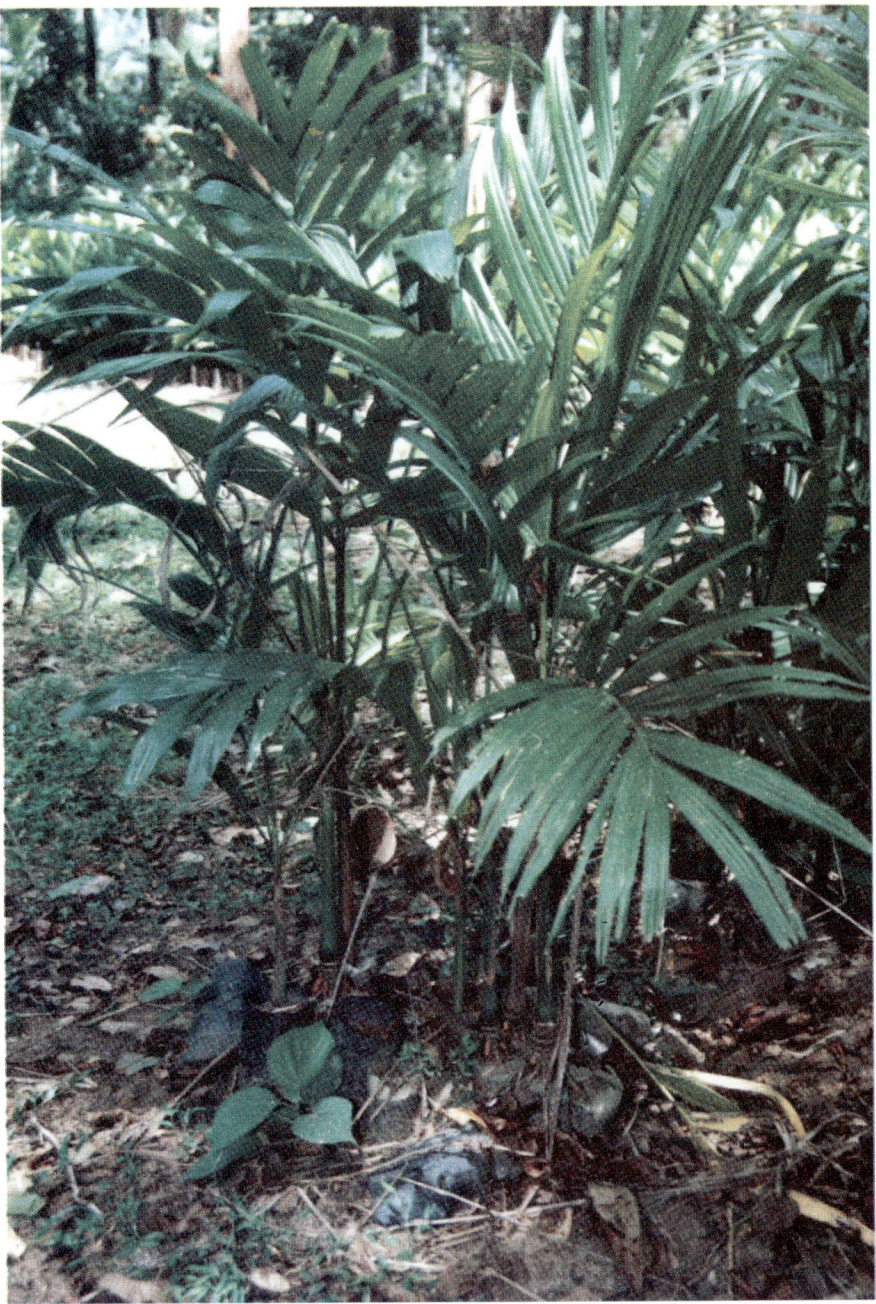

PLATE

14

Areca catechu Linn

ARECACEAE

Common Names

Eng	:	Betel-nut palm, Areca
Hind	:	Supari
Sans	:	Kramuka
Ben	:	Supari, Gua
Tam	:	Kamugu
Mal	:	Pakku

Parts Used

Roots, kernel, seeds, tender leaves

Constituents

The bioactive polyphenolic substance like NF-861, NF-86II, NPF-86IA, NPF-86IB, NPF86IIA, NPF86IIB were isolated from seeds of areca. The reported alkaloids were arecain, arecoline, arecaieline, guvacoline, guvacine, choline, leucocyanidin, avenacines A & B.

Uses

The fatty acid and procynidin from betelnut shows antibacterial activity, and the aqueous extract containing the phenolic compounds prevent the dental caries and gingivitis. It also exhibit activities like Anti implantation, stimulant, astringent increases the flow of saliva, aromatic, decrease in blood pressure.

Classification	
Kingdom	Plantae – Plants
Subkingdom	Tracheobionta – Vascular plants
Superdivision	Spermatophyta – Seed plants
Division	Magnoliophyta – Flowering plants
Class	Liliopsida – Monocotyledons
Subclass	Arecidae –
Order	Arecales –
Family	Arecaceae – Palm family
Genus	Areca L. – areca palm

Artemisia annua Linn

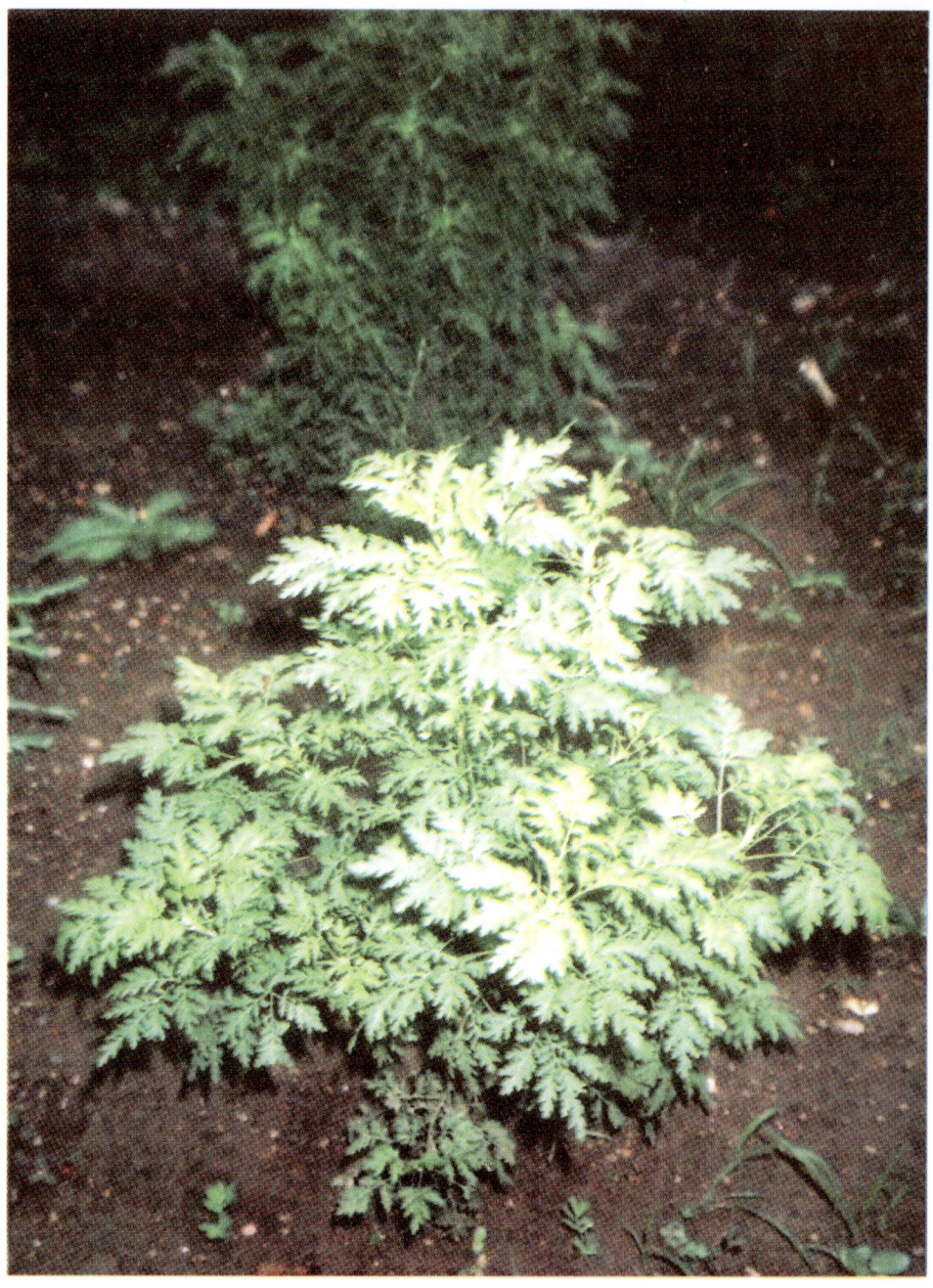

PLATE

15

Artemisia annua Linn

COMPOSITAE

Common Names

Eng : Sweet sagewort
Chi : Quinghao

Parts Used

Leaves

Constituent

Sesquiterpenes- artemisinin.

Uses

Antimalarial, it acts against chloroquine sensitive and resistant malarial parasites.

Classification	
Kingdom	Plantae – Plants
Subkingdom	Tracheobionta – Vascular plants
Superdivision	Spermatophyta – Seed plants
Division	Magnoliophyta – Flowering plants
Class	Magnoliopsida – Dicotyledons
Subclass	Asteridae –
Order	Asterales –
Family	Asteraceae – Aster family
Genus	Artemisia L. – sagebrush

Artocarpus communis JR & Forst

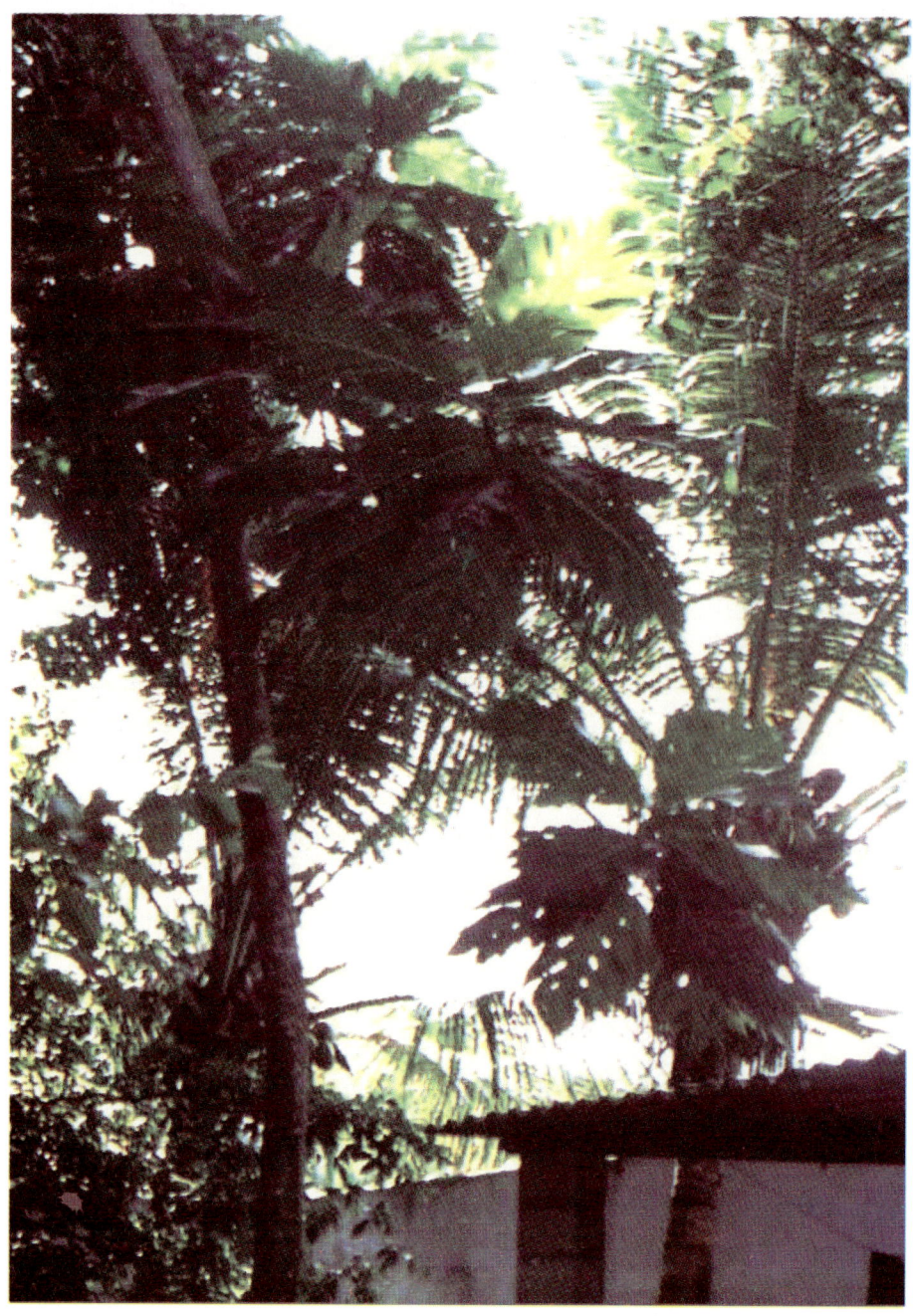

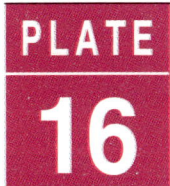

PLATE
16

Artocarpus communis JR & Forst

MORACEAE

Common Names

Eng	:	Bread fruit
Hind	:	Barhal
Ben	:	Dephal
Tam	:	Seema Chakka
Mal	:	Karichakka

Parts Used

Fruits, leaves, latex

Constituents

Prenyl flavones, artonin E, F, isocyclomorusin, isocyclomulberrin, cycloaltilisin, cyclomorusin, cyclomulberrin, artomunoxanthone, dihydrocycloartomunin, β sitosterol.

Uses

Laxative, Cure boils with pus, rheumatism, hernia, antibacterial, antitumour.

Classification	
Kingdom	Plantae – Plants
Subkingdom	Tracheobionta – Vascular plants
Superdivision	Spermatophyta – Seed plants
Division	Magnoliophyta – Flowering plants
Class	Magnoliopsida – Dicotyledons
Subclass	Hamamelidae –
Order	Urticales –
Family	Moraceae – Mulberry family
Genus	Artocarpus Lam. – breadfruit

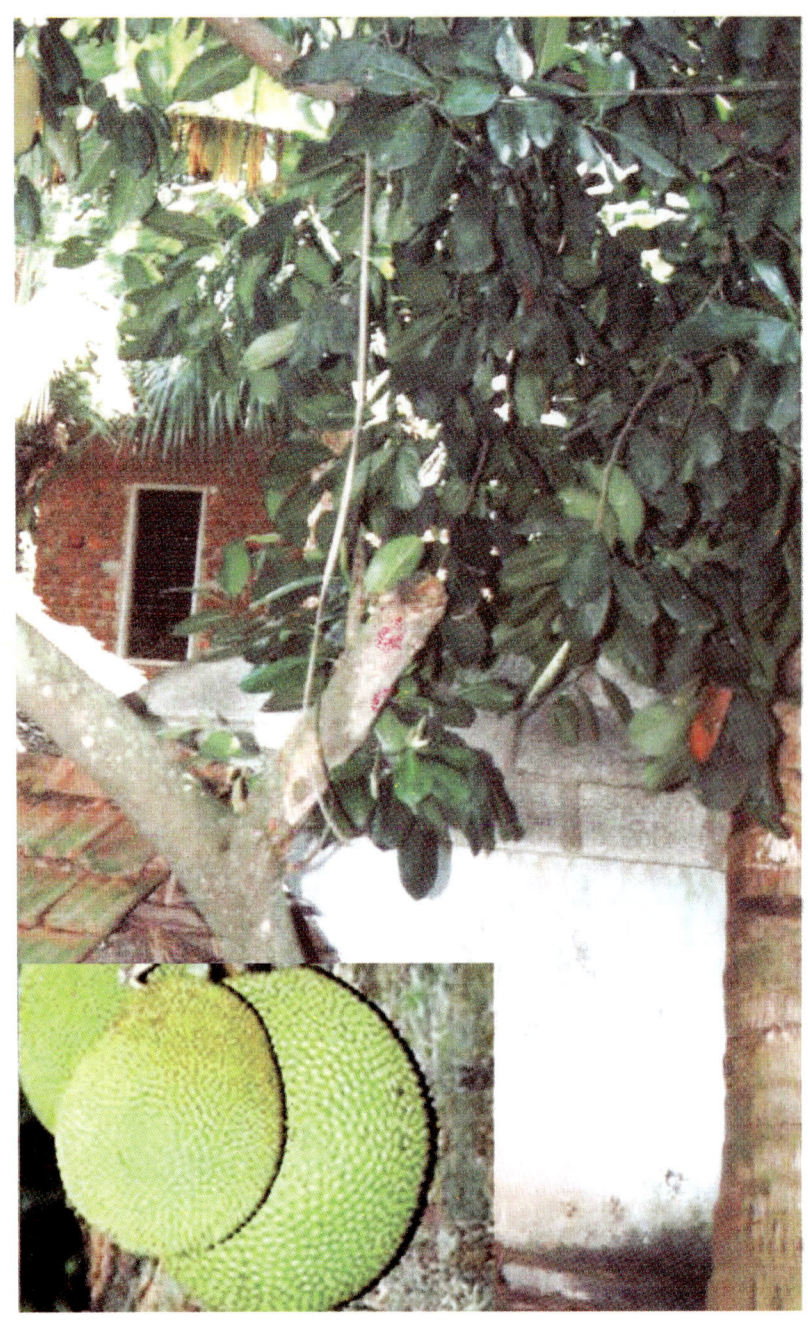

PLATE

17 Artocarpus heterophyllus Lam

MORACEAE

Common Names

Eng	:	Jack fruit
Hind	:	Katel
Ben	:	Katal
Tam	:	Pala palam
Mal	:	Chakka palam

Parts Used

Roots, seeds, pulps.

Constituents

Root bark consists of prenyl flavones, heterophylline, cycloheterophylline, hetero flavonone A & B, artonins A, B, C, D, J, K and L. Pulp contains several volatile flavour constituents like carboxylic acid and carbonyl compounds. Seed is rich in iron and protein.

Uses

Hypoglycemic, demulcent, nutritive, laxative.

Classification	
Kingdom	Plantae – Plants
Subkingdom	Tracheobionta – Vascular plants
Superdivision	Spermatophyta – Seed plants
Division	Magnoliophyta – Flowering plants
Class	Magnoliopsida – Dicotyledons
Subclass	Hamamelidae –
Order	Urticales –
Family	Moraceae – Mulberry family
Genus	Artocarpus Lam. – Jack fruit

Asparagus racemosus Wild

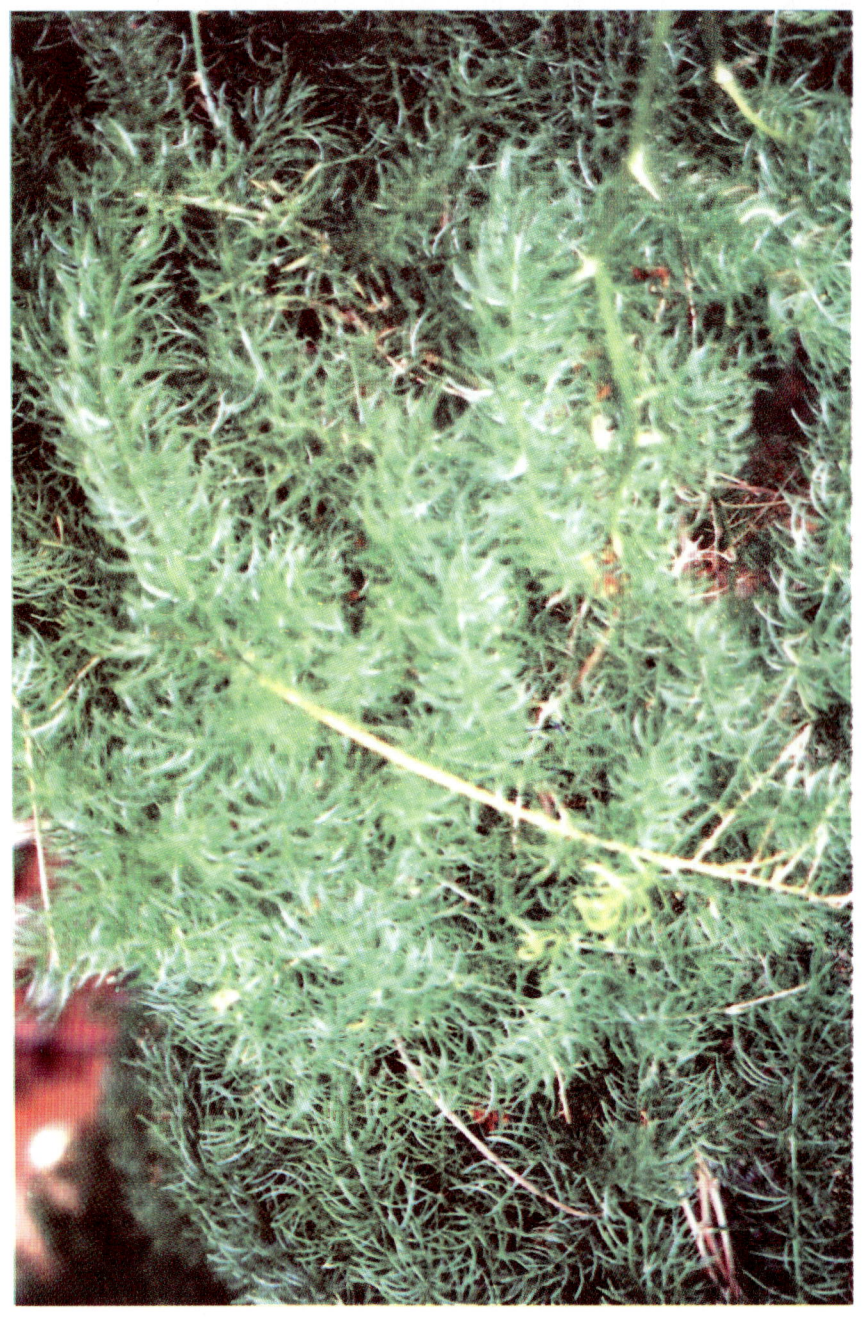

PLATE
18

Asparagus racemosus Wild

LILIACEAE

Common Names

Eng	:	Aparagus
Hind	:	Shakakul, Satavari
Sans	:	Shatavari
Ben	:	Satmuli, Halarru-makkal
Tam	:	Kilavari, Tannir Vittankizhangu
Mal	:	Shatavali

Parts Used

Roots & leaves

Constituents

The dried root contains sitosterol; 4,6- dihydroxy –2-O-(2' hydroxyisobutyl) benzaldehyde and undecanyl cetanoate.Quercetin 3 glucuronide, saccharine & mucilage are also present.

Uses

The root extract shows inhibitory effect on the digestive enzymes, lipase and trypsin and lead to the stoppage in the degredation of food material in the intestinal tract. It also acts as antidiarrhoel, mucilagenous, diuretic, antidysenteric, demulcent, antispasmodic, aphrodisiac.

Classification	
Kingdom	Plantae – Plants
Subkingdom	Tracheobionta – Vascular plants
Superdivision	Spermatophyta – Seed plants
Division	Magnoliophyta – Flowering plants
Class	Liliopsida – Monocotyledons
Subclass	Liliidae –
Order	Liliales –
Family	Liliaceae – Lily family
Genus	Asparagus L. – asparagus

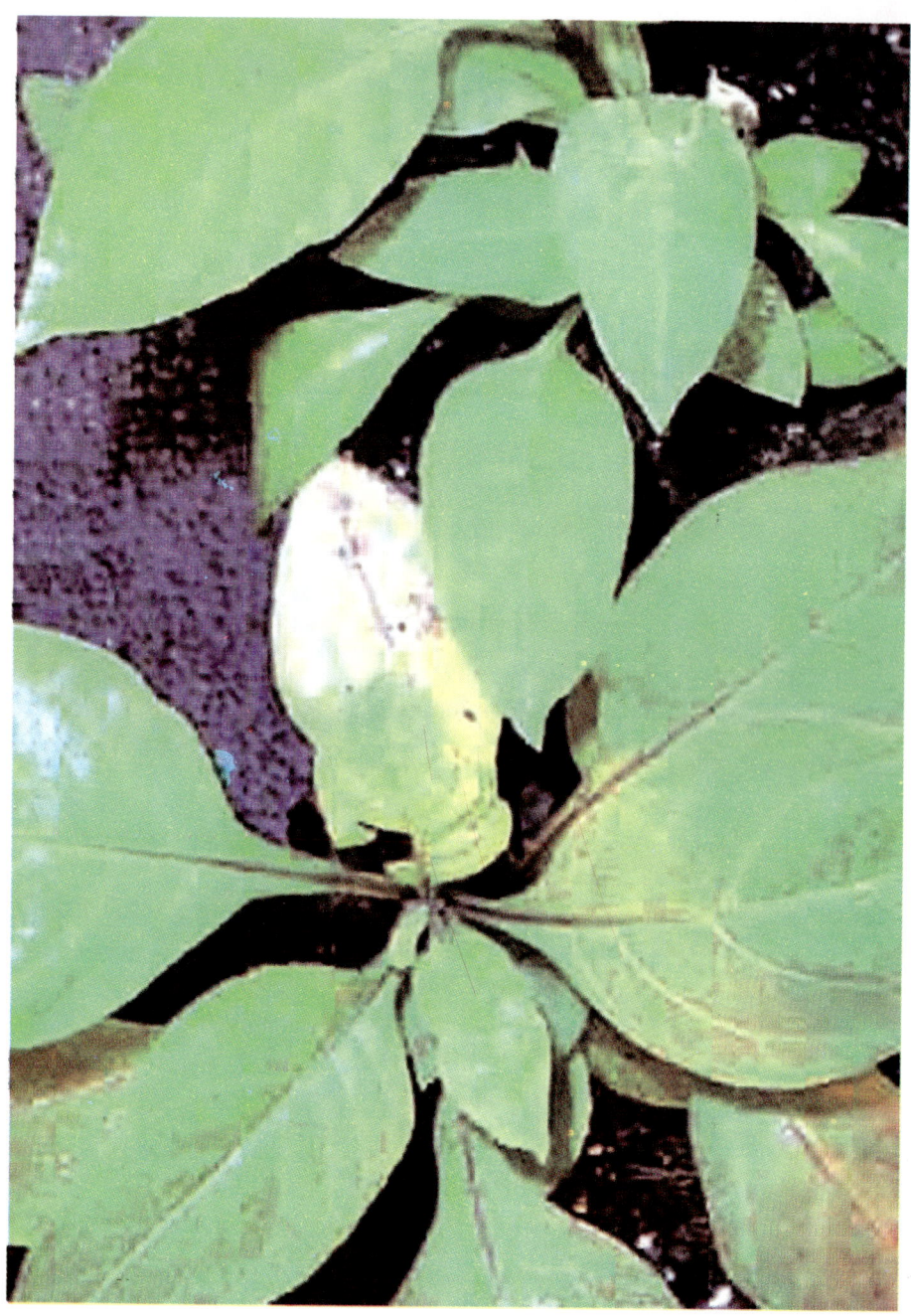

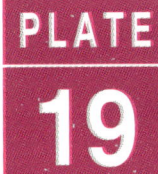

PLATE

19

Atropa belladonna Linn

SOLANACEAE

Common Names

Eng	:	Deadly night shade
Hind	:	Sagangu, angurshefa
Ben	:	Vebruj
Tam	:	Girbuti

Parts Used

Roots, Leaves

Constituents

Acetophenones, acetosyringon, α- hydroxy acetosyringon, acetovanillone, α – hydroxyaceto vanillone and methyl vanillate have been isolated from the plant. alkaloids like, hyoscyamine, belladonine, scopoletin, hyoscine, pyridine are also present.

Uses

Parasysmpatholytic, anticholinergic, antidote in opium and chloral hydrate.

Classification	
Kingdom	Plantae – Plants
Subkingdom	Tracheobionta – Vascular plants
Superdivision	Spermatophyta – Seed plants
Division	Magnoliophyta – Flowering plants
Class	Magnoliopsida – Dicotyledons
Subclass	Asteridae –
Order	Solanales –
Family	Solanaceae – Potato family
Genus	Atropa L. – belladonna

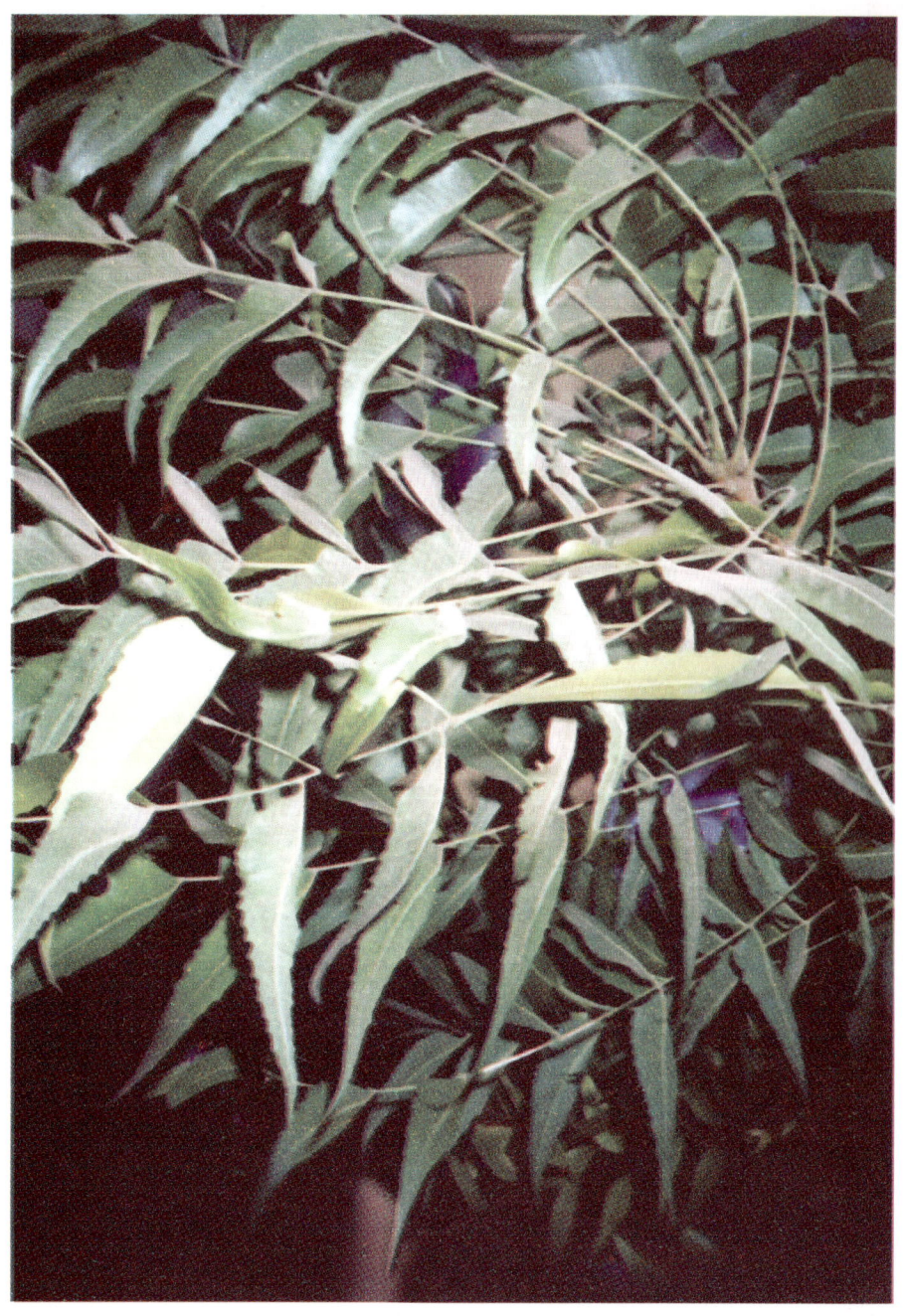

PLATE

20

Azadirachta indica Adr. Juss

MELIACEAE

Common Names

Eng	:	Neem or Margasa
Hind	:	Nim, Nimb
Sans	:	Ravipriya, Vembaka
Ben	:	Nim
Tam	:	Vembu, Veppan
Mal	:	Veppu

Parts Used

Bark, root bark, young fruit, nut, seeds, leaves, flowers, gum

Constituents

Diterpenoids, margolone, nimbonone, nimbonolone, nimbolinin and methylgreillate, two fatty acid derivatives margosinone, and margosinolone, nimbima sulphur, ninbidin, oreophenol-nimbiol are present.

Uses

Antibacterial, anti inflammatory, anti-arthritis, antimalarial, bitter tonic, astringent, anti periodic, antipyretic, antileprotic, and used also in eczema.

Classification	
Kingdom	Plantae – Plants
Subkingdom	Tracheobionta – Vascular plants
Superdivision	Spermatophyta – Seed plants
Division	Magnoliophyta – Flowering plants
Class	Magnoliopsida – Dicotyledons
Subclass	Rosidae –
Order	Sapindales –
Family	Meliaceae – Mahogany family
Genus	Azadirachta Adr. Juss. – Azadirachta

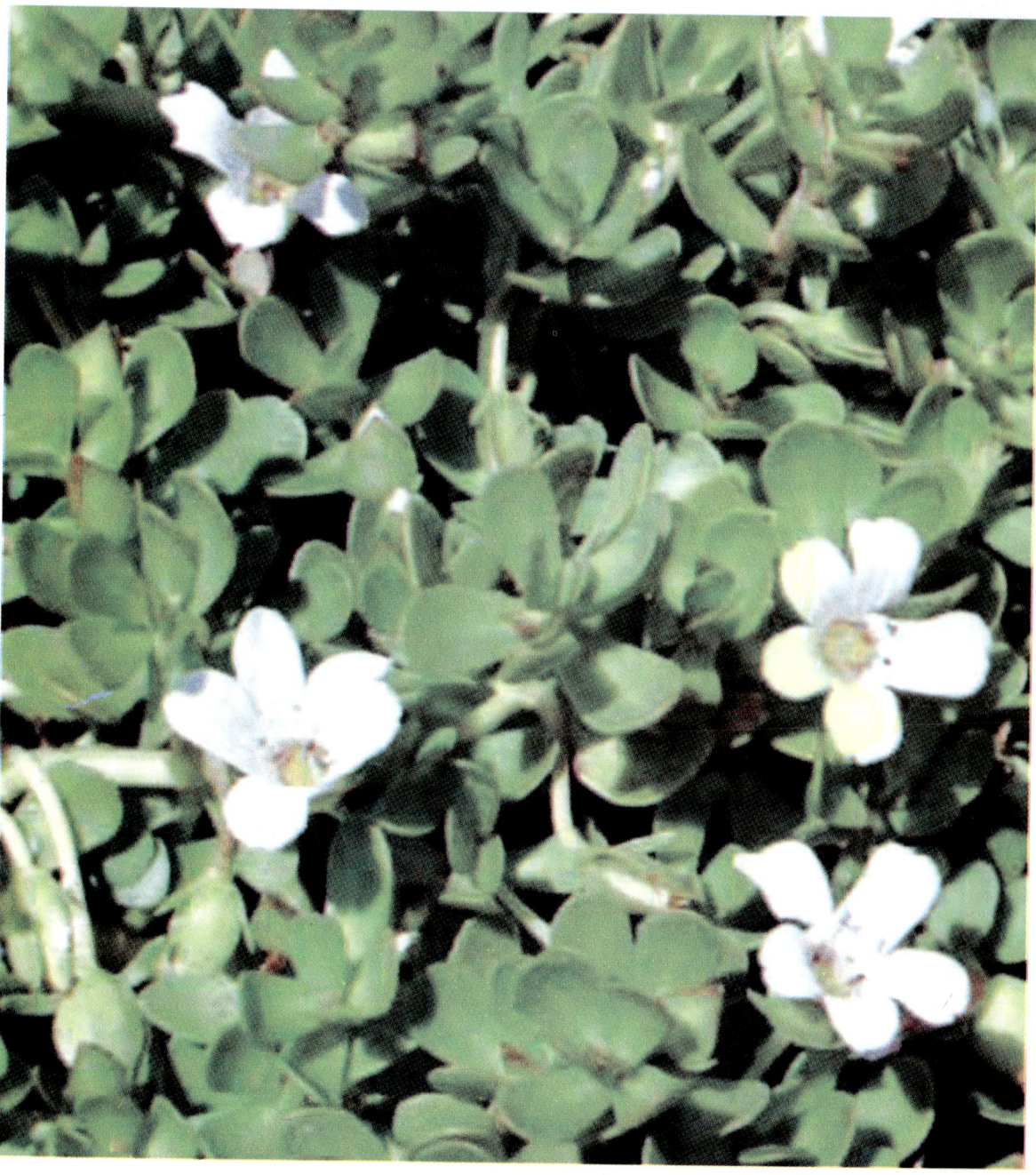

PLATE
21

Bacopa monnieri Linn

SCROPHULARIACEAE

Common Name

Eng	:	Herb of grace
San	:	Nirabrahmi
Hin	:	Brahmi
Ben	:	Brahmisak
Tam	:	Nirbrahmi
Mal	:	Nirbrahmi

Parts Used

Leaves

Constituents

Alkaloids – brahmine, herpestine, saponins mainly bacosides A and B, Butelic acid, stigmasterol, hersaponin.

Uses

Nervine tonic, asthma, epilepsy, insanity, aperients, diuretic. Alcoholic extract has anti tumour activity, bacosides A & B enhances proteinkinase activity and it is also used in the treatment of dementia.

Classification	
Kingdom	Plantae – Plants
Subkingdom	Tracheobionta – Vascular plants
Superdivision	Spermatophyta – Seed plants
Division	Magnoliophyta – Flowering plants
Class	Magnoliopsida – Dicotyledons
Subclass	Asteridae –
Order	Scrophulariales –
Family	Scrophulariaceae – Figwort family
Genus	Bacopa Aubl. – waterhyssop

Boerhavia diffusa Wild

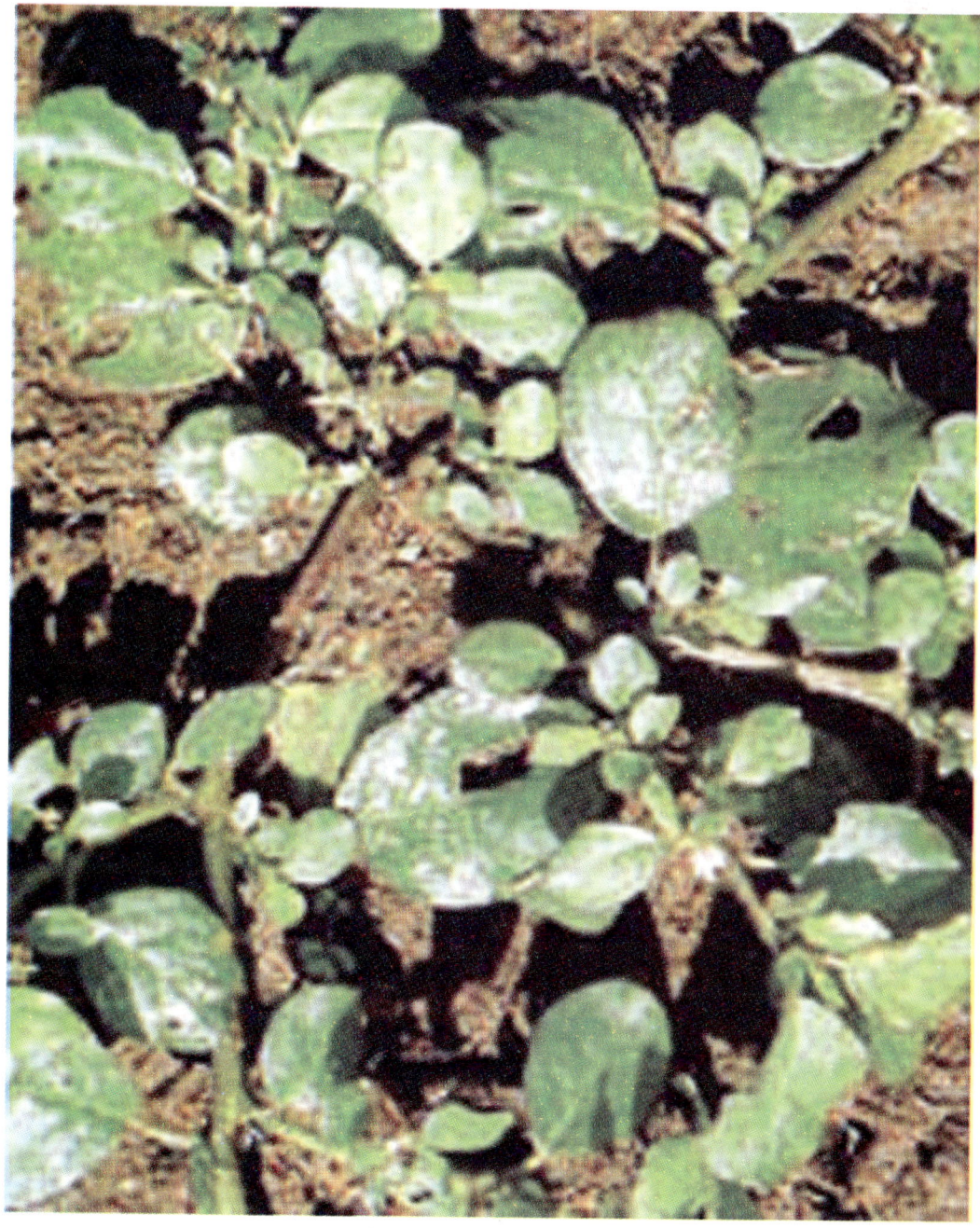

PLATE

22

Boerhavia diffusa Wild

NYCTAGINACEAE

Common Names

Eng	:	Spreading log weed
Hind	:	Beshakopore
Sans	:	Punarnava
Ben	:	Gandhapurna, Swetapoorna
Tam	:	Mukkaratai, Kediyirrattam
Mal	:	Tamilama, Talitama

Parts Used

Whole herb

Constituents

Root contain rotenoids, boeravinones A, B, C, D, E, F besides a dihydroisofurenoxanthone, borhavine, two lignans, liriodendrin and syringararesinol mono- β D- glucoside have been reported. Alkaloids like punarnavine and punernavosides.

Uses

Hepatoprotective, Bitter stomachic, laxative, diuretic, expectorant, diaphoretic, emetic, pugative, anthelmintic, febrifuge, anaemia, cough.

Classification	
Kingdom	Plantae – Plants
Subkingdom	Tracheobionta – Vascular plants
Superdivision	Spermatophyta – Seed plants
Division	Magnoliophyta – Flowering plants
Class	Magnoliopsida – Dicotyledons
Subclass	Caryophyllidae –
Order	Caryophyllales –
Family	Nyctaginaceae – Four o'clock family
Genus	Boerhavia L. Wild – spiderling

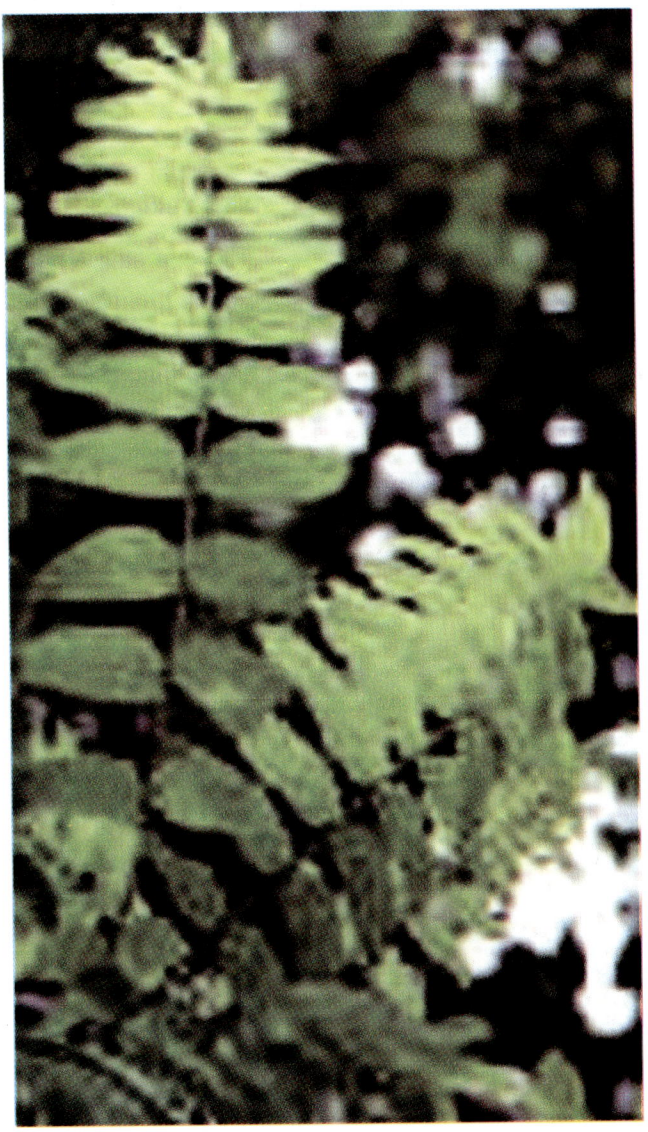

PLATE

23

Boswellia serrata Roxb. ex Colebr.

BURSERACEAE

Common Names

Eng	:	Indian olibenum tree
Hind	:	Luben
Sans	:	Shallaki
Ben	:	Luben. salai
Tam	:	Kungiliam
Mal	:	Vellakuntrikam

Parts Used

Bark

Constituents

The major constituent of essential oil are α-thujene, α-pinine, sabinene, δ-3-carene, α phellandrene, limonene, α – and β thujone and β – bourbonene, oleogum resin containing terpentinic liquid, rosin like resin and gum.

Uses

It is used in the treatment of cough, bronchitis, mouth sore, asthma, jaundice, menstrual and urinary disorders, diaphoretic, diuretic, emmenagougue, anti-inflammatory.

Classification	
Kingdom	Plantae – Plants
Subkingdom	Tracheobionta – Vascular plants
Superdivision	Spermatophyta – Seed plants
Division	Magnoliophyta – Flowering plants
Class	Magnoliopsida – Dicotyledons
Subclass	Rosidae –
Order	Sapindales –
Family	Burseraceae – Frankincense family
Genus	Boswellia Roxb. ex Colebr. – boswellia

Bougainvillea glabra Choisy

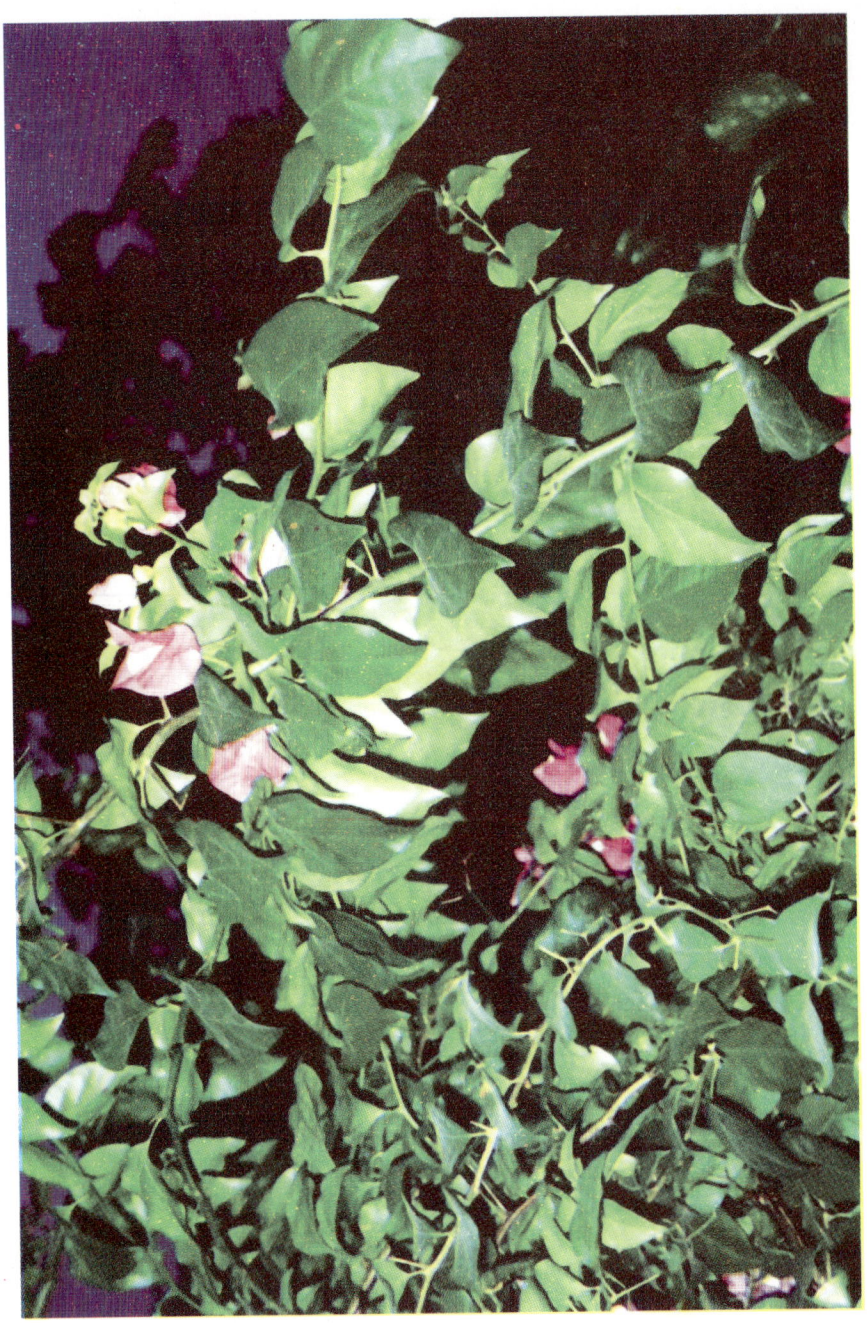

PLATE

24

Bougainvillea glabra Choisy

NYCTAGINACEAE

Common names

Eng	:	Paper flower
Hin	:	Kagaz pool
Tam	:	Thalpoovu
Mal	:	Thalampuvu

Parts used

Leaves, flower, stem

Constituents

Alkaloids, flavanoids, D-pinitol a major carbohydrate is isolated from it, betacynin in bark.

Uses

Anti-inflammatory, insecticidal.

Classification	
Kingdom	Plantae – Plants
Subkingdom	Tracheobionta – Vascular plants
Superdivision	Spermatophyta – Seed plants
Division	Magnoliophyta – Flowering plants
Class	Magnoliopsida – Dicotyledons
Subclass	Caryophyllidae –
Order	Caryophyllales –
Family	Nyctaginaceae – Four o'clock family
Genus	Bougainvillea Choisy. – bougainvillea

Brassica nigra Linn

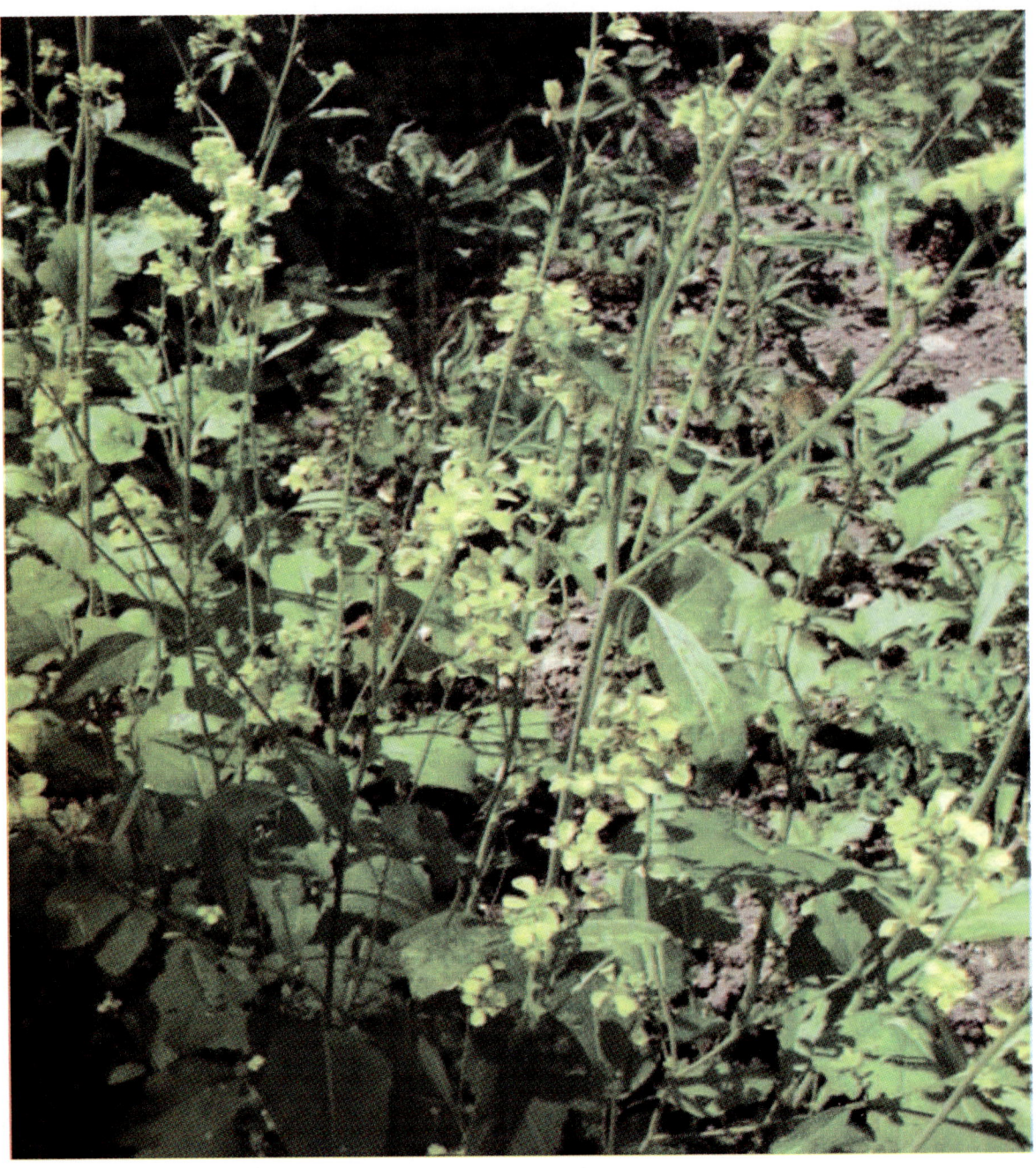

PLATE
25

Brassica nigra Linn

CRUCIFERAE

Common names

Eng	:	Black mustard
Hin	:	Kalorai
San	:	Sarshaph
Ben	:	Krishnrai
Tam	:	Kadugu
Mal	:	Kaduhu

Parts used

Seeds, oils, leaves

Constituents

Fixed oils, proteins, volatile oils, isothiocynates glycoside called sinigrin.

Uses

Condiment, emetic, irritant, rubefacient.

Classification	
Kingdom	Plantae – Plants
Subkingdom	Tracheobionta – Vascular plants
Superdivision	Spermatophyta – Seed plants
Division	Magnoliophyta – Flowering plants
Class	Magnoliopsida – Dicotyledons
Subclass	Dilleniidae –
Order	Capparales –
Family	Brassicaceae – Mustard family
Genus	Brassica L. – mustard

Bryophyllum pinnatum Lam

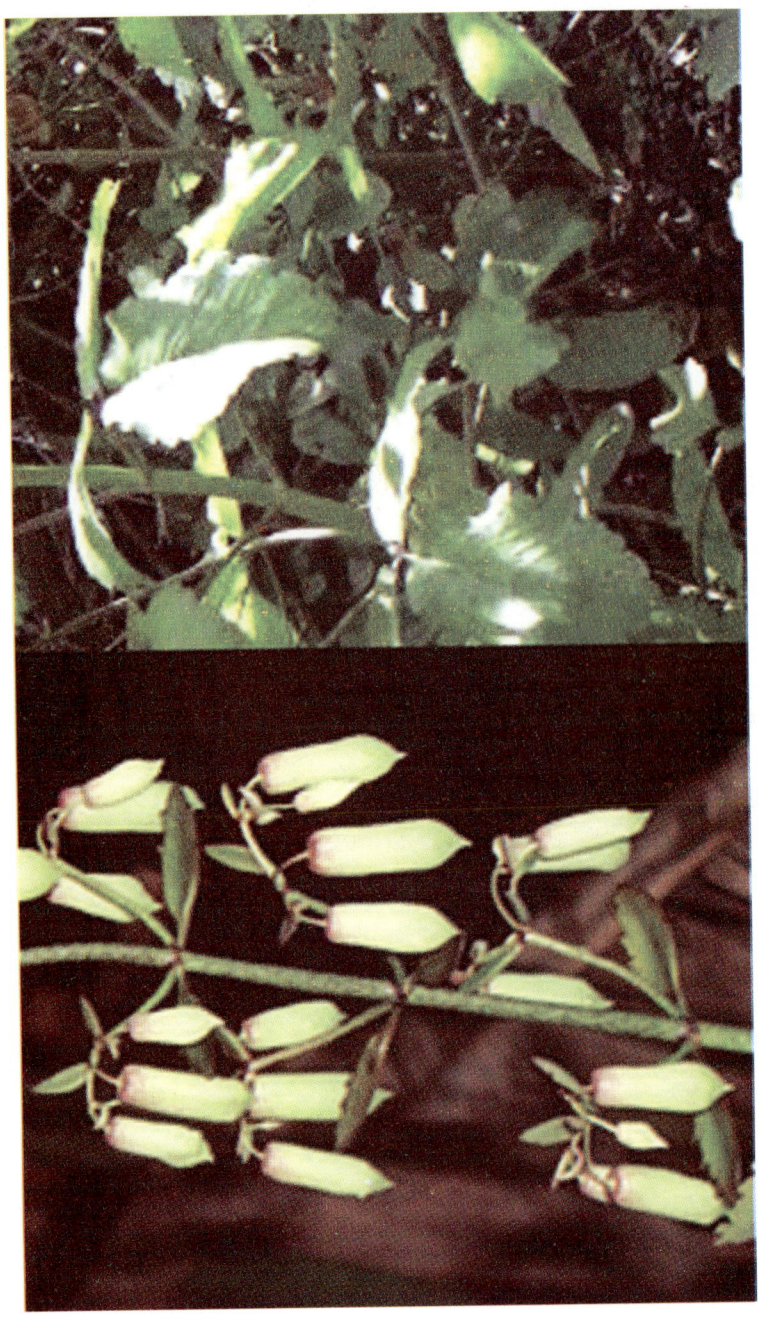

PLATE
26

Bryophyllum pinnatum Lam

CRASSULACEAE

Common Names

Eng	:	Cathedral bells
San	:	Asthibhaksha
Hind	:	Zakhm haiyat
Ben	:	Koppata
Tam	:	Chodaku
Mal	:	Elamarunga

Parts Used

Leaves

Constituents

Quercetin diarabinoside, kaempferal 3 glucoside, ferulic, P-coumaric, fatty acids.

Uses

Applied on wound, boils, insect bites, antiinflammatory, oedema, arthritis.

Classification	
Kingdom	Plantae – Plants
Subkingdom	Tracheobionta – Vascular plants
Superdivision	Spermatophyta – Seed plants
Division	Magnoliophyta – Flowering plants
Class	Magnoliopsida – Dicotyledons
Subclass	Rosidae –
Order	Rosales –
Family	Crassulaceae – Stonecrop family
Genus	Bryophyllum. – widow's-thrill

Butea frondosa Roxb & Koen

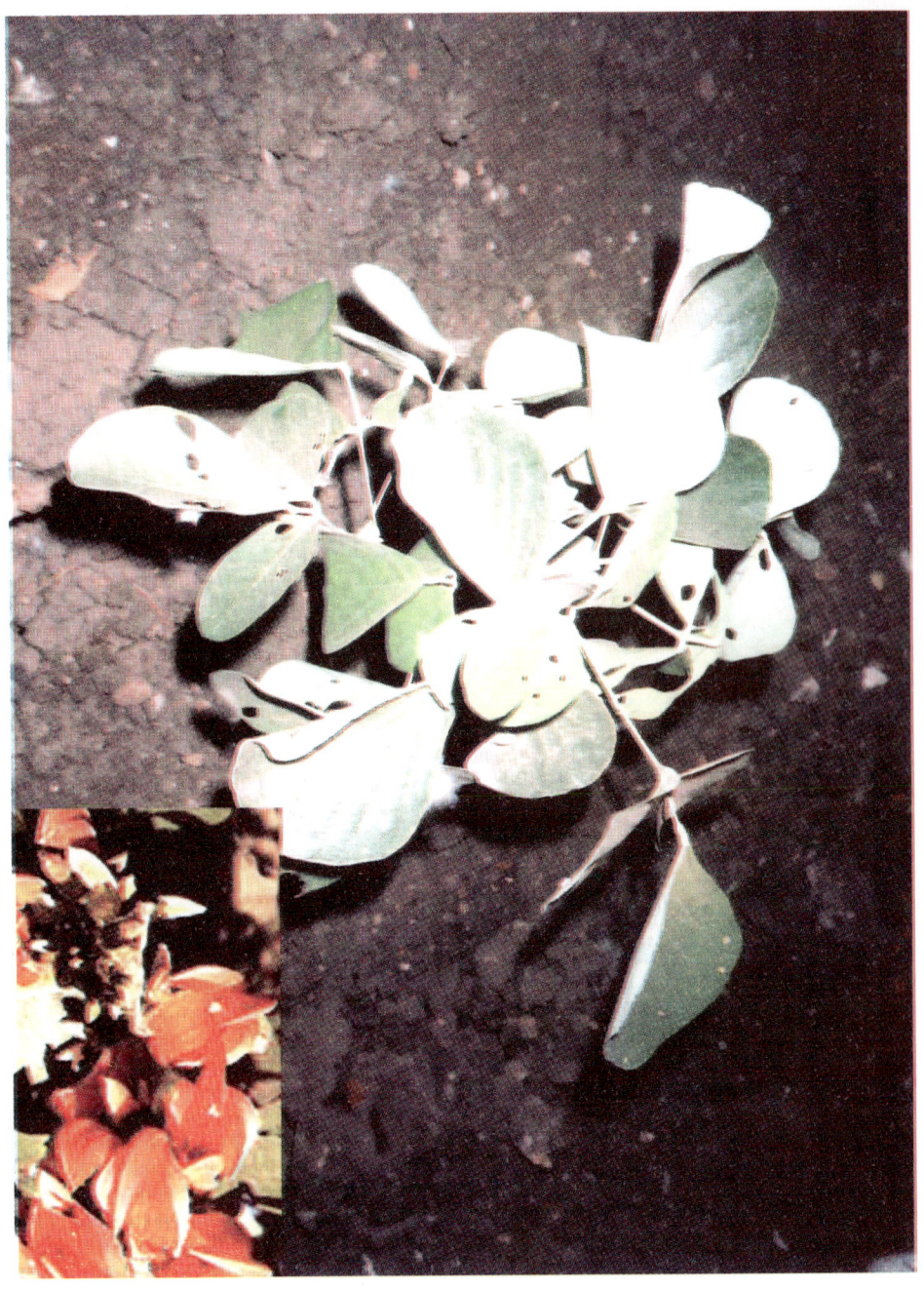

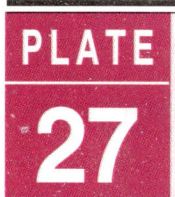

PLATE
27

Butea frondosa Roxb & Koen

PAPILIONACEAE

Common Names

Eng	:	Bastard teak, bengal kino
Hind	:	Palas, Tesu
Sans	:	Kinsuka
Ben	:	Palas
Tam	:	Palasam, Mukampoo
Mal	:	Pilacham, Murukka maram

Parts Used

Leaves, flowers, bark, gums, seeds

Constituents

Kinotannic acid, gallic acid, mucilage, glucoside

Uses

Astringent, laxative, anthelmintic, tonic, aphrodisiac, depurative, diuretic.

Classification	
Kingdom	Plantae – Plants
Subkingdom	Tracheobionta – Vascular plants
Superdivision	Spermatophyta – Seed plants
Division	Magnoliophyta – Flowering plants
Class	Magnoliopsida – Dicotyledons
Subclass	Rosidae –
Order	Fabales –
Family	Fabaceae – Pea family
Genus	Butea Roxb & Koen – butea

Caesalpinia bonduc Roxb

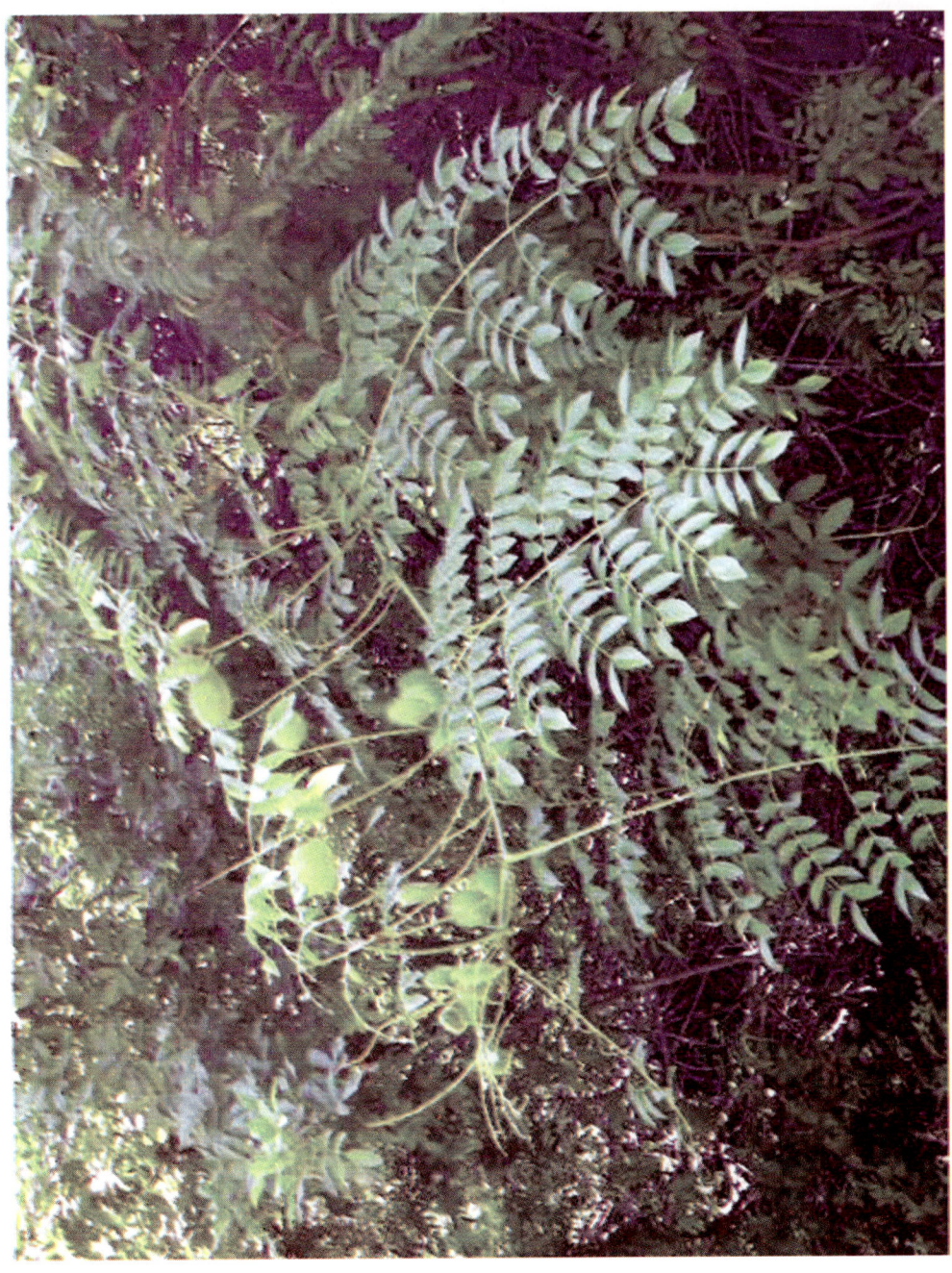

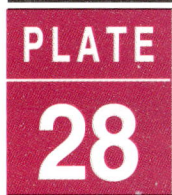

PLATE 28

Caesalpinia bonduc Roxb

CAESALPINIACEAE

Common Names

Eng	:	Yellow nicker
Hind	:	Katkaranj
Sans	:	Latakaranja
Ben	:	Dahara
Tam	:	Kazhar-shikkay
Mal	:	Kalanchikuru

Parts Used

Seeds, roots, barks, leaves

Constituents

Bitter principles - bonducine, fatty oils which consist of glyceryl of palmitic, stearic acids, phytosterols.

Uses

Antiperiodic, antispasmodic, bitter tonic, anthelmintic, febrifuge, leaves are emmenogogue.

Classification	
Kingdom	Plantae – Plants
Subkingdom	Tracheobionta – Vascular plants
Superdivision	Spermatophyta – Seed plants
Division	Magnoliophyta – Flowering plants
Class	Magnoliopsida – Dicotyledons
Subclass	Rosidae –
Order	Fabales –
Family	Fabaceae – Pea family
Genus	Caesalpinia L. – nicker

Calotropis gigantea R.Br.

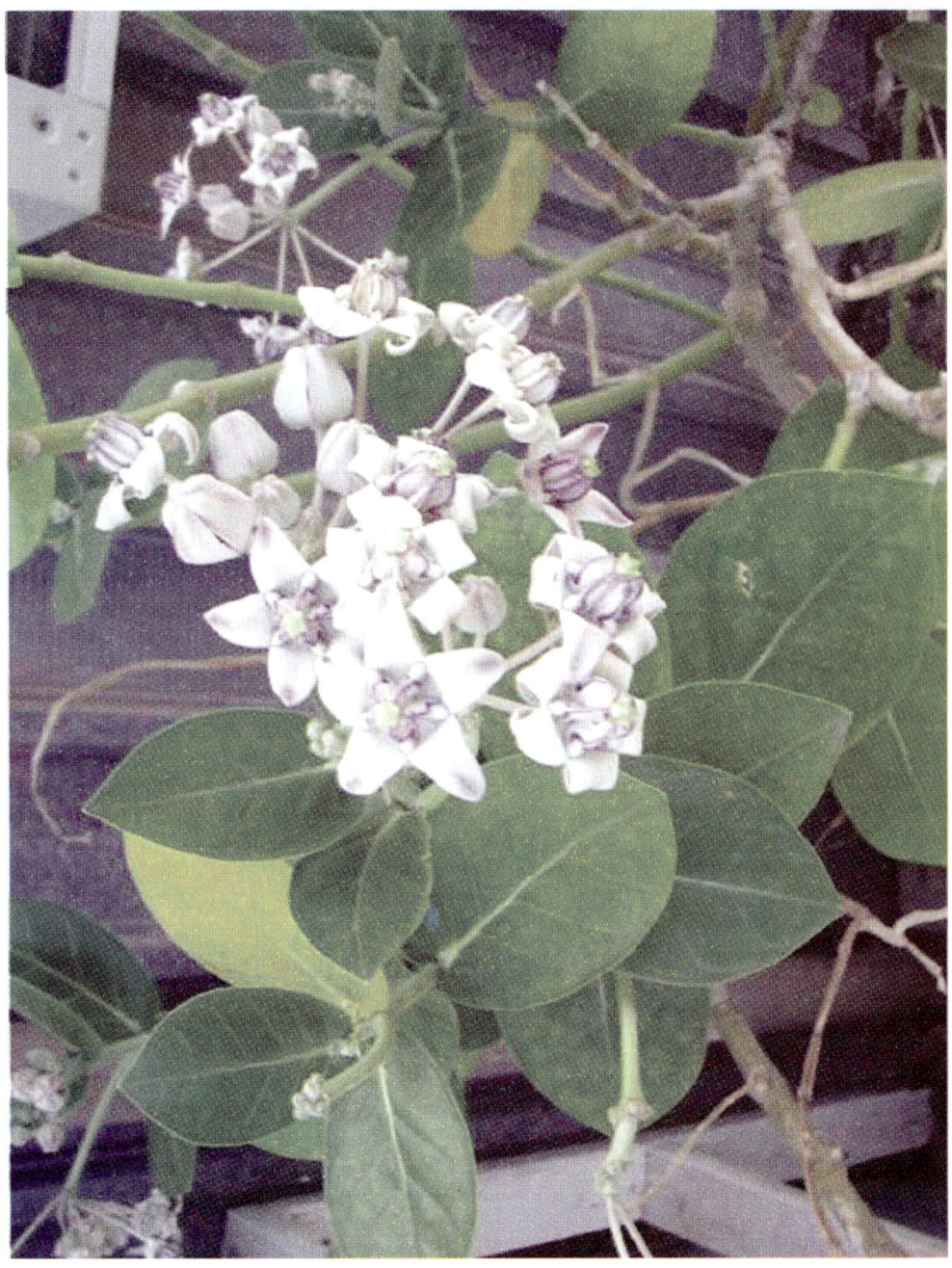

PLATE
29

Calotropis gigantea R.Br.

ASCLEPIADACEAE

Common Names

Eng	:	Gigantic swallow wert, mudar
Hind	:	Madar
Sans	:	Arka, Alarka, Mandara
Ben	:	Akanda
Tam	:	Badabadam, Erukku
Mal	:	Erikka

Parts Used

Root, leaves, flower, juice

Constituents

Root contain cardiac glycoside, several oxypregnane-oligoglycosides, calotroposides A-G, Latex contain α calotropeol, β calotropeal, caoutchouc, akundarin & calotropin.

Uses

Roots are used in the treatment of scabies, hepatoprotective, flower is stomachic digestive & tonic, root bark is tonic, antispasmodic, expectorant and emetic in large dose.

Classification	
Kingdom	Plantae – Plants
Subkingdom	Tracheobionta – Vascular plants
Superdivision	Spermatophyta – Seed plants
Division	Magnoliophyta – Flowering plants
Class	Magnoliopsida – Dicotyledons
Subclass	Asteridae –
Order	Gentianales –
Family	Asclepiadaceae – Milkweed family
Genus	Calotropis R. Br. – calotropis

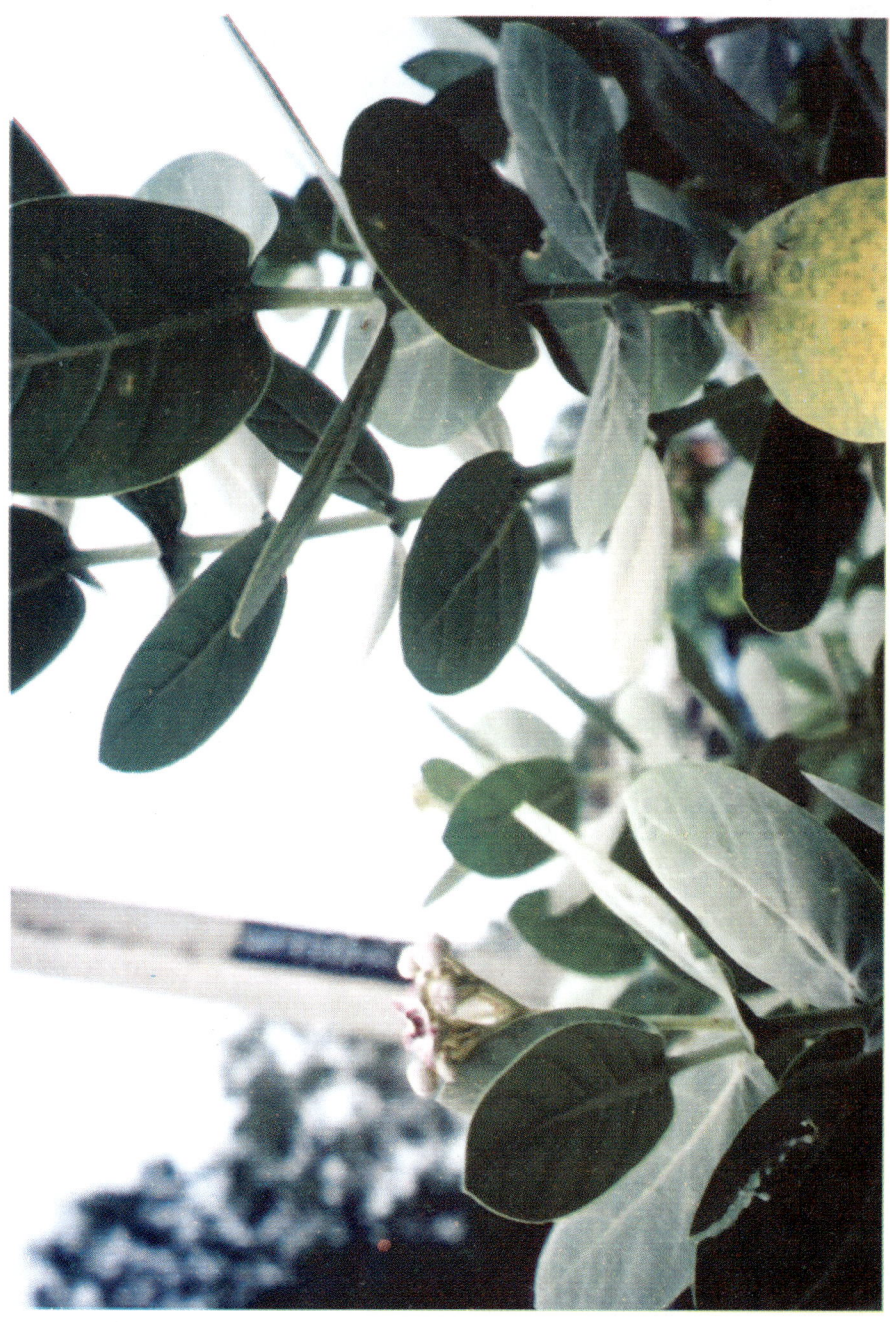

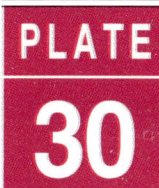

PLATE

30

Calotropis procera R.Br.

ASCLEPIADACEAE

Common Names

Eng	:	Small crown flower
Hind	:	Madar, safed ak
Sans	:	Alarka
Ben	:	Akanda
Tam	:	Vellarukku

Parts Used

Root, leaves, flower, juice

Constituents

Resins, tannins, sterols, glycosides.

Uses

Roots are used in the treatment of dysentery and toothache. Flower is emetic in large dose.

Classification	
Kingdom	Plantae – Plants
Subkingdom	Tracheobionta – Vascular plants
Superdivision	Spermatophyta – Seed plants
Division	Magnoliophyta – Flowering plants
Class	Magnoliopsida – Dicotyledons
Subclass	Asteridae –
Order	Gentianales –
Family	Asclepiadaceae – Milkweed family
Genus	Calotropis R. Br. – calotropis

Camellia sinensis (L.) O. Kuntze

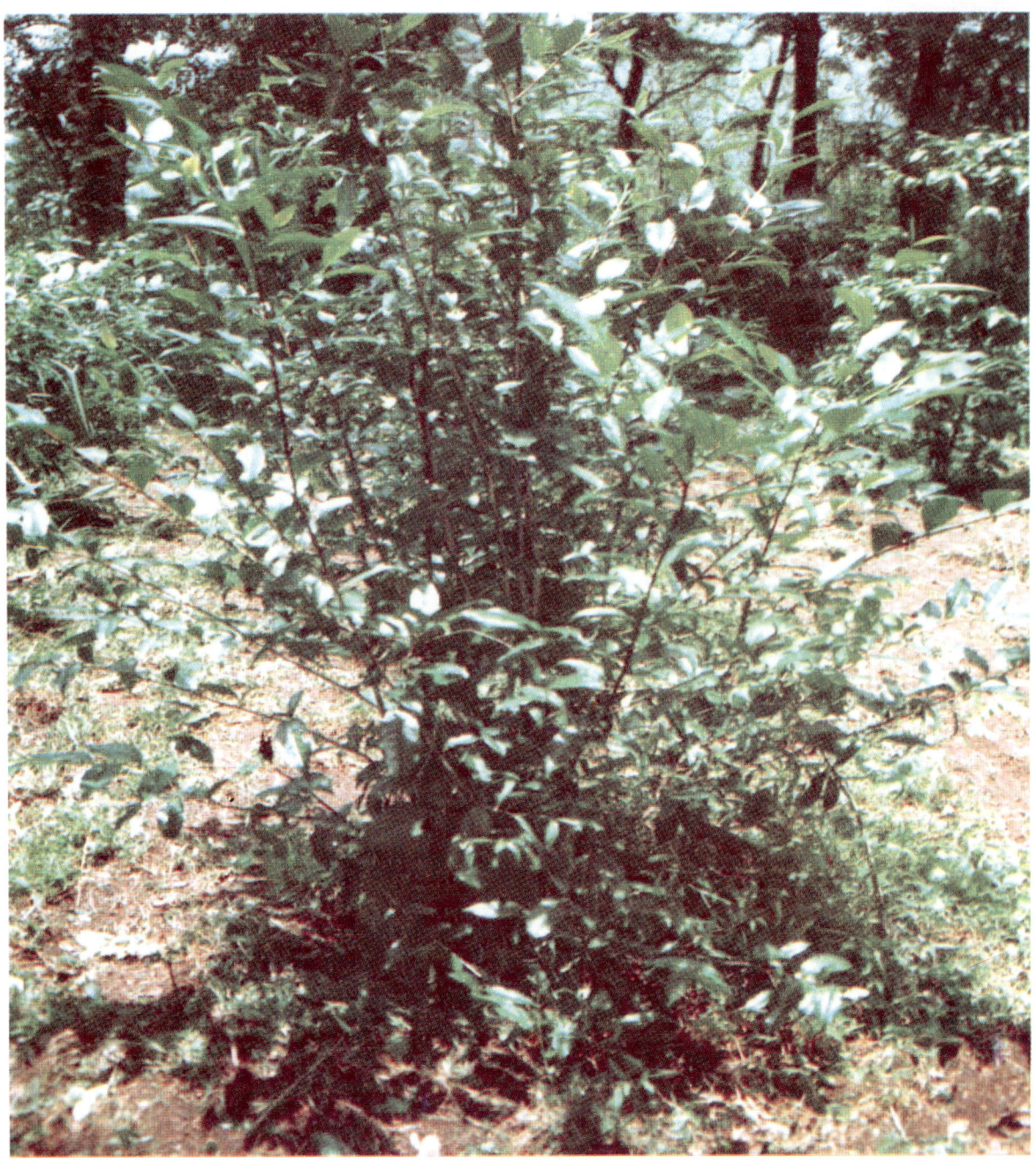

PLATE

31

Camellia sinensis (L.) O. Kuntze

THEACEAE

Common Names

Eng	:	Tea plant
Hin	:	Chha
Ben	:	Chha
Tam	:	Taielai
Mal	:	Chaya

Parts used

Young leaves

Constituent

Volatile oil to which the flavour of the tea is largely due to tannic and gallic acid, querecetin, theine, xanthine, adenine, saponin, theophylline, the active principles are polyphenon with d-catechin, epicatechin, epicatechin gallate, epigallocatechin gallate etc.

Uses

Stimulant, diuretic, astringent. The tea extract exhibits, antitumour, antioxidation, anti mutagenic, antivirus, anti coagulation, serum cholesterol and blood pressure reducing activity.

Classification	
Kingdom	Plantae – Plants
Subkingdom	Tracheobionta – Vascular plants
Superdivision	Spermatophyta – Seed plants
Division	Magnoliophyta – Flowering plants
Class	Magnoliopsida – Dicotyledons
Subclass	Dilleniidae –
Order	Theales –
Family	Theaceae – Tea family
Genus	Camellia L. – camellia

Carica papaya Linn

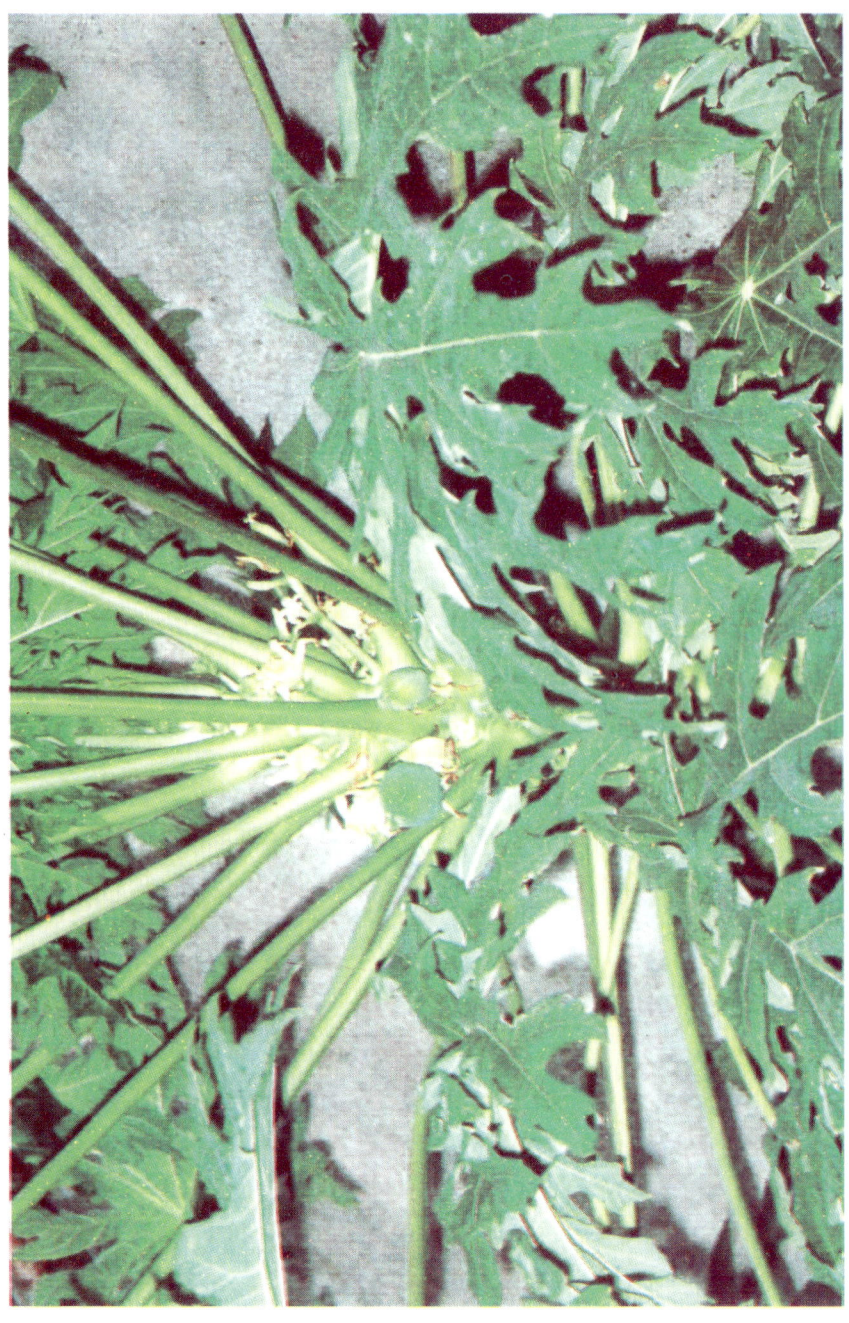

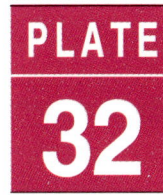

PLATE

32

Carica papaya Linn

CARICACEAE

Common Names

Eng	:	Papaw, Papaya
Hind	:	Popaiyah, Arandak karbuza
Ben	:	Papeya panpe
Tam	:	Poppayi, Pappali
Mal	:	Kappalam, Pappayam

Parts Used

Milky juice, seeds, pulps

Constituents

Papain, malic acid, tartaric acid, citric acid, leaves contain alkaloid known as carpaine and a glucoside known as carposide.

Uses

Juice of green fruit is rubefacient, anthelmintic, laxative, diuretic, ripe fruit is digestive. The latex from green fruit is considered very usefull in constipation, bleeding piles, enlarged liver and spleen, in large dose it accelerates uterine contraction.

Classification	
Kingdom	Plantae – Plants
Subkingdom	Tracheobionta – Vascular plants
Superdivision	Spermatophyta – Seed plants
Division	Magnoliophyta – Flowering plants
Class	Magnoliopsida – Dicotyledons
Subclass	Dilleniidae –
Order	Violales –
Family	Caricaceae – Papaya family
Genus	Carica L. – papaya

Cassia angustifolia Vahl

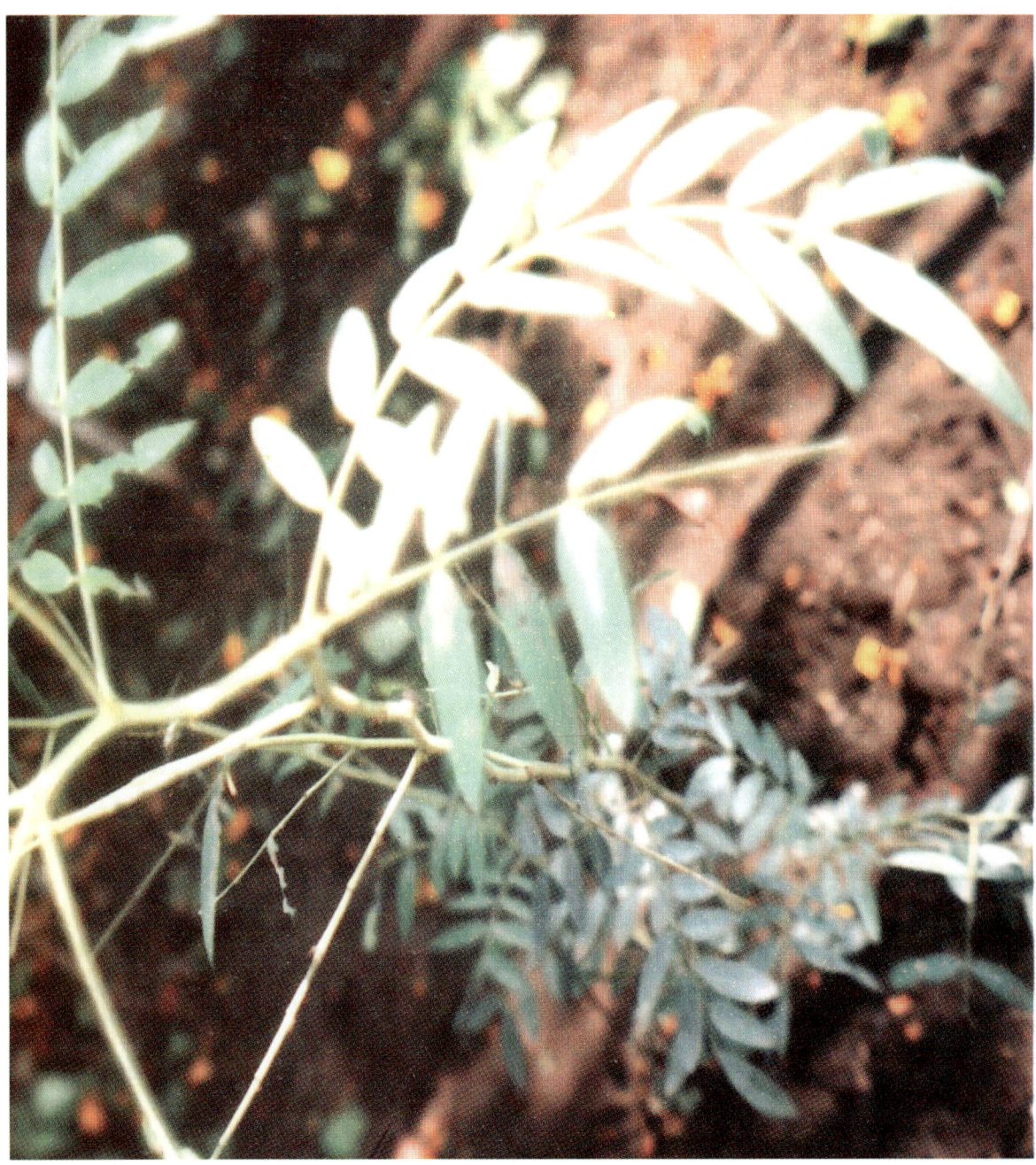

PLATE

33

Cassia angustifolia Vahl

LEGUMINOSAE

Common Names

Eng	:	Indian Senna
Hind	:	Sena-ka-pata
Ben	:	Sona Mukhi
Tam	:	Nilavakai
Mal	:	Nilavaka

Parts Used

Pods & dried leaves

Constituents

Anthraquinone glycosides- sennosides A, B, C, D, cathartin, emodin.

Uses

Purgative, stimulate intestinal peristalsis.

Classification	
Kingdom	Plantae – Plants
Subkingdom	Tracheobionta – Vascular plants
Superdivision	Spermatophyta – Seed plants
Division	Magnoliophyta – Flowering plants
Class	Magnoliopsida – Dicotyledons
Subclass	Rosidae –
Order	Fabales –
Family	Fabaceae – Pea family
Genus	Cassia Vahl. – senna

Cassia fistula L.

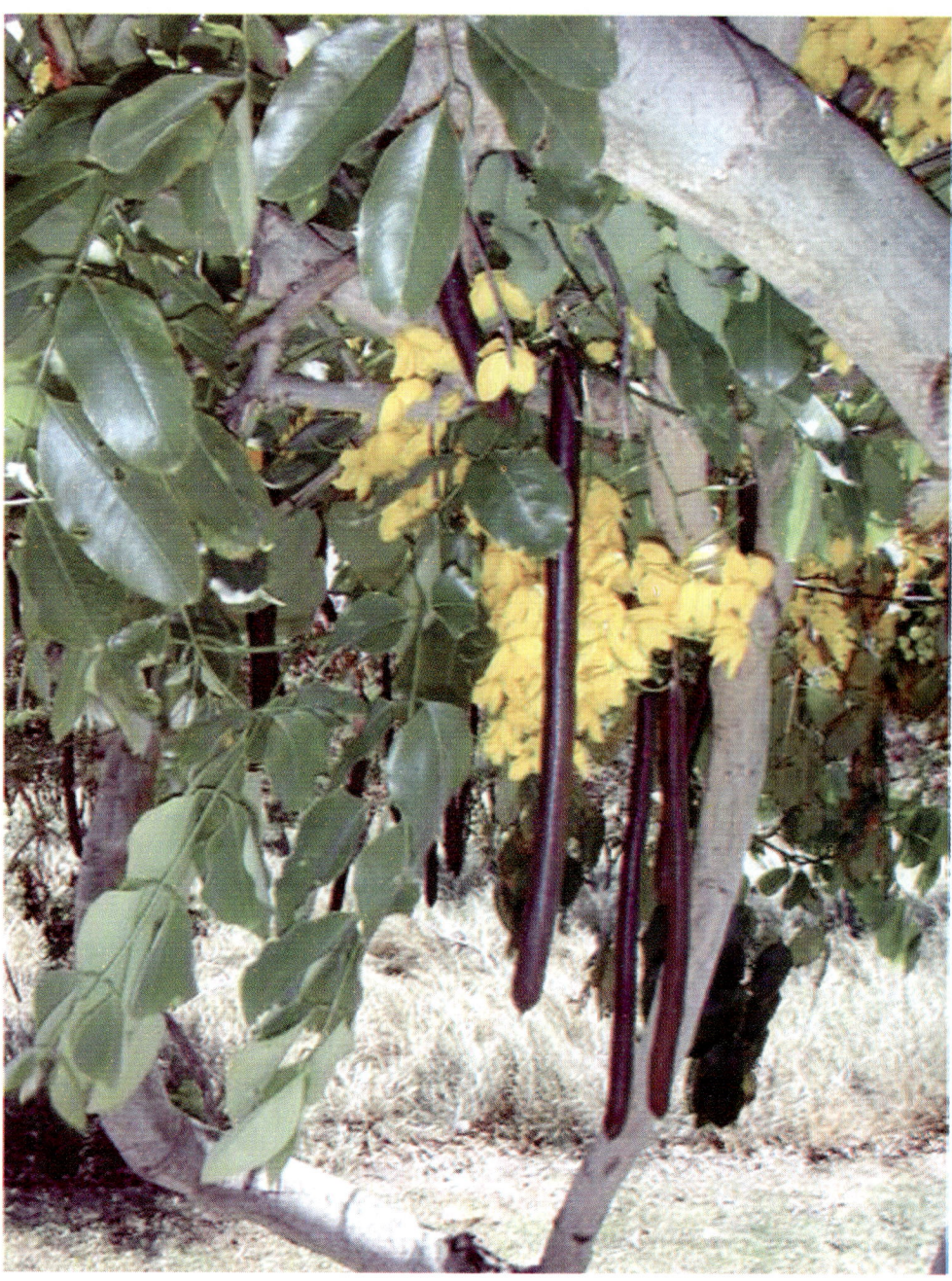

PLATE

34

Cassia fistula L.

FABACEAE

Common Names

Eng	:	Indian ladurnum
Hin	:	Sonhali
San	:	Naripadruma
Ben	:	Bundarlati
Tam	:	Konai
Mal	:	Konna

Parts used

Pulp, root barks, flowers, pods, roots

Constituents

Bark contain flavanol glycoside and xanthone glycoside, the pods contain procyanidin B-2, epicatechin, epiafzelechin, seed oil contain cyclopropenoid, fatty acid like vernolic, malvalic, sterculic acid.

Uses

Roots used in chest pain, jointpains, migraine, dysentery, Stem bark used against amenorrhoea, swelling, Aqueous extract of flower inhibit the ovarian function and stimulates the uterine function, seeds are antisecretory.

Classification	
Kingdom	Plantae – Plants
Subkingdom	Tracheobionta – Vascular plants
Superdivision	Spermatophyta – Seed plants
Division	Magnoliophyta – Flowering plants
Class	Magnoliopsida – Dicotyledons
Subclass	Rosidae –
Order	Fabales –
Family	Fabaceae – Pea family
Genus	Cassia L. – cassia

Catharanthus roseus G.Don/Linn

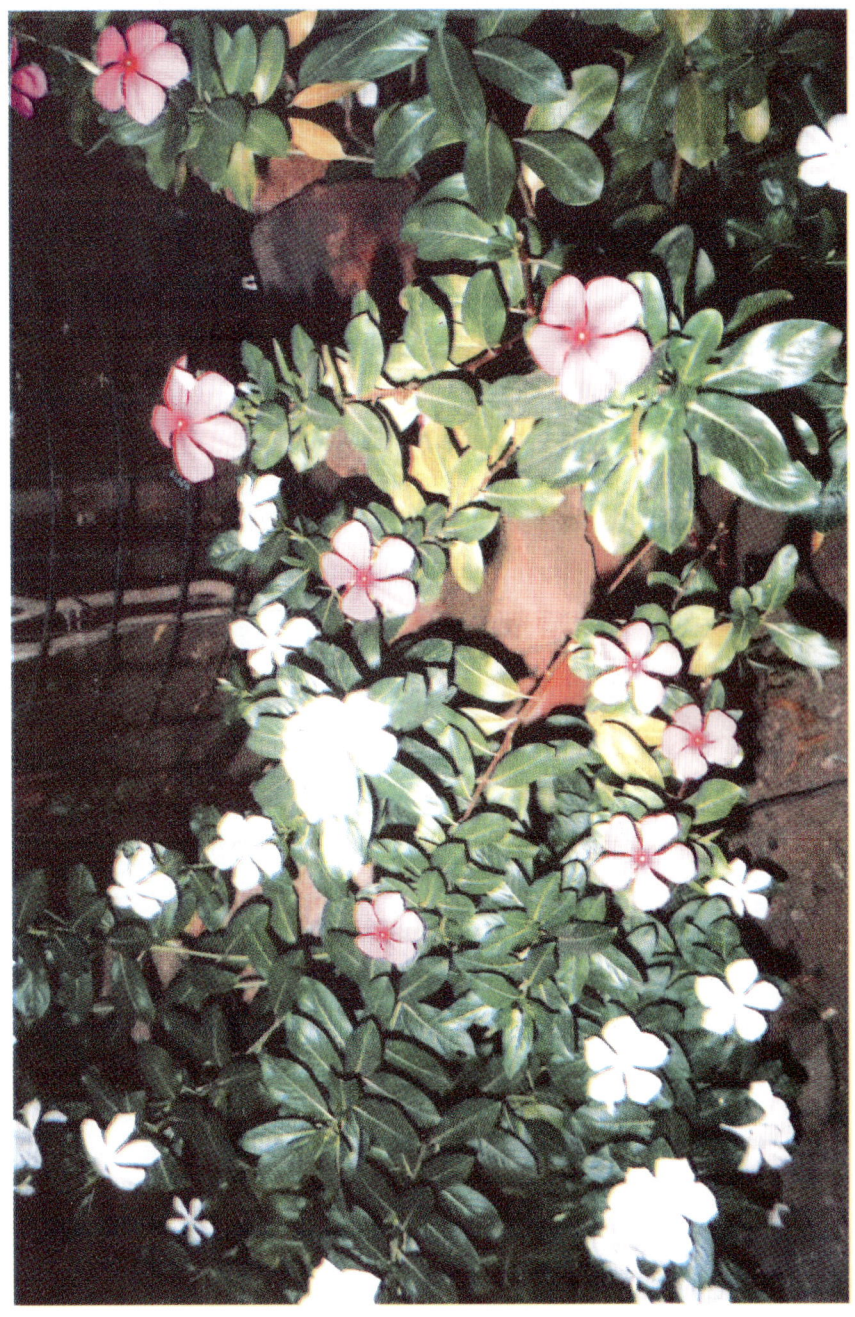

PLATE 35

Catharanthus roseus G.Don/Linn

APOCYNACEAE

Common Names

Eng : Vinca, Periwinkle
Hind : Sadabahar
Ben : Nayantara
Tam : Nithya kalyani
Mal : Kasithumpa

Parts Used

Whole plant

Constituents

The plant contain alkaloids coronaridine, 11-methoxytabersonine, tetrahydroalstonine, ajmalicine, vindorosine, catharanthine, mitraphylline, vindoline, vincristine, vinblastin, urosolic acid, leurosine, Iso leurosine, previne.

Uses

Vincristine and vinblastine are used in the treatment of human neoplasma, while ajmalicine is used in the treatment of circulatory disorders, hypertension, diabetes, and as antibacterial.

Classification	
Kingdom	Plantae – Plants
Subkingdom	Tracheobionta – Vascular plants
Superdivision	Spermatophyta – Seed plants
Division	Magnoliophyta – Flowering plants
Class	Magnoliopsida – Dicotyledons
Subclass	Asteridae –
Order	Gentianales –
Family	Apocynaceae – DogBene family
Genus	Catharanthus G. Don – periwinkle

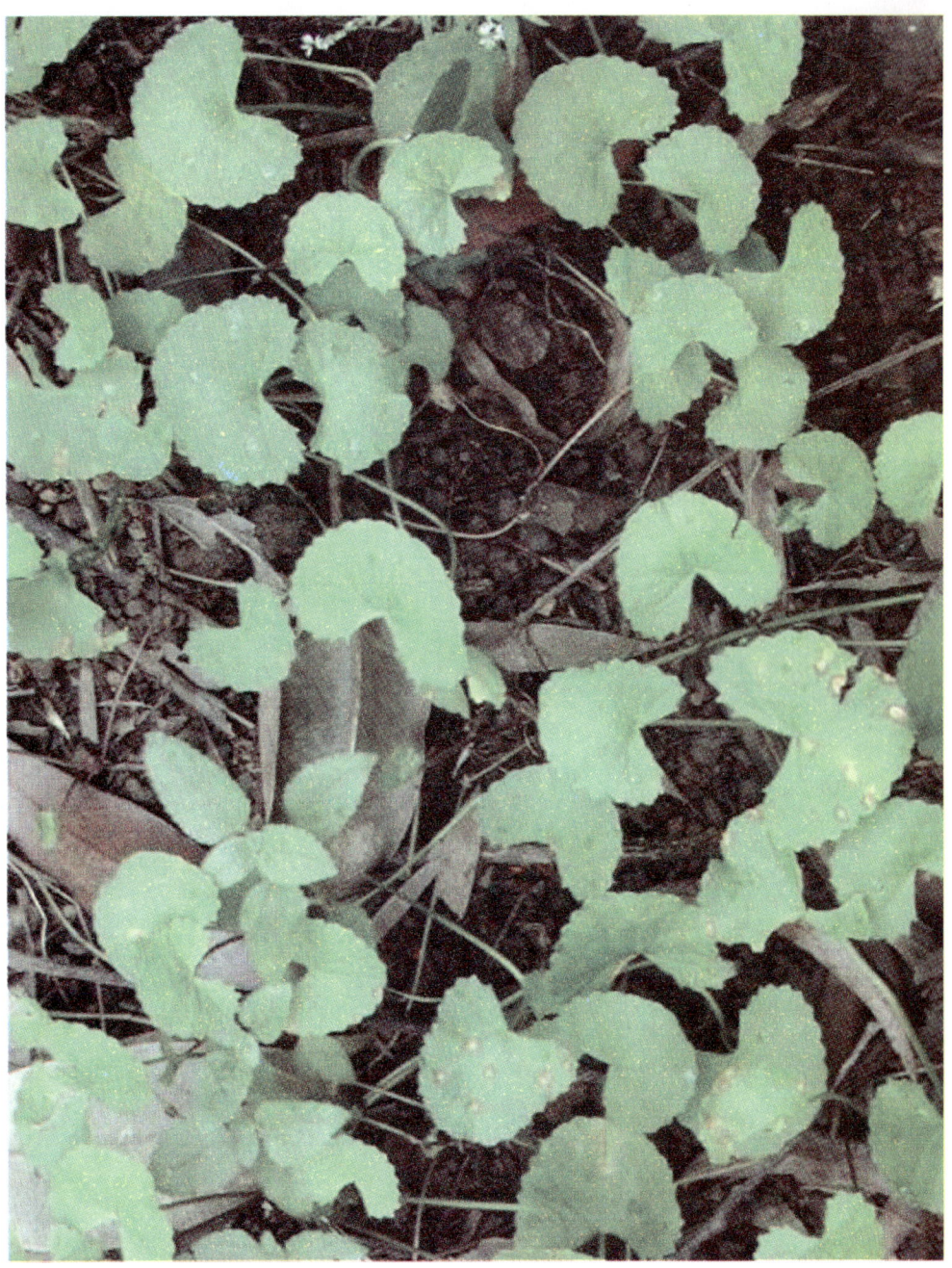

PLATE
36

Centella asiatica Linn

APIACEAE

Common Names

Eng	:	Indian penny wert
Hind	:	Khulakudi, Brahma marduki
Sans	:	Brahmi
Ben	:	Tholkuri, Brahma Marduki
Tam	:	Vallarai, Batassa
Mal	:	Kutakam

Parts Used

Whole plant

Constituents

Asiaticosides, Vellarin, thankunic acid, triterpene glycoside thankuniside, asiatic acid.

Uses

Plant has an antispasmodic effect, used in the treatment of leprosy, antifertility activity is shown by the expressed juice, tonic, diuretic, stimulant, emmenagogue.

Classification	
Kingdom	Plantae – Plants
Subkingdom	Tracheobionta – Vascular plants
Superdivision	Spermatophyta – Seed plants
Division	Magnoliophyta – Flowering plants
Class	Magnoliopsida – Dicotyledons
Subclass	Rosidae –
Order	Apiales –
Family	Apiaceae – Carrot family
Genus	Centella L. – centella

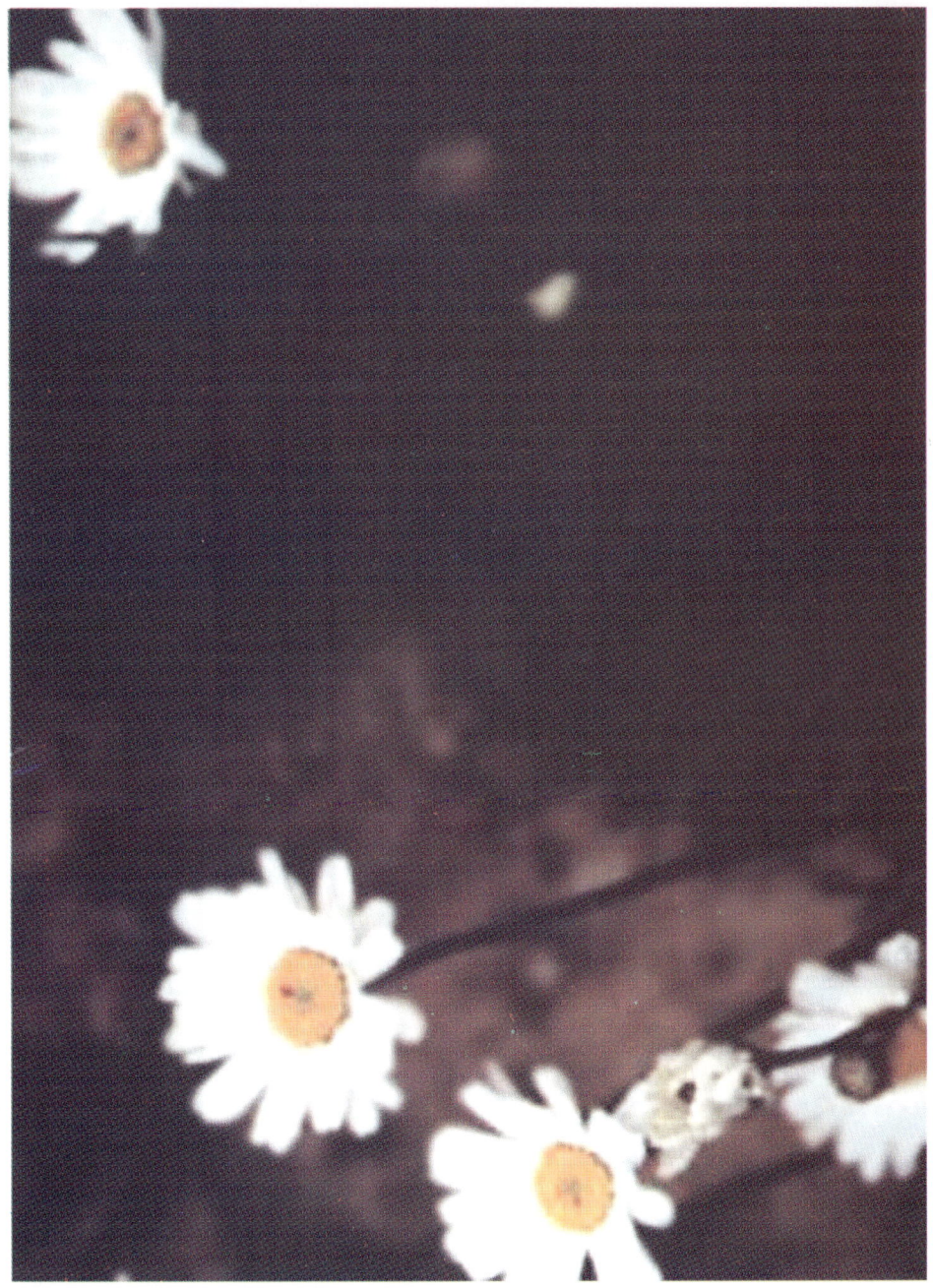

PLATE
37

Chrysanthemum cinerariaefolium (Trevir.) Vis.

ASTERACEAE

Common Name

Eng : Pyrethrum

Parts used

Flowers

Constituents

Geraniol, chrysanthemyl alcohol, chrysanthemic acid, chrysanthemum dicarboxylic acids, pyrethrins, cinerins.

Uses

Flower heads is effective molluscide against bulinus species.

Classification	
Kingdom	Plantae – Plants
Subkingdom	Tracheobionta – Vascular plants
Superdivision	Spermatophyta – Seed plants
Division	Magnoliophyta – Flowering plants
Class	Magnoliopsida – Dicotyledons
Subclass	Asteridae –
Order	Asterales –
Family	Asteraceae – Aster family
Genus	Chrysanthemum L. – daisy

Cinchona calisaya Wedd

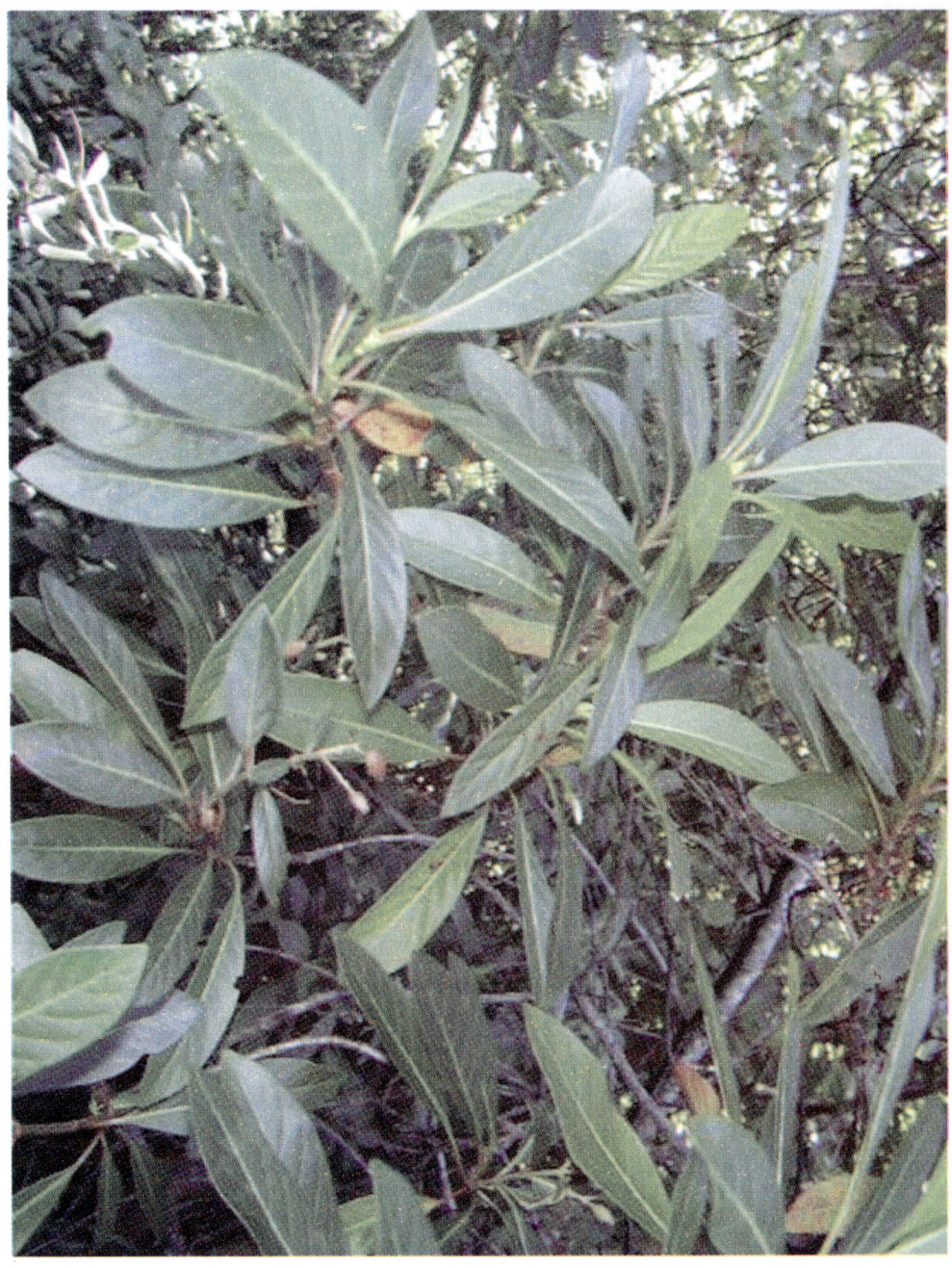

PLATE

38

Cinchona calisaya Wedd

RUBIACEAE

Common Names

Eng   :   Jesuits bark, Cinchona

Parts Used

Barks, fruits

Constituents

Alkaloid of quinoline groups quinine, quinidine, cinchonine, cinchonidine, the alkaloids of less importance are quinicine, cinchonicine, hydroquinine, hydrocinchonicine, homocinchonidine, quinine and quinidine are stereoisomers, tannins essential oil, quinovin are also present.

Uses

Anti-malarial, Bitter stomachic, antipyretic, arrhythmias.

Classification	
Kingdom	Plantae – Plants
Subkingdom	Tracheobionta – Vascular plants
Superdivision	Spermatophyta – Seed plants
Division	Magnoliophyta – Flowering plants
Class	Magnoliopsida – Dicotyledons
Subclass	Asteridae –
Order	Rubiales –
Family	Rubiaceae – Madder family
Genus	Cinchona L. – cinchona

Cinnamomum zeylanicum Nees

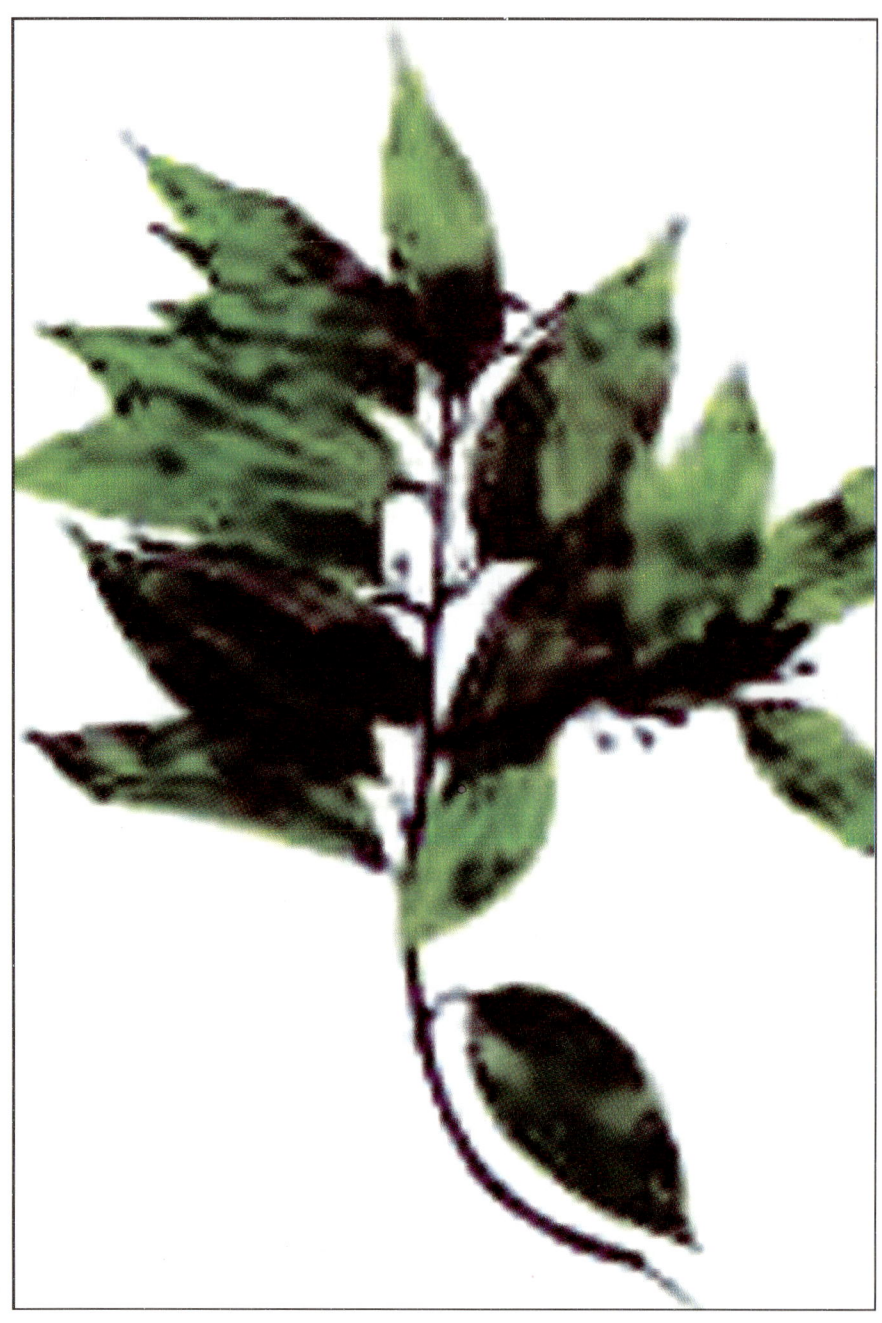

PLATE
39

Cinnamomum zeylanicum Nees

LAURACEAE

Common Names

Eng	:	True cinnamon
Hind	:	Dalchini
Sans	:	Gudatvak
Ben	:	Dalchini
Tam	:	Lowangapattai
Mal	:	Lowangapatta

Parts Used

Dried inner bark.

Constituents

Volatile oil, cinnamic acid, resin, tannin, starch, mucilage, caryophyllene, eugenol, cinamaldehyde, cuminaldehyde, other terpenes like phellandrene, pinene, cymene, caryophyllene.

Uses

Carminative, antispasmodic, aromatic, stimulant, haemostatic, astringent, antiseptic, stomachic, germicide.

Classification	
Kingdom	Plantae – Plants
Subkingdom	Tracheobionta – Vascular plants
Superdivision	Spermatophyta – Seed plants
Division	Magnoliophyta – Flowering plants
Class	Magnoliopsida – Dicotyledons
Subclass	Magnoliidae –
Order	Laurales –
Family	Lauraceae – Laurel family
Genus	Cinnamomum – cinnamon

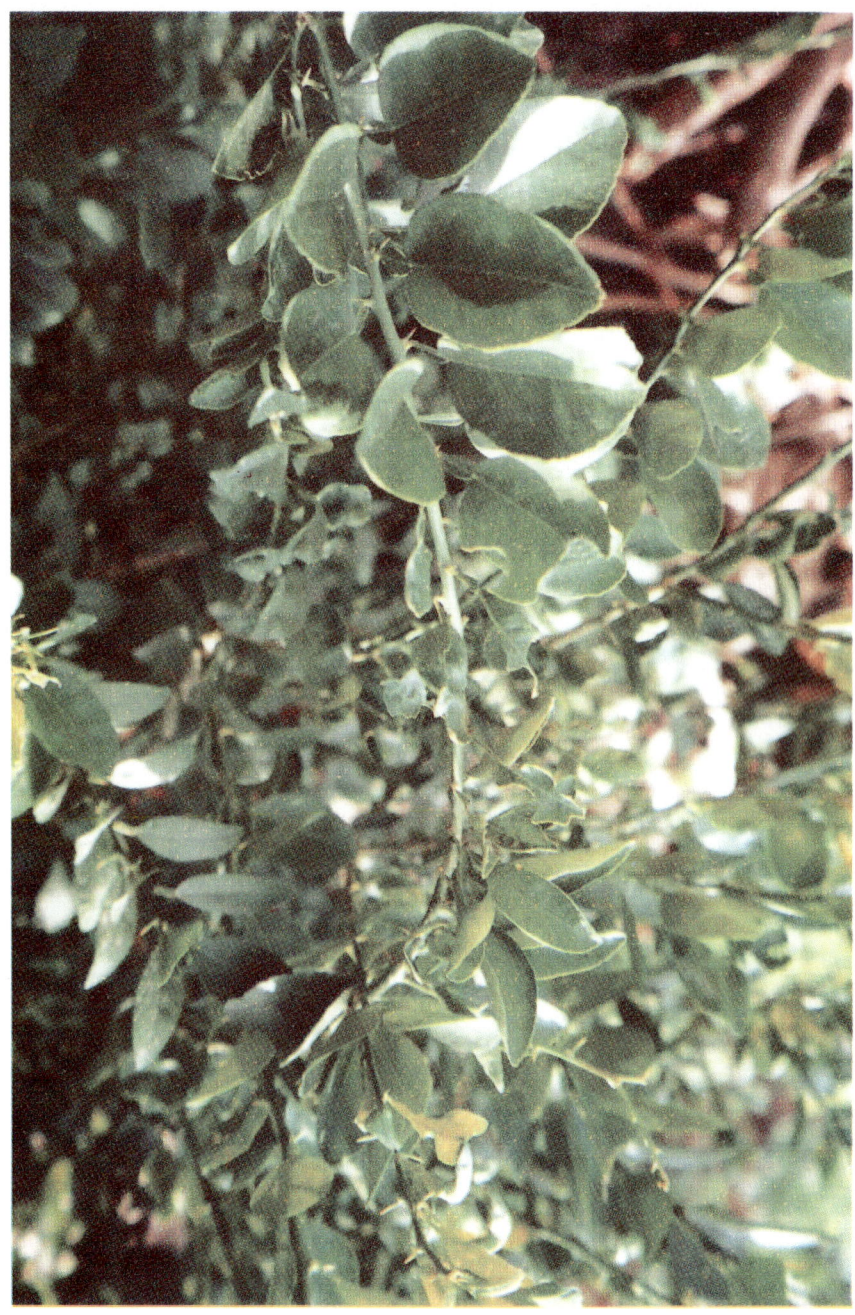

PLATE
40

Citrus limonum Linn

RUTACEAE

Common Names

Eng	:	Lemon
Hin	:	Pahadi Nimbu
Sans	:	Limpaka
Ben	:	Karnanebu
Tam	:	Periya elimichcham
Mal	:	Naranga

Parts used

Ripe fruit, root, leaves

Constituents

Limonoid glycosides, ichangin 4-β-glucopyranoside, nomilinic acid, 4-β glucopyranoside are reported on peel. Essential oil of leaves contains neral, geranial, limonene as the major constituent.

Uses

Rind is stomachic, carminative, lemon oil is bitter, aromatic, stomachic, peel is used as cosmetic as a hair rinse and mouth freshner, root is used as anthelmintic.

Classification	
Kingdom	Plantae – Plants
Subkingdom	Tracheobionta – Vascular plants
Superdivision	Spermatophyta – Seed plants
Division	Magnoliophyta – Flowering plants
Class	Magnoliopsida – Dicotyledons
Subclass	Rosidae –
Order	Sapindales –
Family	Rutaceae – Rue family
Genus	Citrus L. – citrus

Clerodendrum inerme (L). Gaertn

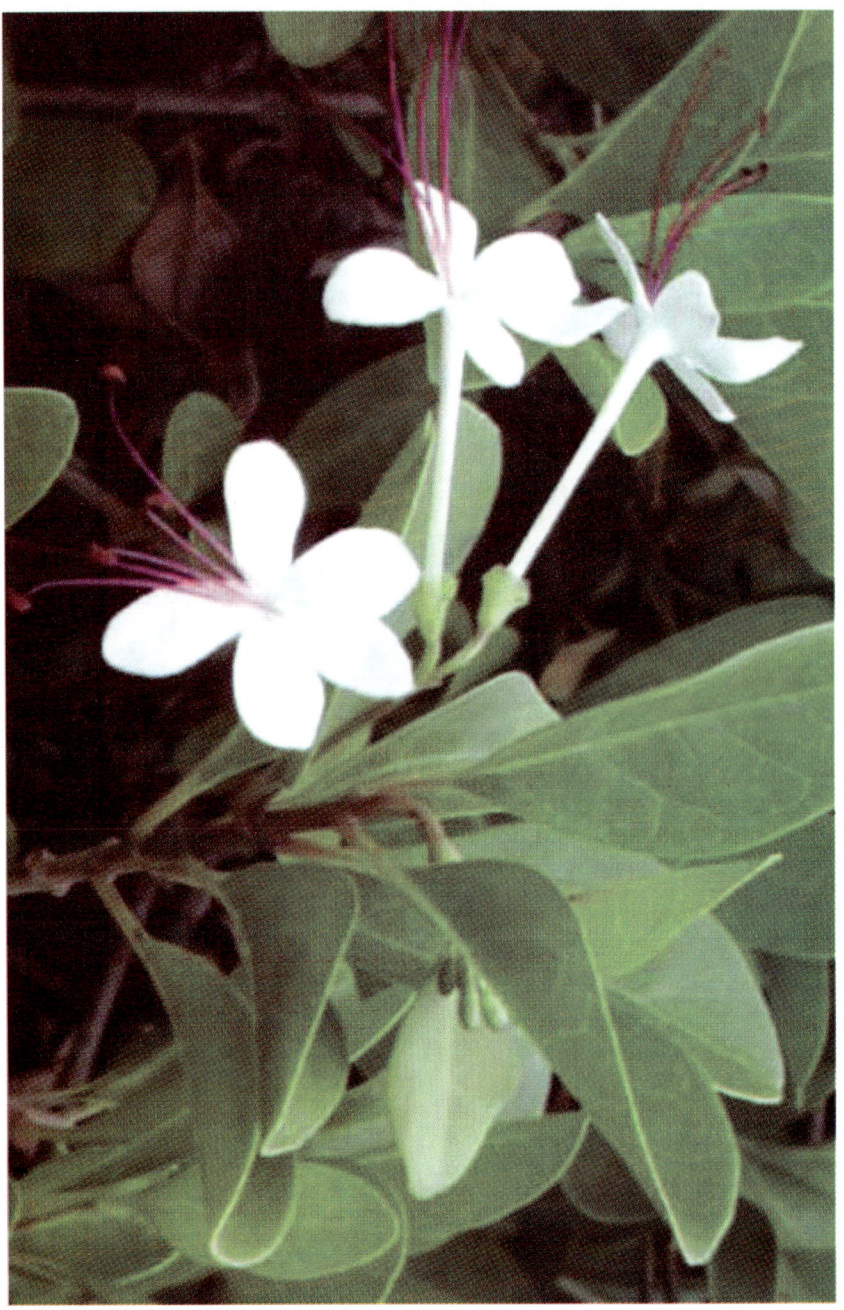

PLATE

41

Clerodendrum inerme (L). Gaertn

VERBENACEAE

Common Names

Eng	:	Garden quinine
Hin	:	Binjoam
Sans	:	Kandali
Ben	:	Benjoi
Tam	:	Pinasangal-koppi
Mal	:	Nirnotijin

Parts used

Leaves, roots

Constituents

Bitter principles, resins, gums, triterpenoids, sterols, brown coloring matter.

Uses

Tonic, febrifuge, mucilagous, bitter, fragrant, analgesic, antimicrobial, and in veneral diseases.

Classification	
Kingdom	Plantae – Plants
Subkingdom	Tracheobionta – Vascular plants
Superdivision	Spermatophyta – Seed plants
Division	Magnoliophyta – Flowering plants
Class	Magnoliopsida – Dicotyledons
Subclass	Asteridae –
Order	Lamiales –
Family	Verbenaceae – Verbena family
Genus	Clerodendrum L. – glorybower

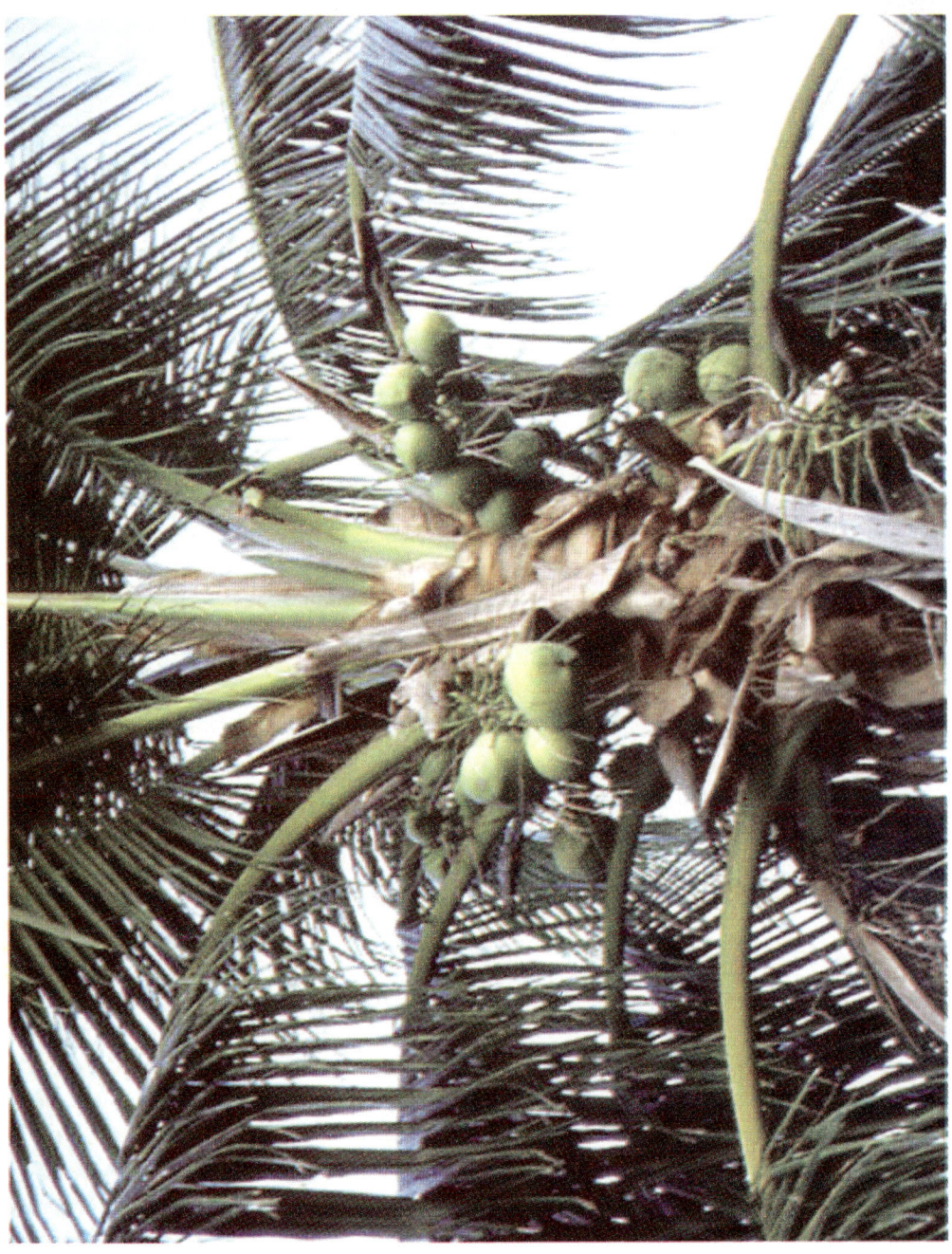

PLATE

42

Cocos nucifera. Linn

ARECACEAE

Common Names

Eng	:	Coconut
Hind	:	Nariyal
Sans	:	Tranaraj
Ben	:	Narikel
Tam	:	Tennai maram
Mal	:	Tengu

Parts Used

Leaves, flowers, barks, gum, seeds.

Constituents

Protamine, albumine, amino acid, rhizomes are rich in starch, fibre, oil contain pinocarveol, cadinene, cineol p-methoxy benzophenone, carvacrol.

Uses

Refrigerant, nutrient, aperients diuretic, anthelmintic, coconut water is demulcent mucilaginous and used as astringent, tonic, anthelmintic, abortificant, aphrodisiac, in cold, cough, pneumonia, stomach trouble, rheumatism, dropsy, urinary infection, the fresh juice is purgative and also applied in leprosy, leaves are antifungal.

Classification	
Kingdom	Plantae – Plants
Subkingdom	Tracheobionta – Vascular plants
Superdivision	Spermatophyta – Seed plants
Division	Magnoliophyta – Flowering plants
Class	Liliopsida – Monocotyledons
Subclass	Arecidae –
Order	Arecales –
Family	Arecaceae – Palm family
Genus	Cocos L. – coconut palm

Coffea arabica Linn

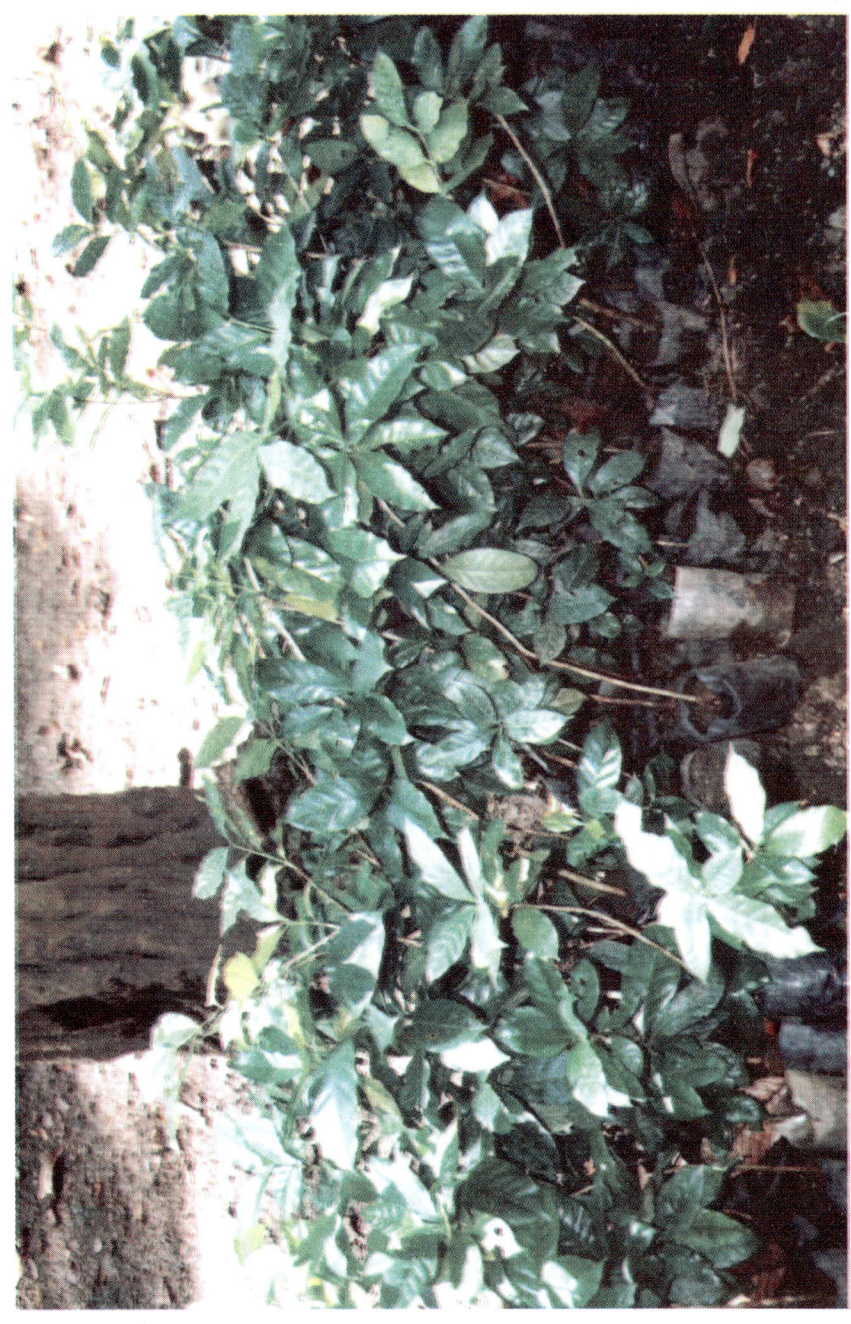

PLATE

43

Coffea arabica Linn

RUBIACEAE

Common Names

Eng	:	Arabian coffee
Kan	:	Kapi-bija
Hin	:	Caphi, Pilu
Tel	:	Kapi-vittulu, Kappi
Tam	:	Kapi
Mal	:	Kappi

Parts Used

Ripe seeds

Constituents

Caffeine, tannin, fixed oil, protein.

Uses

Stimulant, diuretic.

Classification	
Kingdom	Plantae – Plants
Subkingdom	Tracheobionta – Vascular plants
Superdivision	Spermatophyta – Seed plants
Division	Magnoliophyta – Flowering plants
Class	Magnoliopsida – Dicotyledons
Subclass	Asteridae –
Order	Rubiales –
Family	Rubiaceae – Madder family
Genus	Coffea L. – coffee

Colchicum autumnale L.

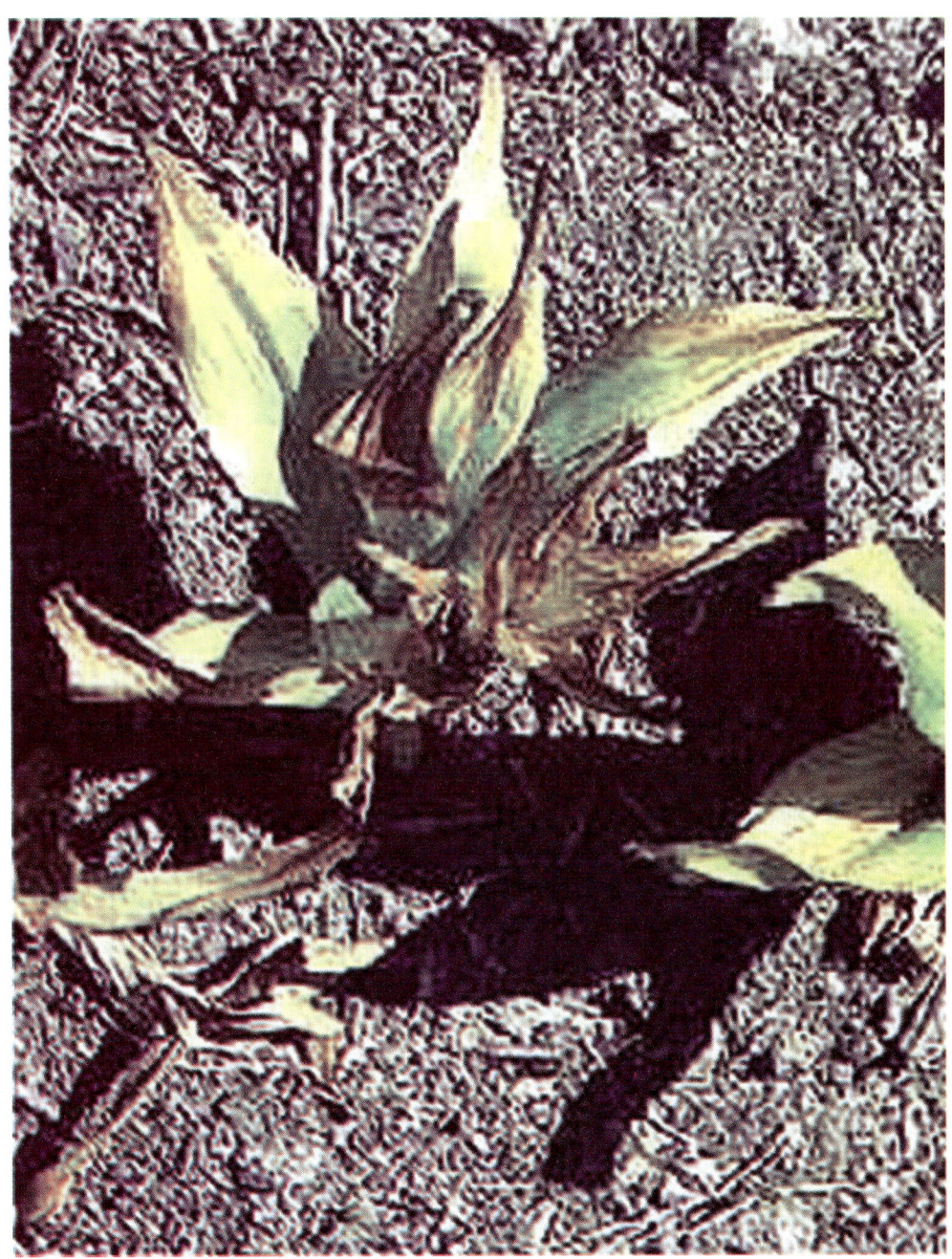

PLATE

44

Colchicum autumnale L.

LILIACEAE

Common Name

End   :   Meadow saffron seeds

Parts Used

Ripe seeds

Constituents

Amino alkaloids, colchicines, demecolcine.

Uses

In the treatment of gout, rheumatism and tumour.

Classification	
Kingdom	Plantae – Plants
Subkingdom	Tracheobionta – Vascular plants
Superdivision	Spermatophyta – Seed plants
Division	Magnoliophyta – Flowering plants
Class	Liliopsida – Monocotyledons
Subclass	Liliidae –
Order	Liliales –
Famil	Liliaceae – Lily family
Genus	Colchicum L. – colchicum

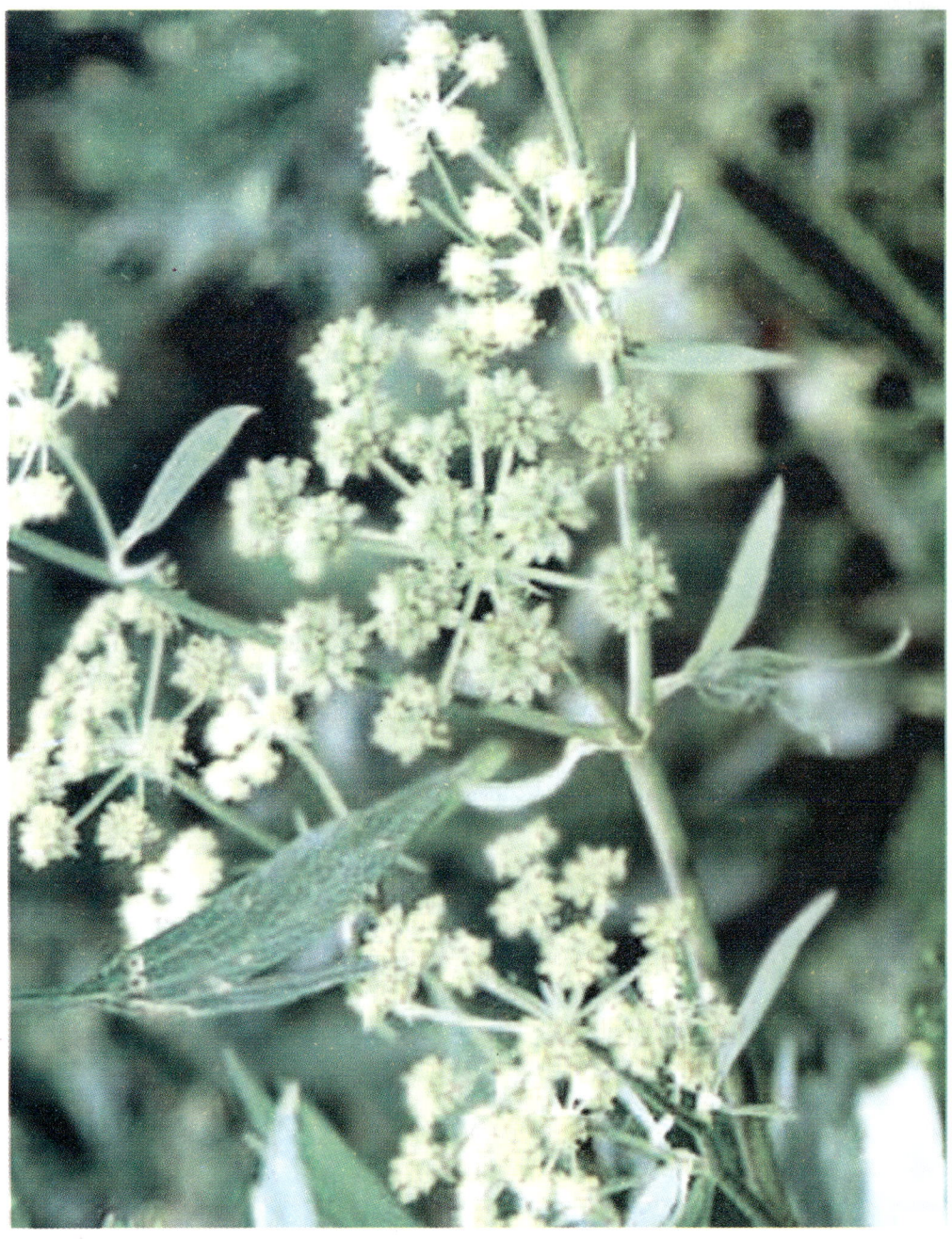

PLATE
45

Coriandrum sativum Linn

UMBELLIFERAE

Common Names

Eng	:	Coriander
Hind	:	Dhaniya/Kottamir
Sans	:	Kustumbari
Ben	:	Dhane
Tam	:	Kottamalli
Mal	:	Kottampalari

Parts Used

Fruit

Constituents

Volatile oil, fixed oil, protein, D-Linalool, coriandryl, L-borneal, geraniol, pinene, camphene, limonene, linalool oxide, terpinolene, linalool, camphor, borneol, terpineol, geraniol.

Uses

The fruits including seeds are stimulant, pectoral, antipyretic, anthelmintic. Infusion of the fruit is used in flatulence, indigestion, vomiting and other intestinal disorder, also used in bleeding piles, rheumatism, neuralgia, cephalagia, locally in eye infection, fruits are given in spermatorrhoea, leucorrhoea and rheumatic fever. Aromatic, carminative, stimulant, flavoring agents.

Classification	
Kingdom	Plantae – Plants
Subkingdom	Tracheobionta – Vascular plants
Superdivision	Spermatophyta – Seed plants
Division	Magnoliophyta – Flowering plants
Class	Magnoliopsida – Dicotyledons
Subclass	Rosidae –
Order	Apiales –
Family	Apiaceae – Carrot family
Genus	Coriandrum L. – coriander

Costus speciosus Sm

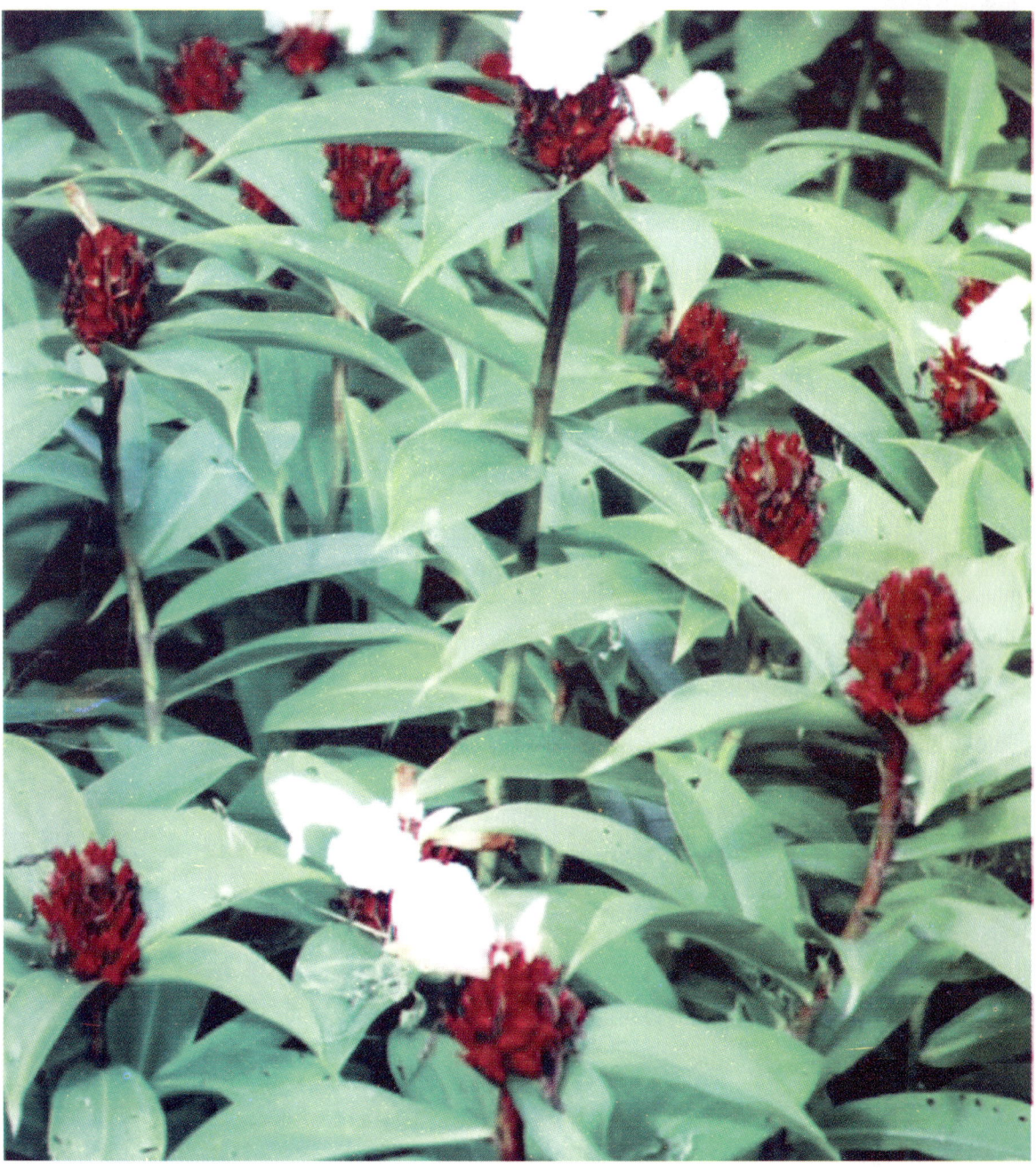

PLATE

46

Costus speciosus Sm

COSTACEAE

Common Names

Eng	:	Canereed
Hind	:	Keu, Kust
Sans	:	Pashakea
Ben	:	Keu Kura
Tam	:	Koestam
Mal	:	Narunchana

Parts Used

Roots & tubers

Constituents

Saponins, tigoginin, diosgenin, α-amyrin sterate, β-amyrin and lupeol palmitatis

Uses

Astringent, stimulant, digestive, anthelmintic, depurative, aphrodisiac.

Classification	
Kingdom	Plantae – Plants
Subkingdom	Tracheobionta – Vascular plants
Superdivision	Spermatophyta – Seed plants
Division	Magnoliophyta – Flowering plants
Class	Liliopsida – Monocotyledons
Subclass	Zingiberidae –
Order	Zingiberales –
Family	Costaceae – Costus family
Genus	Costus L. – costus

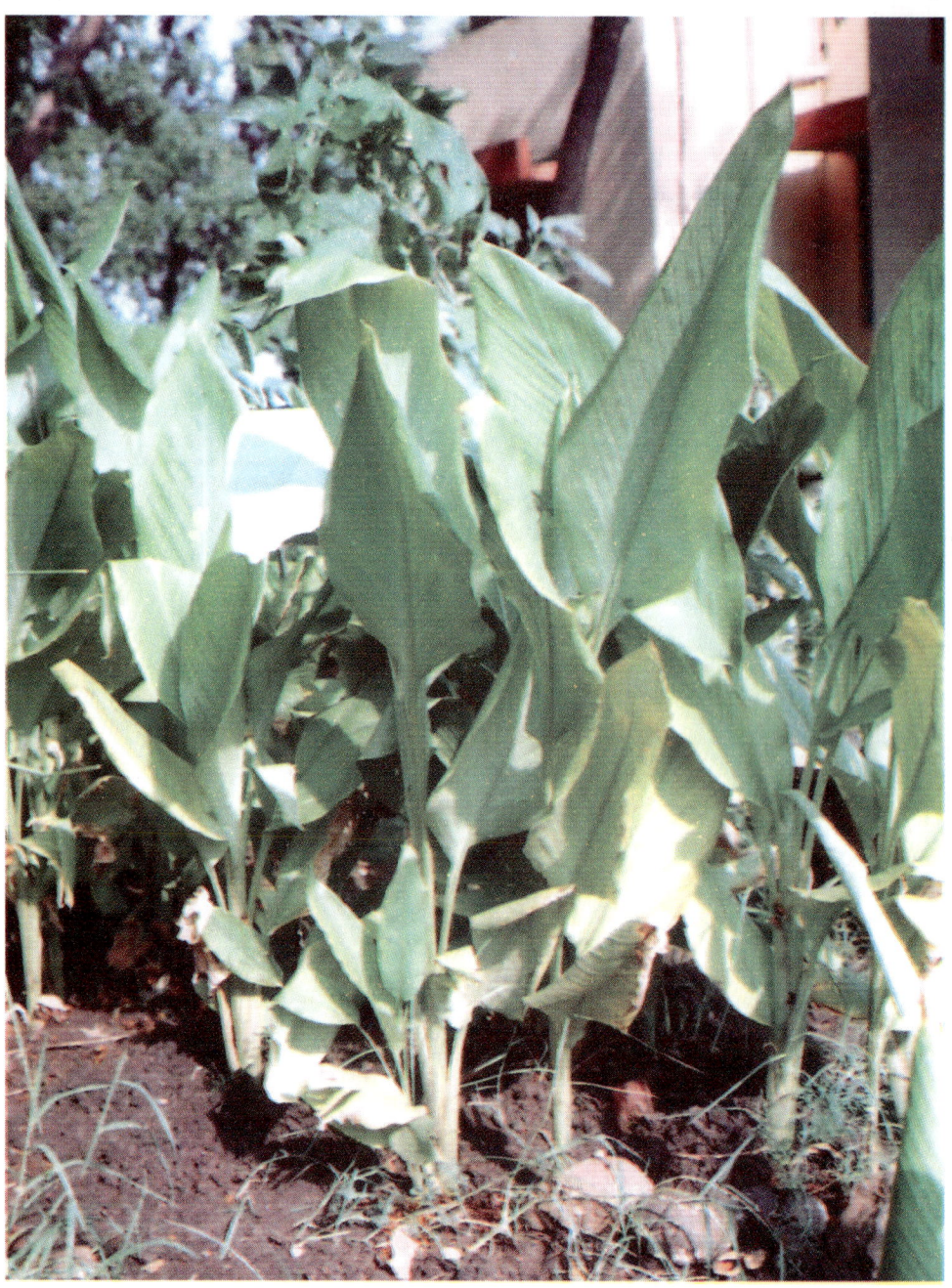

PLATE
47

Curcuma longa Linn

ZINGIBERACEAE

Common Names

Eng	:	Turmeric
Hind	:	Haldi
Sans	:	Rajani, Gauri
Ben	:	Halud
Tam	:	Manjal
Mal	:	Manjal

Parts Used

Tubers & rhizomes

Constituents

Essential oil, Protein, crystalline coloring matter known as curcumin curcuminoids, demethoxy curcumin, bis-demethoxy curcumin, 5 methoxycurcumin dehydrocurcumin, other curcuminoid isolated is cyclocurcumin, fresh rhizome contain curcumin related phenolics, several sesquiterpenes.

Uses

Antioxidant, anti-inflammatory, aromatic. stimulant, tonic, carminative, anthelmintic, antifertility.

Classification	
Kingdom	Plantae – Plants
Subkingdom	Tracheobionta – Vascular plants
Superdivision	Spermatophyta – Seed plants
Division	Magnoliophyta – Flowering plants
Class	Liliopsida – Monocotyledons
Subclass	Zingiberidae –
Order	Zingiberales –
Family	Zingiberaceae – Ginger family
Genus	Curcuma L. – curcuma

Curcuma zedoaria Rosc or Zerumber

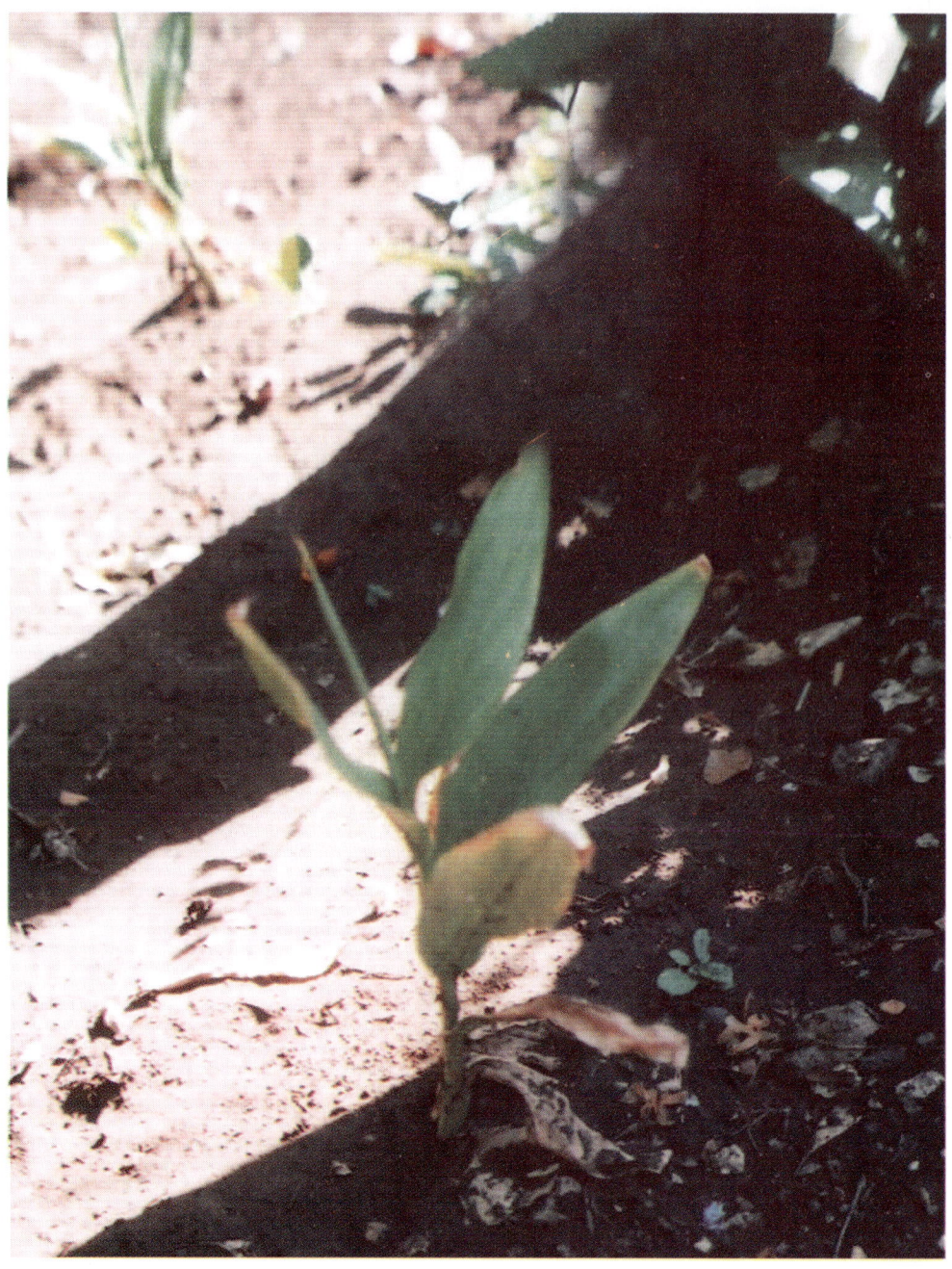

PLATE
48

Curcuma zedoaria Rosc or Zerumber

ZINGIBERACEAE

Common Names

Eng	:	Round zeodary
Hind	:	Gandamasti
Sans	:	Kachura
Ben	:	Sutha
Tam	:	Kastoori manjal
Mal	:	Pulan kizhanna

Parts Used

Tubers & leaves

Constituents

Essential oil, phenolic compounds, gum, resins.

Uses

Aromatic, stimulant, tonic, carminative, expectorant, demulcent, diuretic, etc.

Classification	
Kingdom	Plantae – Plants
Subkingdom	Tracheobionta – Vascular plants
Superdivision	Spermatophyta – Seed plants
Division	Magnoliophyta – Flowering plants
Class	Liliopsida – Monocotyledons
Subclass	Zingiberidae –
Order	Zingiberales –
Family	Zingiberaceae – Ginger family
Genus	Curcuma L. – curcuma

Cymbopogon citratus Stapf

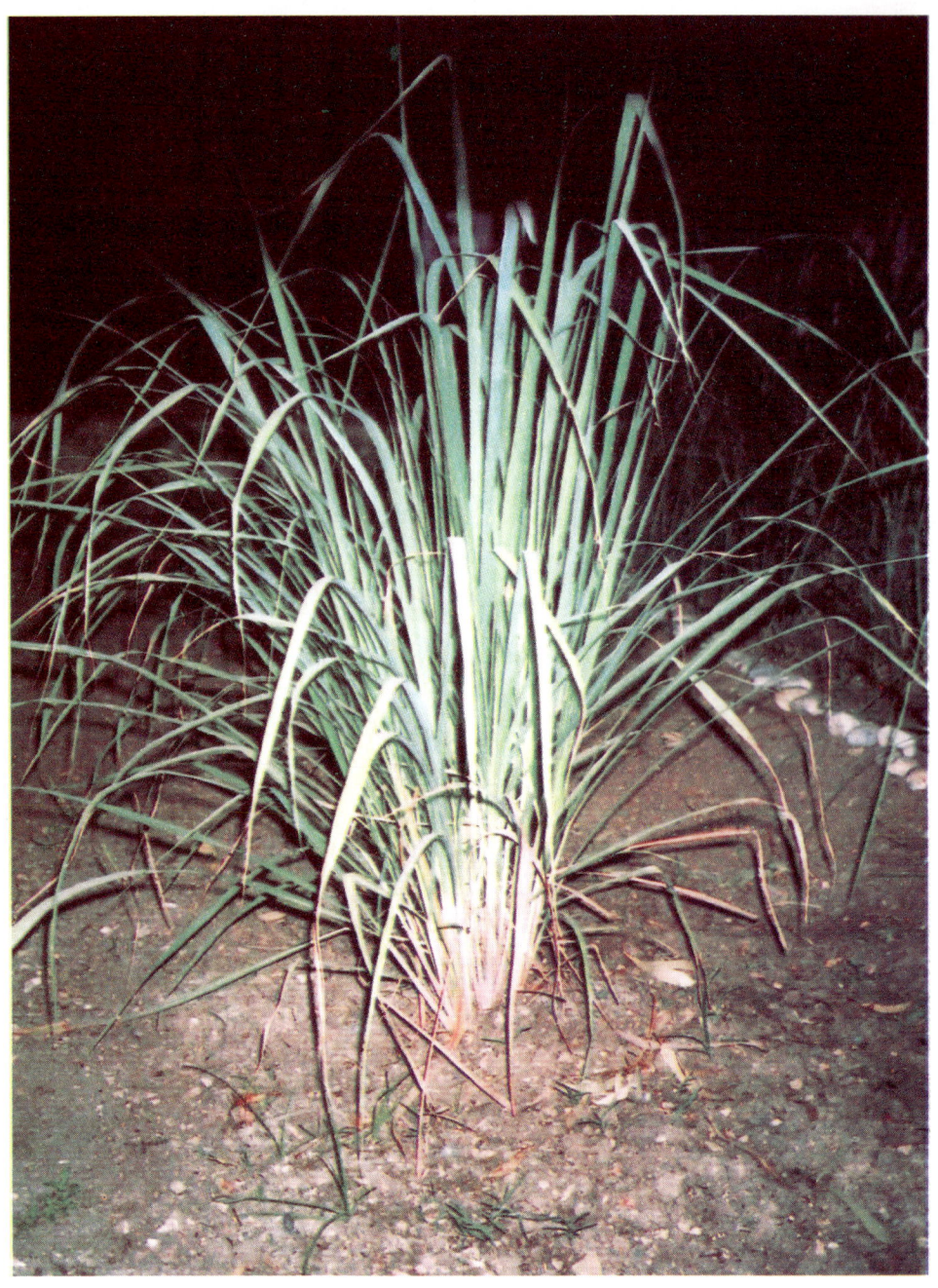

PLATE

49

Cymbopogon citratus Stapf

POACEAE

Common Name

Eng	:	lemon grass
San	:	Bhustrina
Ben	:	Gandhabena
Mal	:	Vasanappulla
Tam	:	Vasanappillu
Tel	:	Nimmagaddi

Parts used

Leaves

Constituents

Leaves contain limonene, geraniol, flavones, luteolin, iso-orientin, caffeic acid, p- coumaric acid, fructose, and sucrose.

Uses

Antibacterial, analgesic, anticarcinogenic.

Classification	
Kingdom	Plantae – Plants
Subkingdom	Tracheobionta – Vascular plants
Superdivision	Spermatophyta – Seed plants
Division	Magnoliophyta – Flowering plants
Class	Liliopsida – Monocotyledons
Subclass	Commelinidae –
Order	Cyperales –
Family	Poaceae – Grass family
Genus	Cymbopogon Spreng. – lemon grass

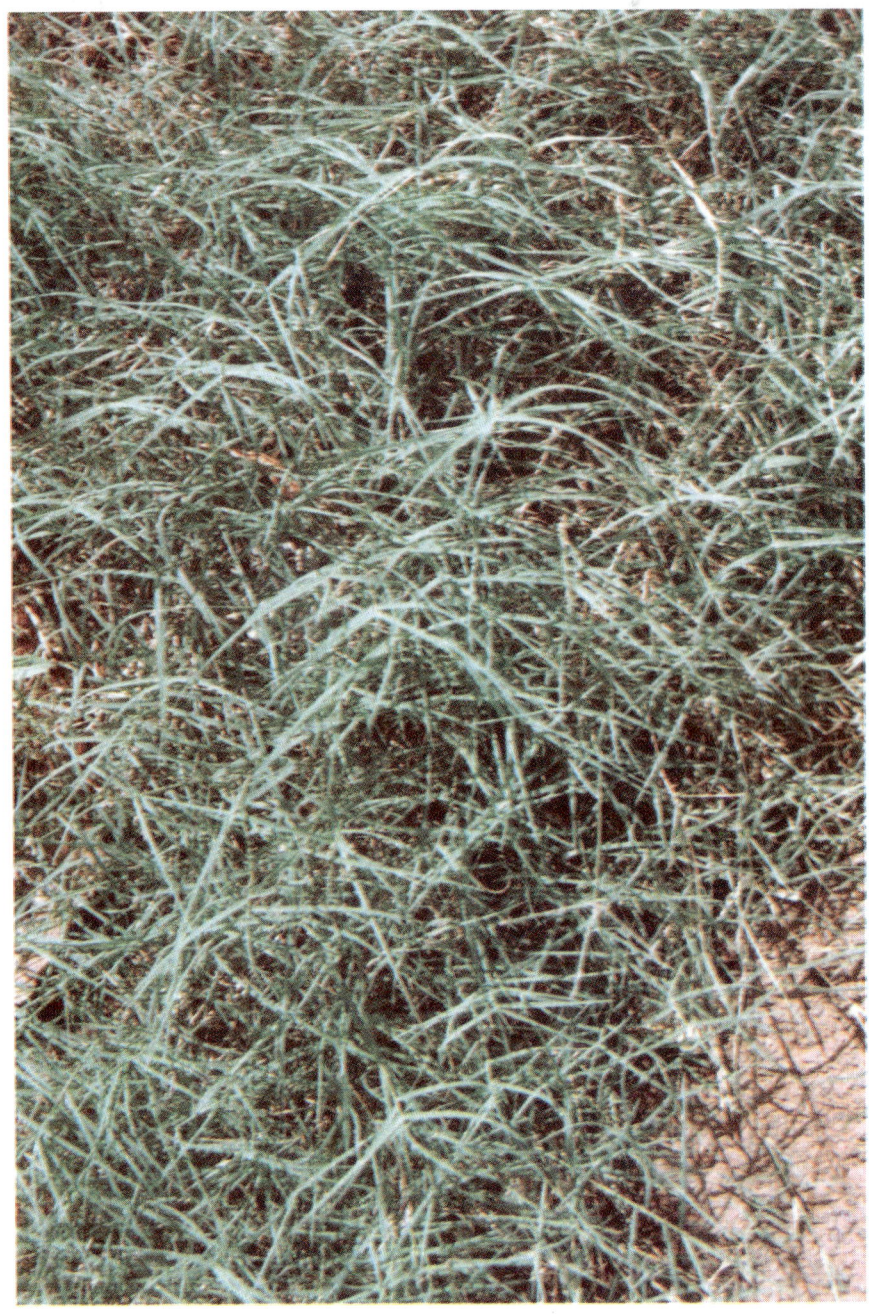

PLATE

50

Cynodon dactylon Pers

GRAMINEAE

Common Names

Eng	:	Bermuda Grass
Hin	:	Doorva
San	:	Granthi
Ben	:	Durba
Tam	:	Arugu
Mal	:	Karuka pulla

Parts used

Whole plant

Constituents

Aromatic acids, arundoin, ferfural, ferfural alcohol, β-ionone, phytol, β-sitosterol-D-glucoside, stigmasterol acetate, phytone, xanthophylls, carotene. Presence of glycosides saponins, tannins, flavonoids and carbohydrates are also reported.

Uses

Haematuresis, in vomiting, fresh juice is used for dropsy anasarca, chronic diarrhea, dysentery, cold infusion of grass stops bleeding from piles, demulcent, astringent, diuretic, laxative.

Classification	
Kingdom	Plantae – Plants
Subkingdom	Tracheobionta – Vascular plants
Superdivision	Spermatophyta – Seed plants
Division	Magnoliophyta – Flowering plants
Class	Liliopsida – Monocotyledons
Subclass	Commelinidae –
Order	Cyperales –
Family	Poaceae – Grass family
Genus	Cynodon L.C. Rich. – Bermudagrass

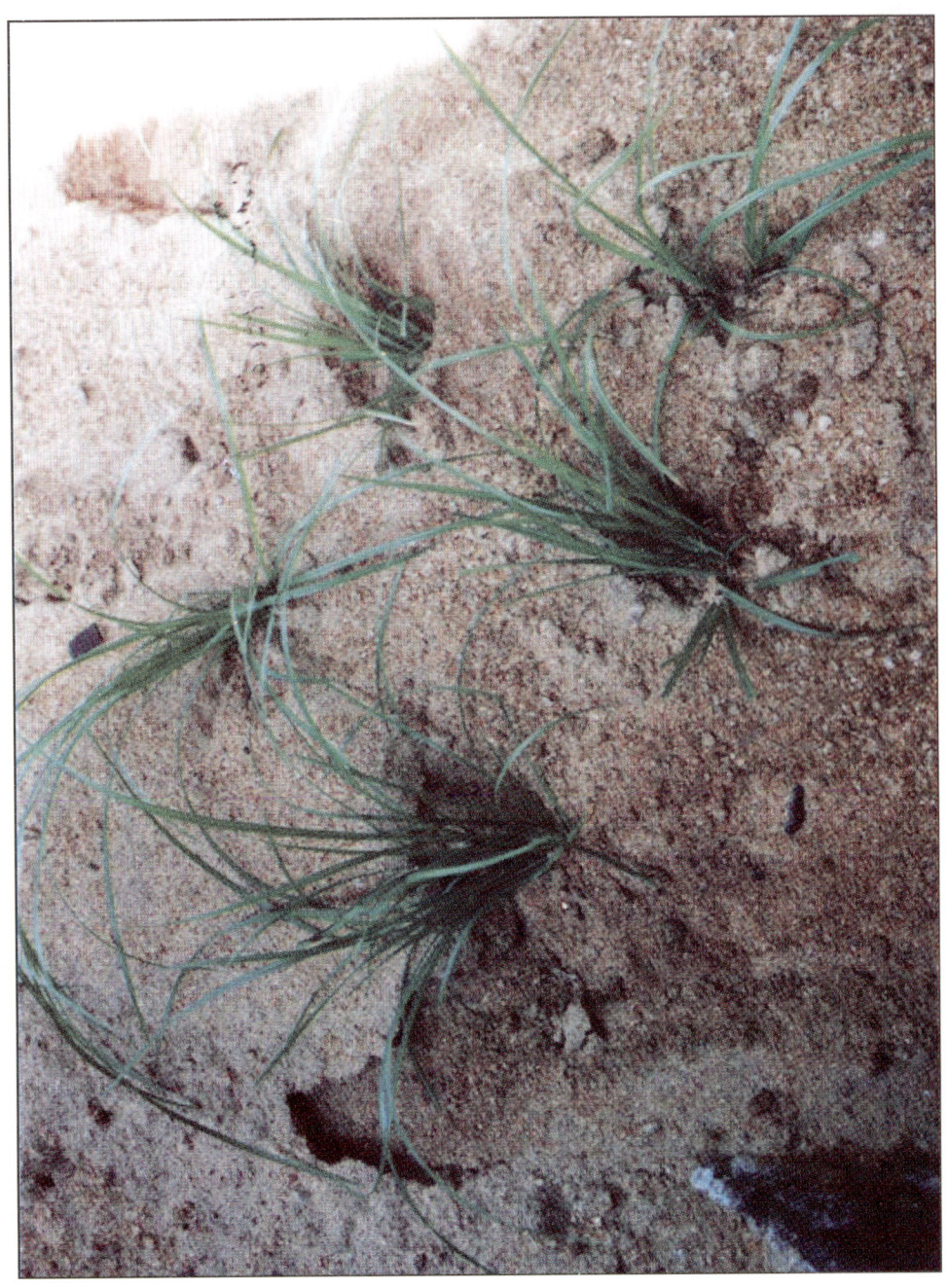

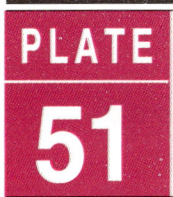

PLATE
51

Cyperus rotundus Linn

CYPERACEAE

Common Names

Eng	:	Nutgrass
Hind	:	Kurehi Jhal
Sans	:	Mustra, Mustaka
Ben	:	Moothoo
Tam	:	Korai kizhanghu
Mal	:	Kari muttan

Parts Used

Tubers & Bulbous Roots

Constituents

Fat, sugar, gum, carbohydrate, essential oil, β-sitosterol, cyperene, sespquiterperoid.

Uses

Stimulant, tonic, demulcent, diuretic, anthelmintic, stomachic carminative, diaphoretic, astringent, emmenagogue, vermifuge.

Classification	
Kingdom	Plantae – Plants
Subkingdom	Tracheobionta – Vascular plants
Superdivision	Spermatophyta – Seed plants
Division	Magnoliophyta – Flowering plants
Class	Liliopsida – Monocotyledons
Subclass	Commelinidae –
Order	Cyperales –
Family	Cyperaceae – Sedge family
Genus	Cyperus L. – flatsedge

Datura inoxia P. Mill.

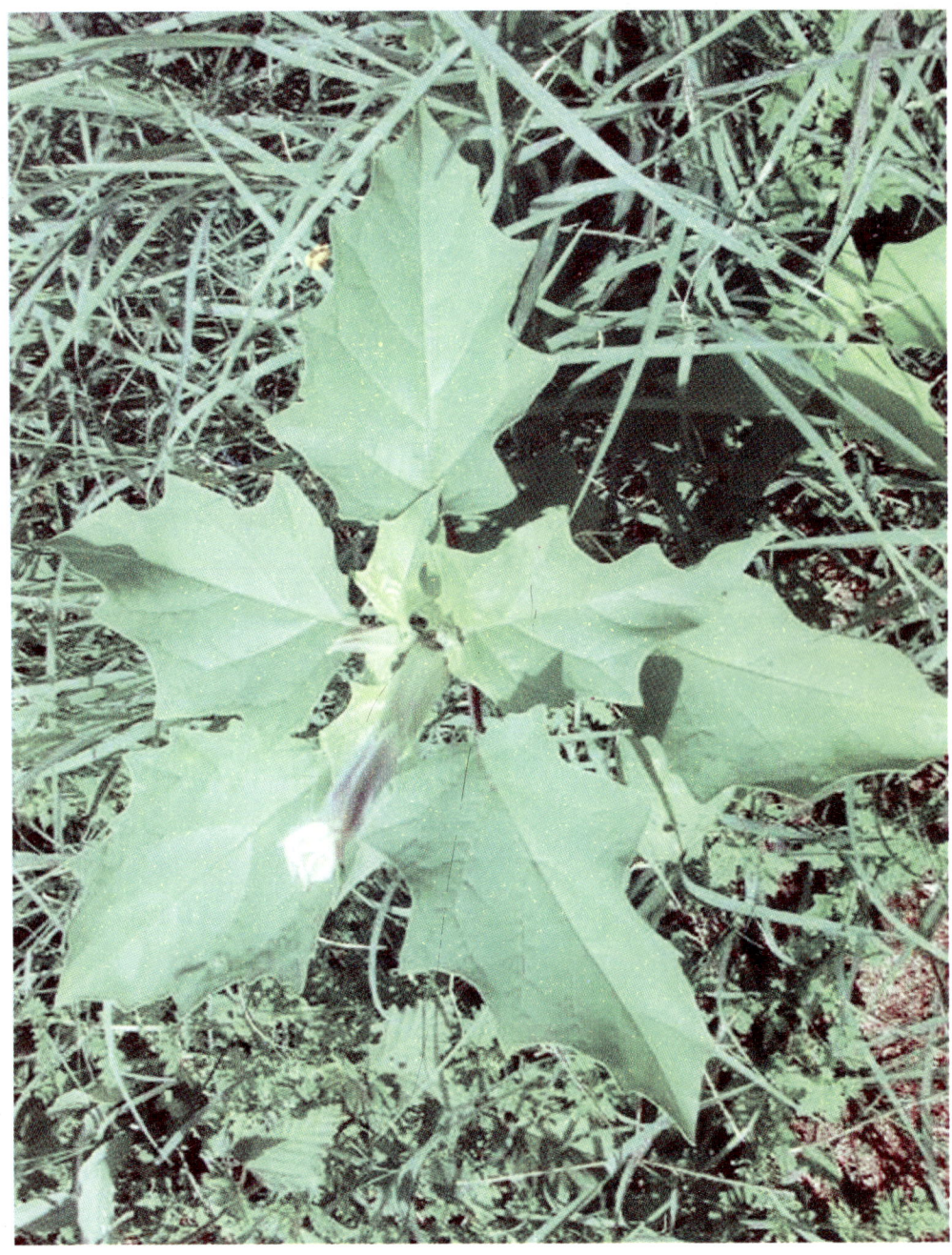

PLATE
52

Datura inoxia P. Mill.

SOLANACEAE

Common Names

Eng	:	Pricklyburr
San	:	Dhustura
Ben	:	Dhatura
Mal	:	Ummatta
Tam	:	Vellummattai
Tel	:	Dutturamu

Parts Used

Leaves and flowering tops

Constituents

The major tropane alkaloid are atropine, hyoscine, hyoscyamine, scopolamine, leaves have flavonoids.

Uses

It controls salivation, muscular rigidity and its sedative property enables it to be used in the control of motion sickness.

Classification	
Kingdom	Plantae – Plants
Subkingdom	Tracheobionta – Vascular plants
Superdivision	Spermatophyta – Seed plants
Division	Magnoliophyta – Flowering plants
Class	Magnoliopsida – Dicotyledons
Subclass	Asteridae –
Order	Solanales –
Family	Solanaceae – Potato family
Genus	Datura L. – jimsonweed

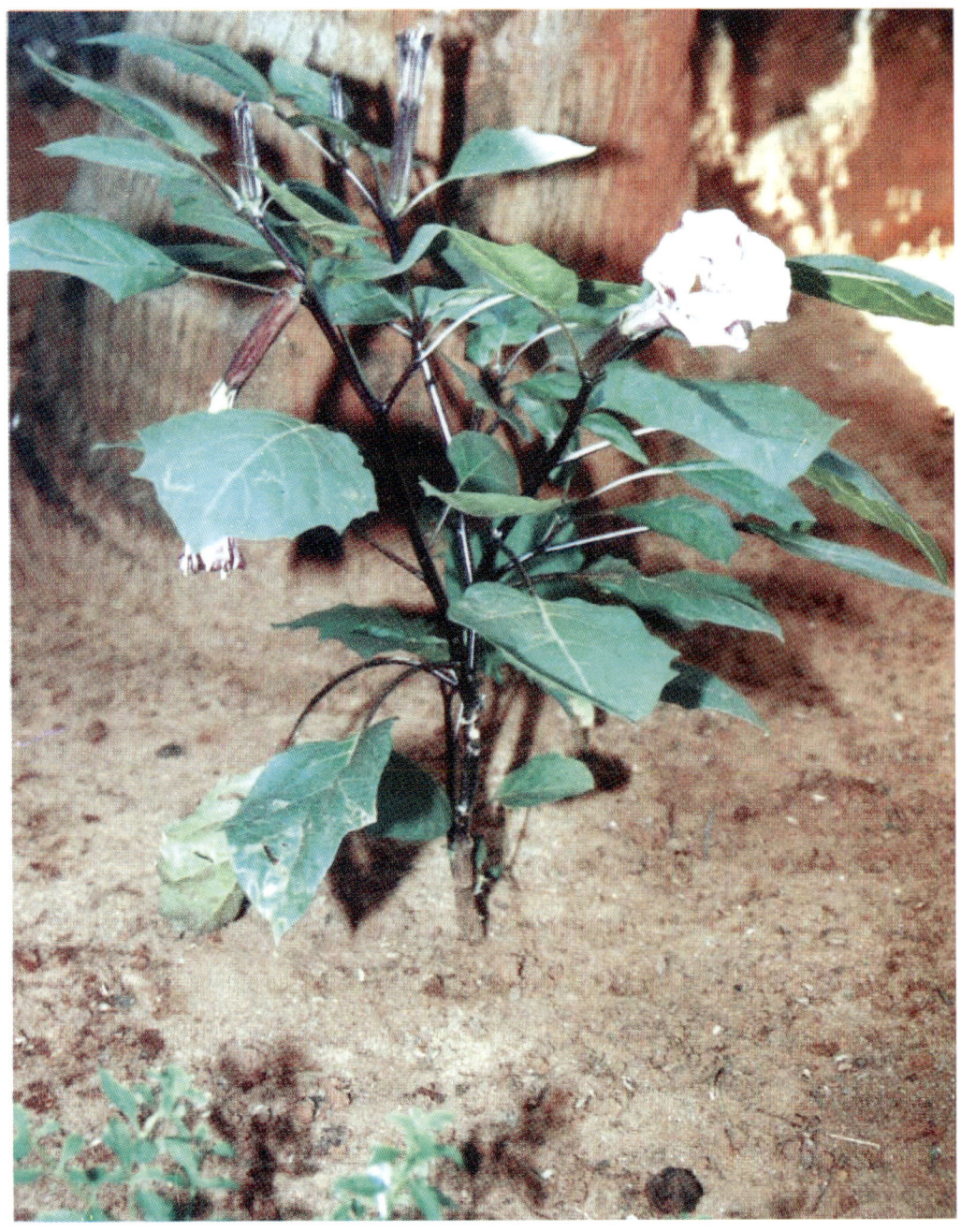

PLATE

53

Datura metal L.

SOLANACEAE

Common Name

Eng   :   Downy Dartura
Tam   :   Karuumattai

Parts Used

Leaves

Constituents

The main alkaloids are hyoscyamine, belladonine, scopoletin, hyoscine, pyridine.

Uses

It has parasympatholytic with anticholinergic property, it reduce the secretion, it is also an antidote in opium and chloralhydrate.

Classification	
Kingdom	Plantae – Plants
Subkingdom	Tracheobionta – Vascular plants
Superdivision	Spermatophyta – Seed plants
Division	Magnoliophyta – Flowering plants
Class	Magnoliopsida – Dicotyledons
Subclass	Asteridae –
Order	Solanales –
Family	Solanaceae – Potato family
Genus	Datura L. – Downy Datura

Datura stramonium Linn

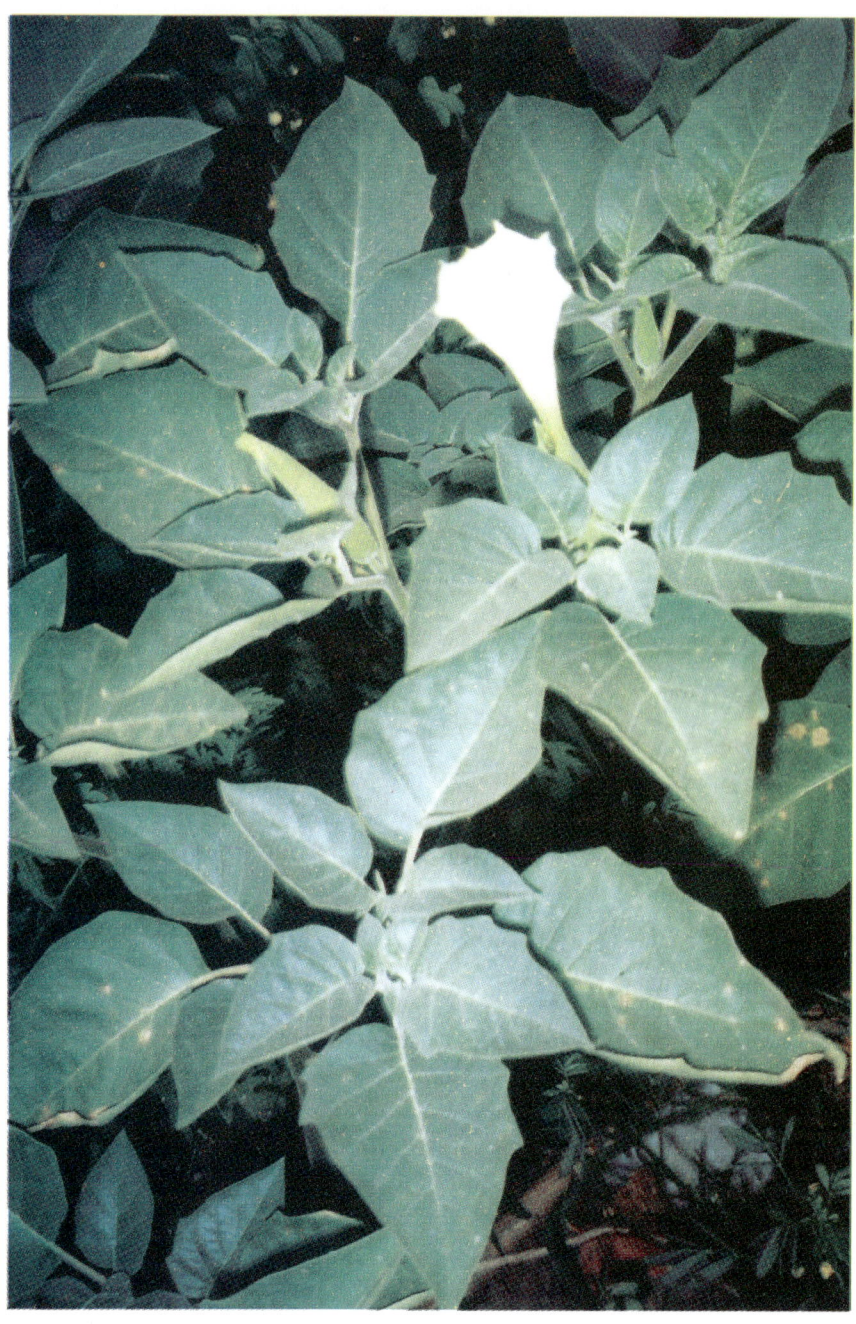

PLATE

54

Datura stramonium Linn

SOLANACEAE

Common Names

Eng	:	Jimsonweed
Ben	:	Sada dhatura
Tam	:	Umatai
Mal	:	Umattu

Parts Used

Leaves and flowering tops

Constituents

The major tropane alkaloid are atropine, hyoscine, hyoscyamine, scopolamine, leaves have flavonoids, chrysin, liquiritigenin, naringenin, kaempferol, quercetin and also it contains withanolide, withastramonolide.

Uses

It controls salivation, muscular rigidity, it is used in the treatment of asthma and its sedative property enables it to be used in the control of motion sickness.

Classification	
Kingdom	Plantae – Plants
Subkingdom	Tracheobionta – Vascular plants
Superdivision	Spermatophyta – Seed plants
Division	Magnoliophyta – Flowering plants
Class	Magnoliopsida – Dicotyledons
Subclass	Asteridae –
Order	Solanales –
Family	Solanaceae – Potato family
Genus	Datura L. – jimsonweed

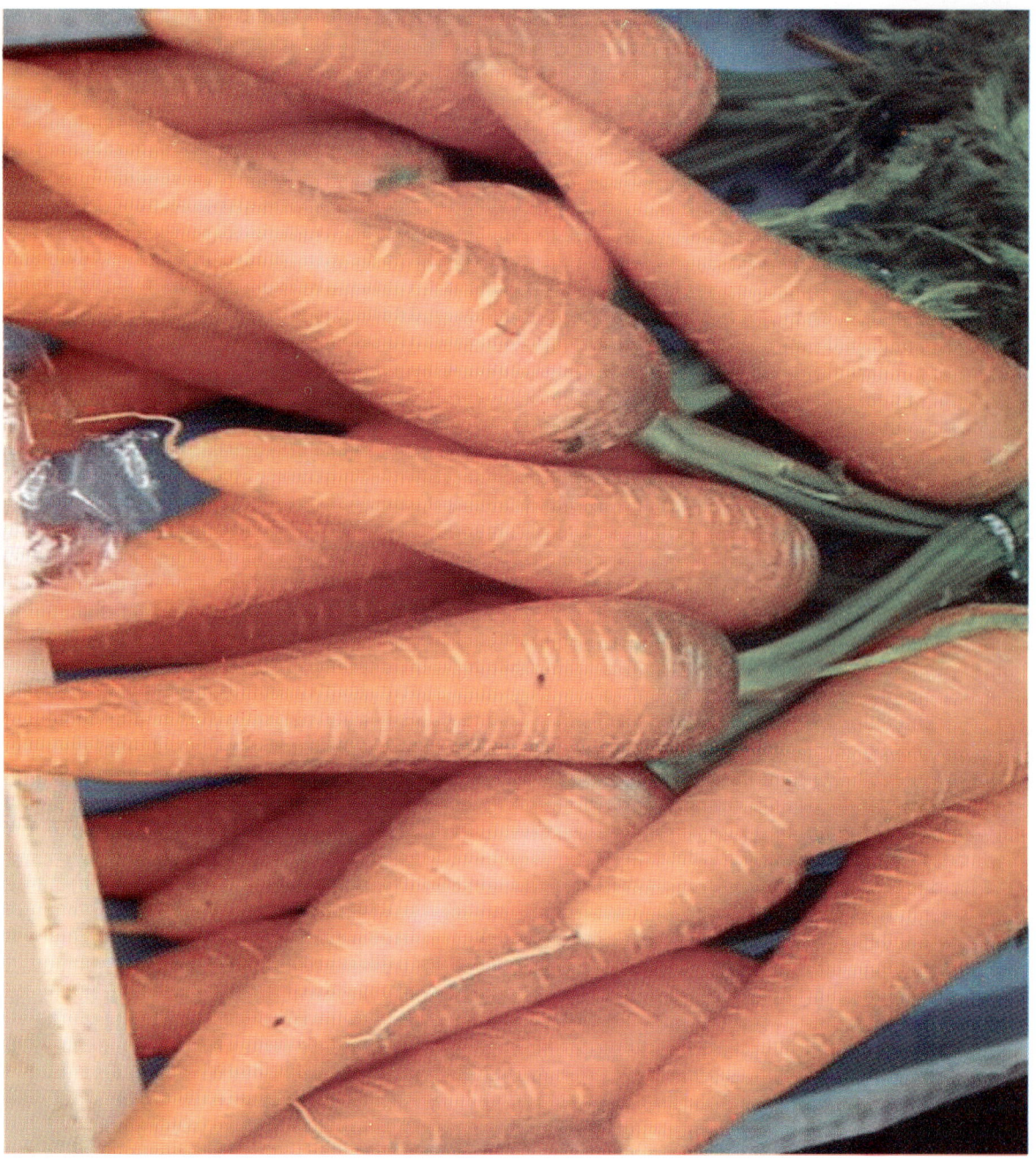

PLATE
55

Daucus carota Linn

UMBELLIFERAE

Common Names

Eng	:	The carrot
Hind	:	Gajar
Sans	:	Shikha mulam
Ben	:	Gajar
Tam	:	Gajjara kilangu

Parts Used

Roots and fruits

Constituents

Leaves and flower contain cyanidin glycoside like 3-O- lathyroside, cynidine 3-O-(2" – O – β – D-xylopranosyl – 6" O – β D glucopyranosyl , D-galactopyranoside, Root contain carotene, hydrocarotin, sugar. starch, protein, malic acid, lignin, albumin, volatile oil. Fruit has both volatile and fixed oil.

Uses

Antiseptic, beneficial influence on kindney, aphrodisiac, tonic, cleans blood. Seeds are aromatic, abortificiant, stimulant and carminative.

Classification	
Kingdom	Plantae – Plants
Subkingdom	Tracheobionta – Vascular plants
Superdivision	Spermatophyta – Seed plants
Division	Magnoliophyta – Flowering plants
Class	Magnoliopsida – Dicotyledons
Subclass	Rosidae –
Order	Apiales –
Family	Apiaceae – Carrot family
Genus	Daucus L. – wild carrot

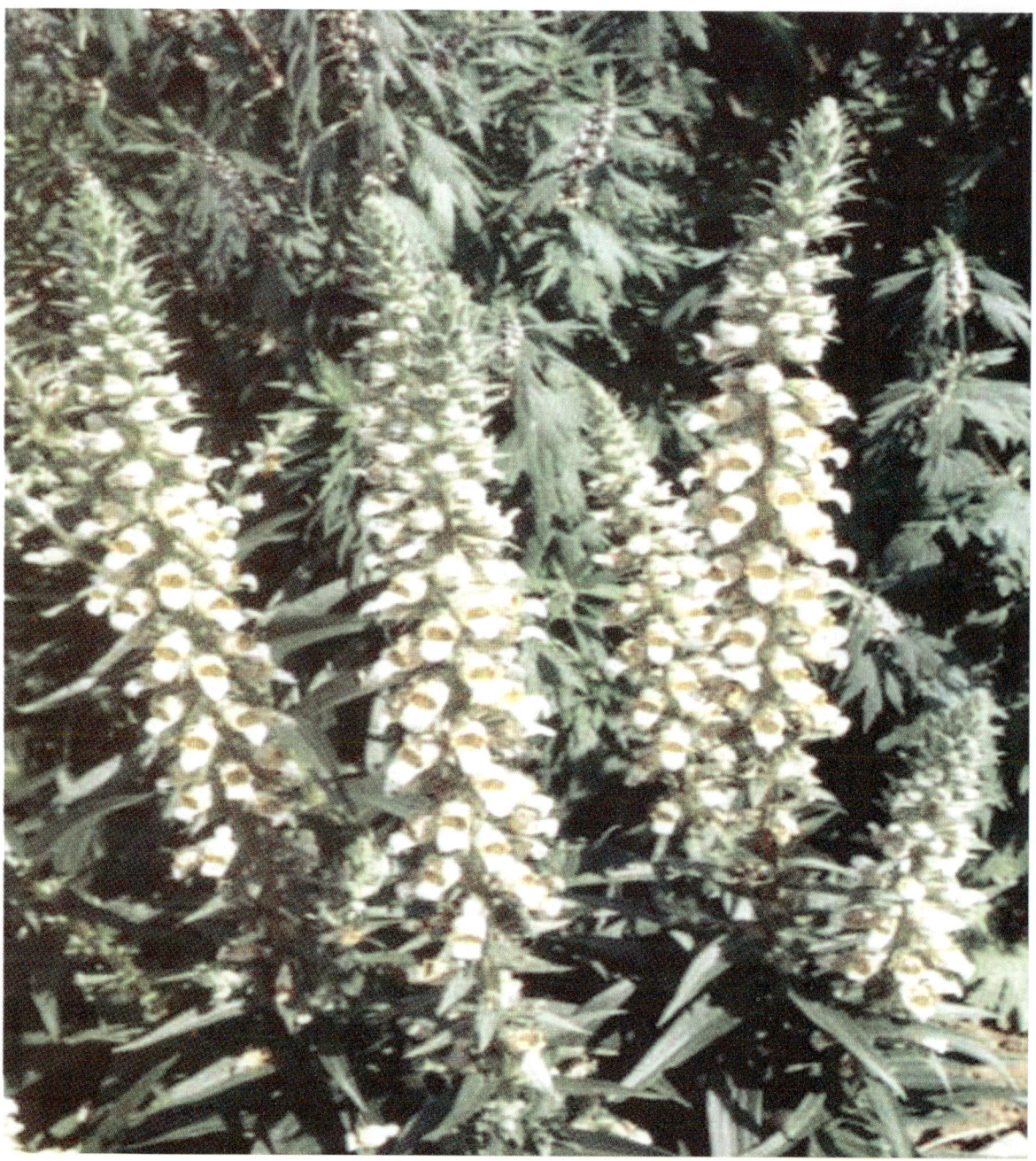

PLATE

56

Digitalis lanata Ehrh.

SCROPHULARIACEAE

Common Name

Eng   :   Grecian Fox glove

Parts Used

Leaves

Constituents

It contain five primary glycoside and in all about 70 cardiac glycoside. The primary glycoside identified are lanatoside A,B,C,D and E.

Uses

Its commercial source for digoxin, lanatoside A, C and a mixture of lanatoside, in congestive heart failure, auricular fibrillatrion.

Classification	
Kingdom	Plantae – Plants
Subkingdom	Tracheobionta – Vascular plants
Superdivision	Spermatophyta – Seed plants
Division	Magnoliophyta – Flowering plants
Class	Magnoliopsida – Dicotyledons
Subclass	Asteridae –
Order	Scrophulariales –
Family	Scrophulariaceae – Figwort family
Genus	Digitalis L. – foxglove

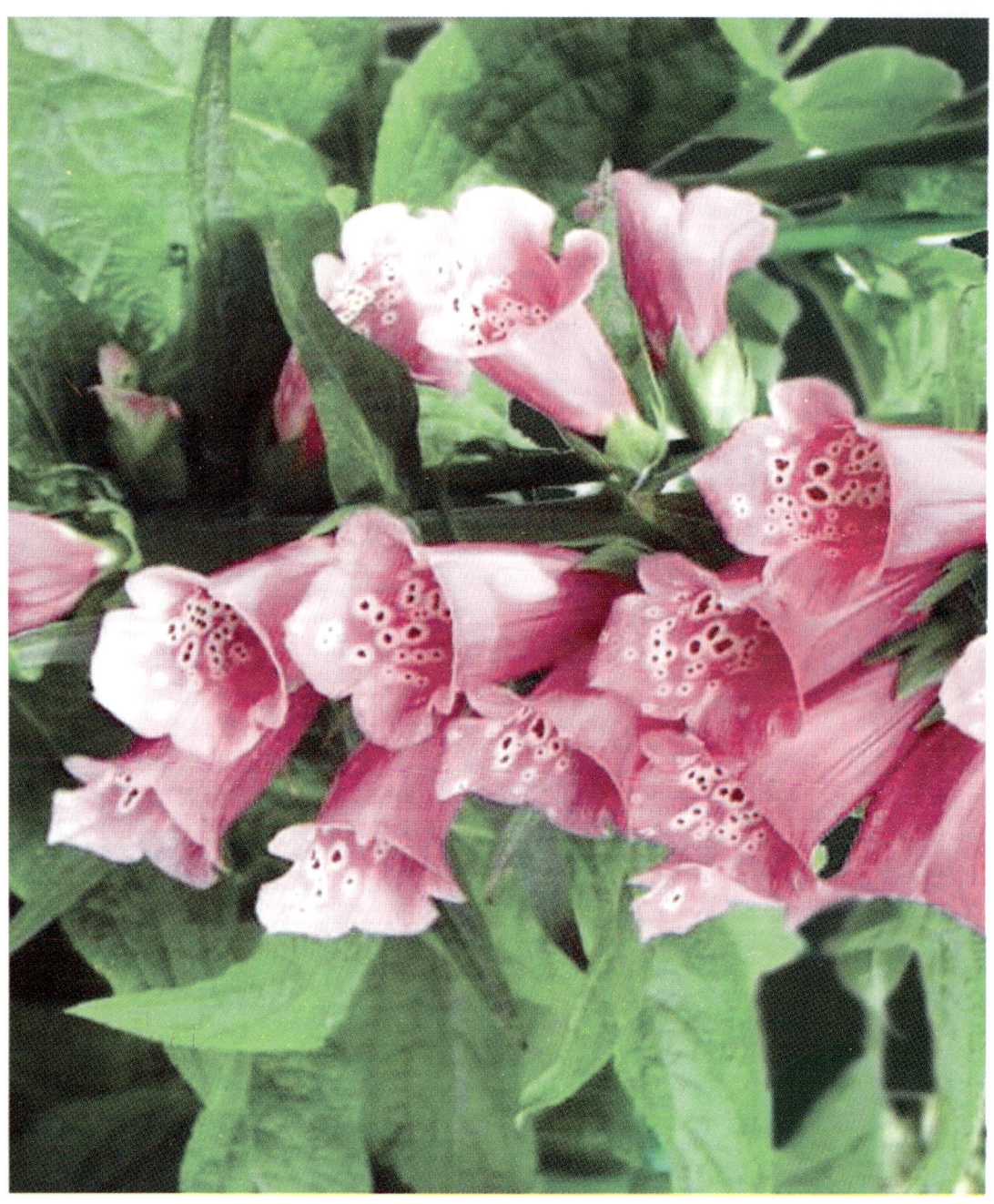

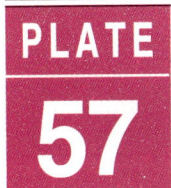

PLATE 57

Digitalis purpurea Linn

SCROPHULARIACEAE

Common Names

Eng : Fox glove
Sans : Tilapuspi
Tam : Nilapukaiyilai

Parts Used

Leaves

Constituents

Cardiac glycosides, digitoxin, gitoxin, gitaloxin, strospeside, phenolic glycosides, desrhamnosyl acetoside, purpureosides A, B.

Uses

Treatment of congestive heart failure, febrifuge, enzyme that catalyst the conversion of progesterone.

Classification	
Kingdom	Plantae – Plants
Subkingdom	Tracheobionta – Vascular plants
Superdivision	Spermatophyta – Seed plants
Division	Magnoliophyta – Flowering plants
Class	Magnoliopsida – Dicotyledons
Subclass	Asteridae –
Order	Scrophulariales –
Family	Scrophulariaceae – Figwort family
Genus	Digitalis L. – foxglove

Eclipta prostrata L

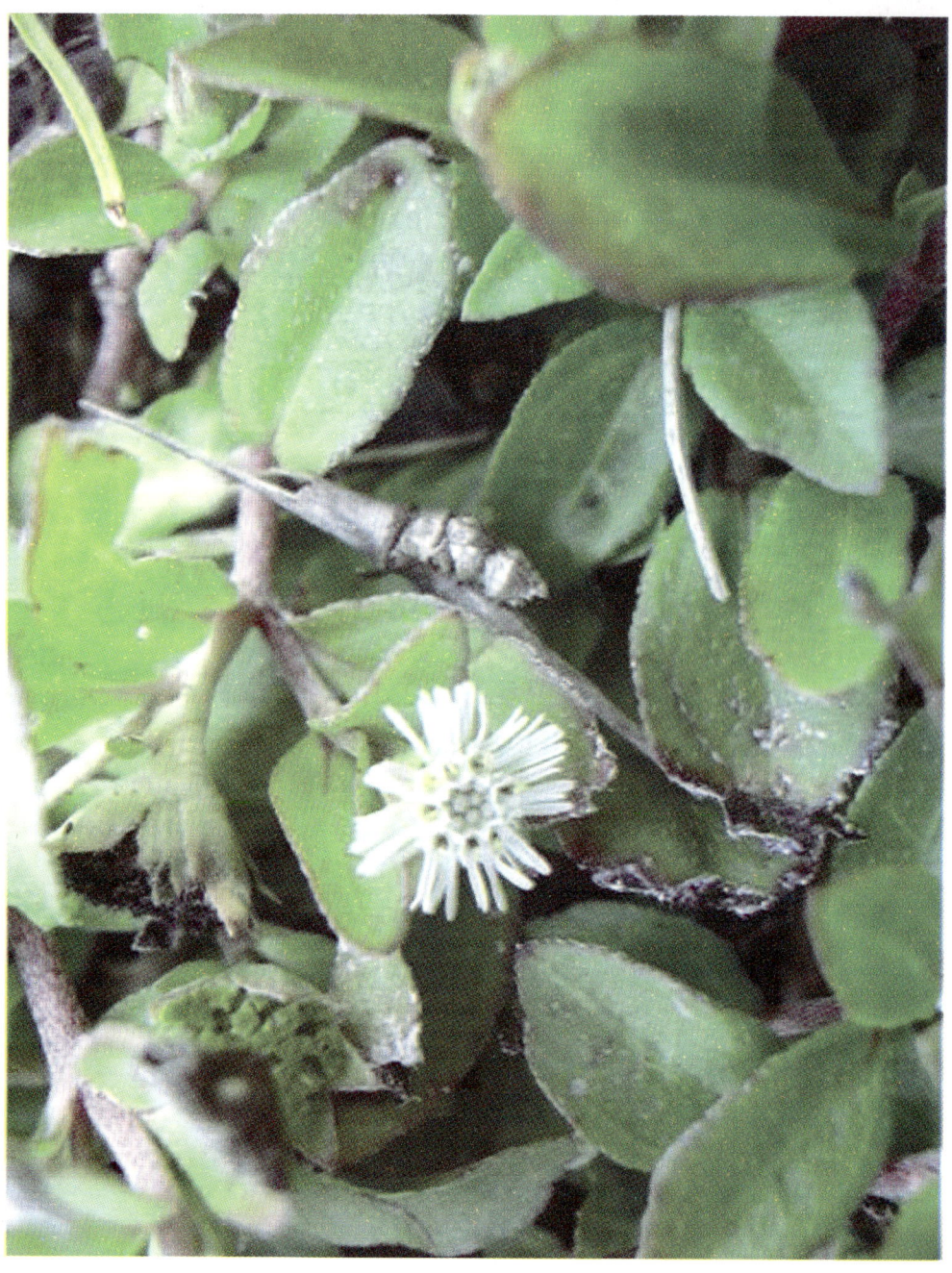

PLATE
58

Eclipta prostrata L

COMPOSITAE

Common Names

Eng	:	False daisy
Hind	:	Mochkard
Sans	:	Kesharaja
Ben	:	Kesuria
Tam	:	Kaikeshi, Karisha-langanni

Parts Used

Aerial parts

Constituents

Reducing sugars and sterols have been detected. From leaves and stems, wedelolactone has been isolated in crystalline form. Stigmasterol and L-terthienyl methanol have been identified,b amyrin and 7-desmethyl wedelolactone- 7 - glucoside have also been isolated. Wedelic acid, apigenin, luteolin and the glucosides of the latter two have been isolated.

Uses

Hepatoprotective property, significantly increase the appetite and body weight in patients of tuberculosis, Immunomodulatory activity is also been reported, and it's also used in the treatment of peptic ulcer.

Classification	
Kingdom	Plantae – Plants
Subkingdom	Tracheobionta – Vascular plants
Superdivision	Spermatophyta – Seed plants
Division	Magnoliophyta – Flowering plants
Class	Magnoliopsida – Dicotyledons
Subclass	Asteridae –
Order	Asterales –
Family	Asteraceae – Aster family
Genus	Eclipta L. – eclipta

Elettaria cardamomum Maton

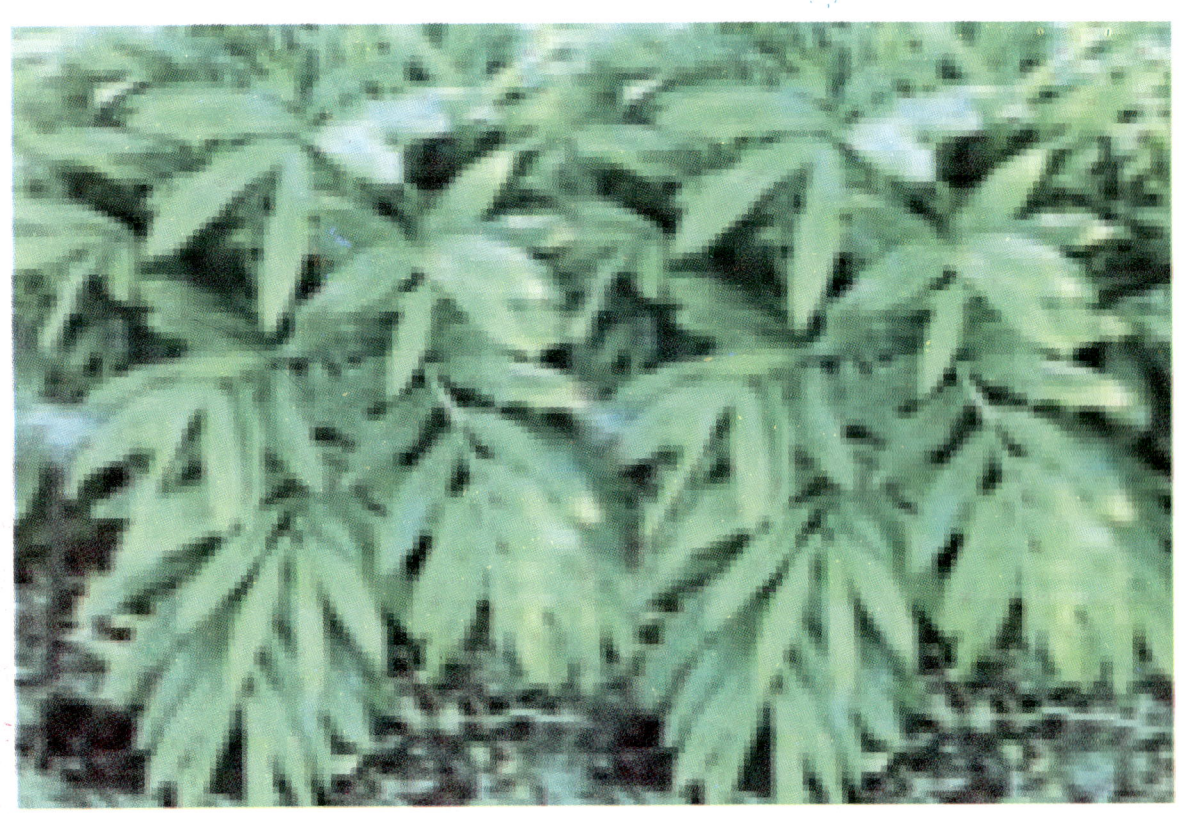

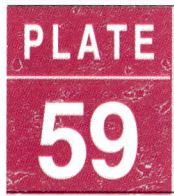

PLATE

59

Elettaria cardamomum Maton

ZINGIBERACEAE

Common Names

Eng	:	Cardamom
Hind	:	Chhoti Elachi
Sans	:	Ela truti
Ben	:	Garate
Tam	:	Elakaya
Mal	:	Elaka

Parts Used

Ripe seeds

Constituents

Fixed oil, essential oil, containing cineole, terpineol, limonene. It is rich in zinc.

Uses

The volatile component of cardamom exhibits antimicrobial activity, aromatic, stimulant, carminative, stomachic, diuretic, for stomach complaints. The fixed oil present act as a fixative for aroma and contribute to flavour properties. Cardamom is chewed slowly to sweeten the breath, as aphrodisiac, to sooth digestion, stimulate appetite, used against flatulence, colic, and often combined with purgative to offset griping.

Classification	
Kingdom	Plantae – Plants
Subkingdom	Tracheobionta – Vascular plants
Superdivision	Spermatophyta – Seed plants
Division	Magnoliophyta – Flowering plants
Class	Liliopsida – Monocotyledons
Subclass	Zingiberidae –
Order	Zingiberales –
Family	Zingiberaceae – Ginger family
Genus	Elettaria Maton – elettaria

Ephedra gerardiana Linn

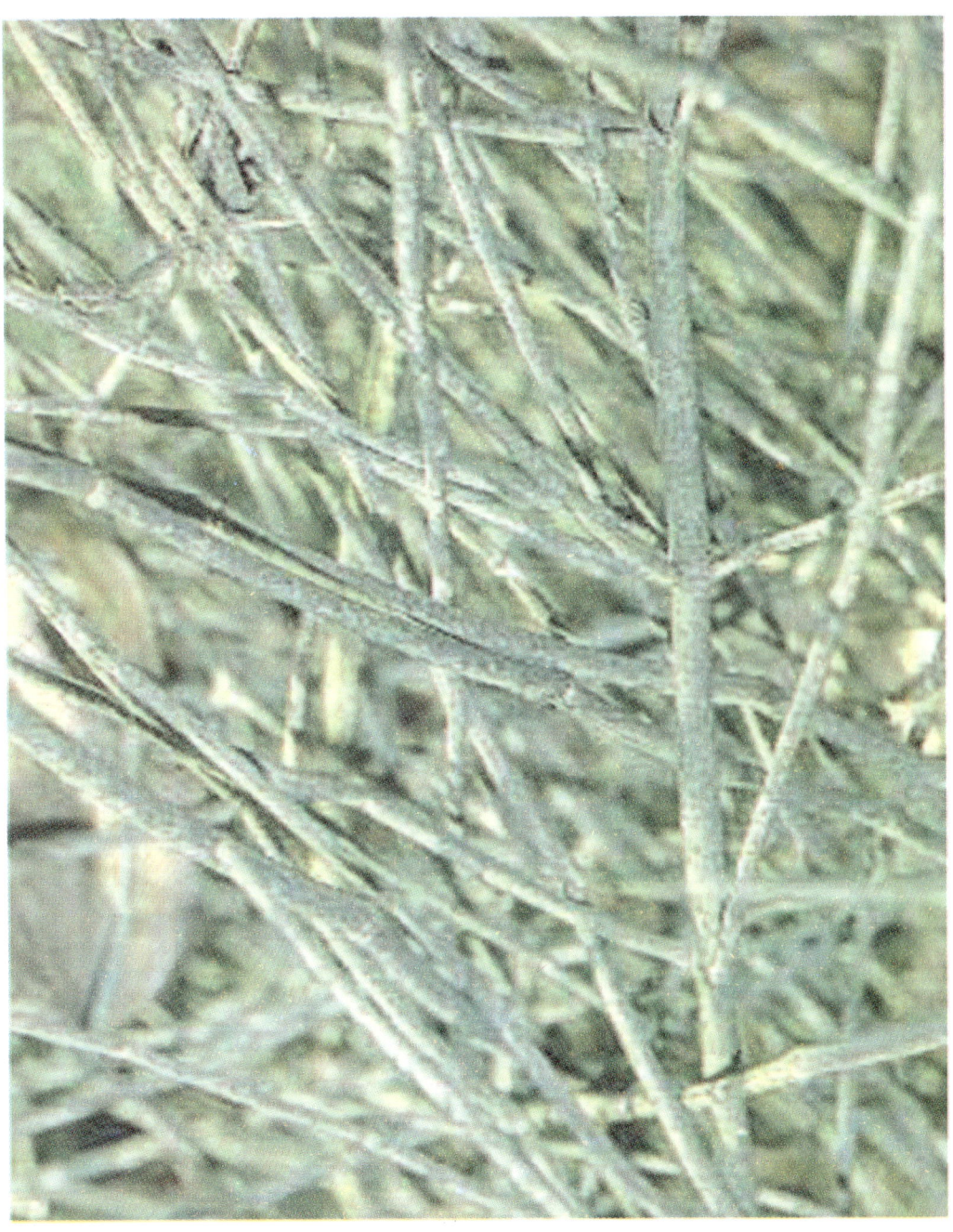

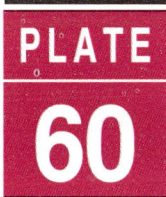

PLATE

60

Ephedra gerardiana Linn

GNETACEAE

Common Names

Eng	:	Ephedra
Ladak	:	Trans
Pun	:	Butsherit
Sutlej	:	Phok

Parts used

Root & dried branches

Constituents

Alkaloids obtained from stems are ephedrine, pseudo-ephedrine, norephedrine, methylphedrine, 3 p-coumaroylamino acid, p-coumaroyl –D-valine, p-coumaroyl –D-serine acid, p-coumaroyl-D-threonine.

Uses

Diuretic, stomachic, tonic, antitumour.

Classification	
Kingdom	Plantae – Plants
Subkingdom	Tracheobionta – Vascular plants
Superdivision	Spermatophyta – Seed plants
Division	Gnetophyta – Mormon tea and other gnetophytes
Class	Gnetopsida –
Order	Ephedrales –
Family	Ephedraceae – Mormon-tea family
Genus	Ephedra L. – jointfir

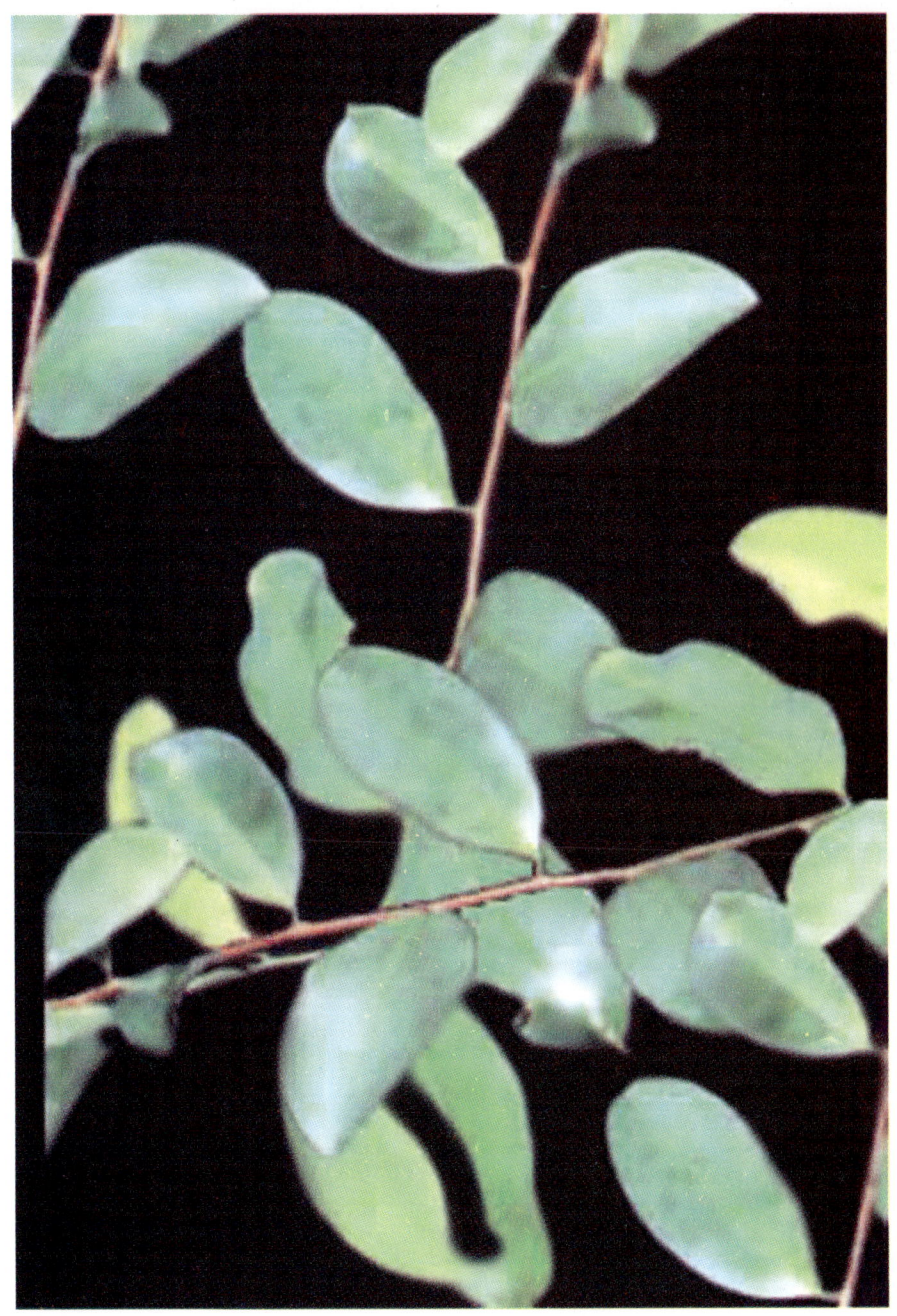

PLATE

61

Erythroxylum coca Lam

ERYTHROXYLACEAE

Common Names

Eng	:	Coca leaves
Latin	:	Folio cocae
Tam	:	Sivadari
French	:	Coca

Part used

Leaves

Constituents

Leaves contain several alkaloid, the most important alkaloid are cocaine with other alkaloids like cinnamyl cocaine, a-truxilline, B-truxilline, benzoyl -ecgonine, tropa-cocaine, hygriene, cuscohygrine, the major component of leaf wax is hentria contane, the dihydro benzaldehydes.

Uses

Leaves are stimulant, carminative, restorative, sialgogue, expectorant, aphrodisiac, emmenagogue, alkaloid cocaine is local anaesthetic it produce mydriasis, nerve stimulant. It is antidote for alcohol, opium and tobacco habits.

Classification	
Kingdom	Plantae – Plants
Subkingdom	Tracheobionta – Vascular plants
Superdivision	Spermatophyta – Seed plants
Division	Magnoliophyta – Flowering plants
Class	Magnoliopsida – Dicotyledons
Subclass	Rosidae –
Order	Linales –
Family	Erythroxlaceae – Coca family
Genus	Erythroxylum P. Br. – coca

Eucalyptus globulus Labill

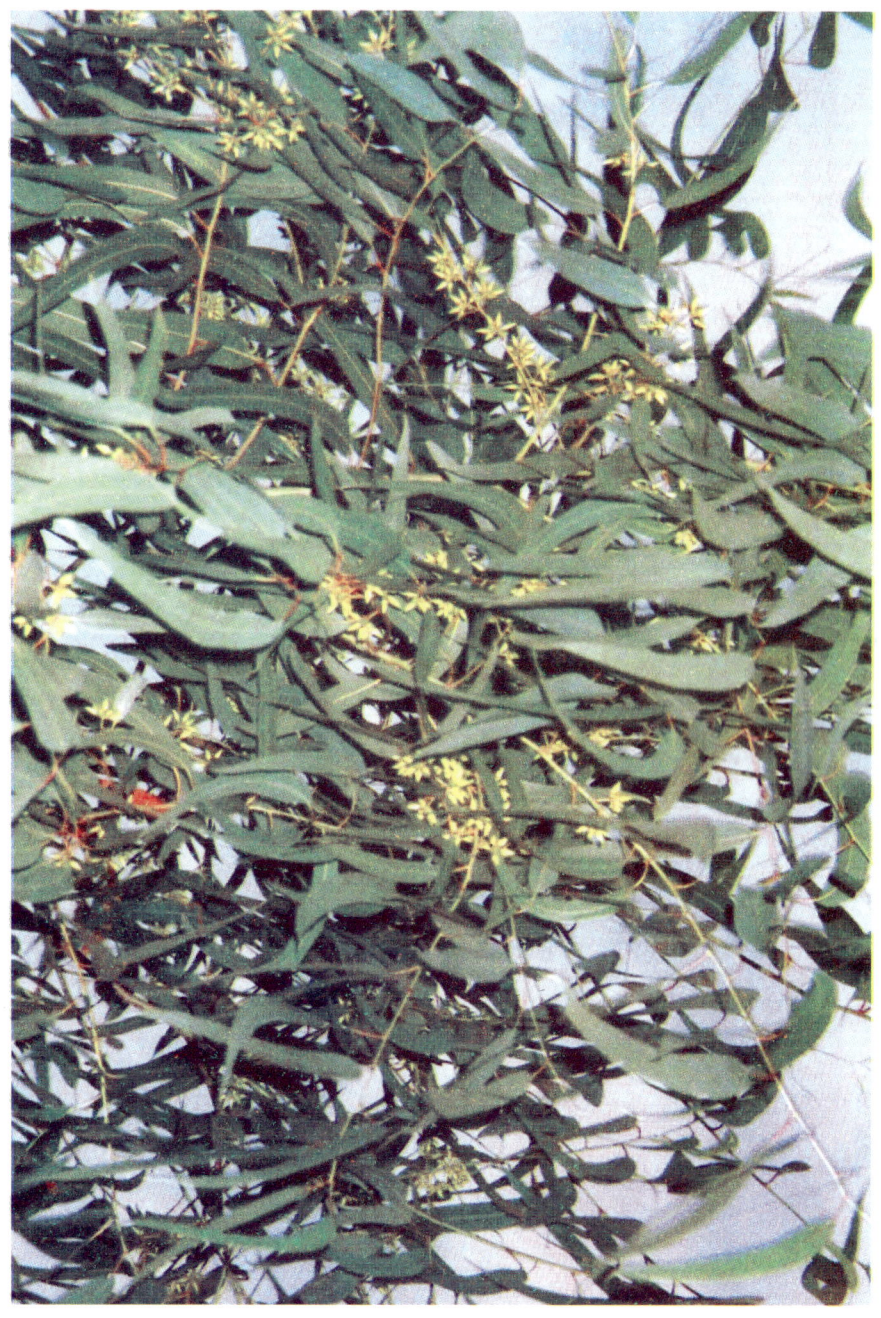

PLATE

62

Eucalyptus globulus Labill

MYRTACEAE

Common Names

Eng	:	Blue gum
Hin	:	Neelgeri
Kan	:	Taila
Tam	:	Karpura maram
Mal	:	Karpura maram

Parts Used

Leaves, gums, exudates.

Constituents

Volatile oil, tannins, cerylic alcohol, cineole(eucalyptol), alcohols like eraniol, eudesmol, aldehydes like crytal, cinol, valeraldehyde, sesquiterpene like aronadendrene.

Use

Febrifuge, carminative, stimulant, expectorant, diaphoretic, antiseptic, antimalarial, antiseptic, disinfectant, it increases the flow of saliva, gastric and intestinal juices, increases the appetite, digestion, large dose is irritant to alimentary canal, produce nausea and vomiting.

Classification	
Kingdom	Plantae – Plants
Subkingdom	Tracheobionta – Vascular plants
Superdivision	Spermatophyta – Seed plants
Division	Magnoliophyta – Flowering plants
Class	Magnoliopsida – Dicotyledons
Subclass	Rosidae –
Order	Myrtales –
Family	Myrtaceae – Myrtle family
Genus	Eucalyptus L'Hér. – gum

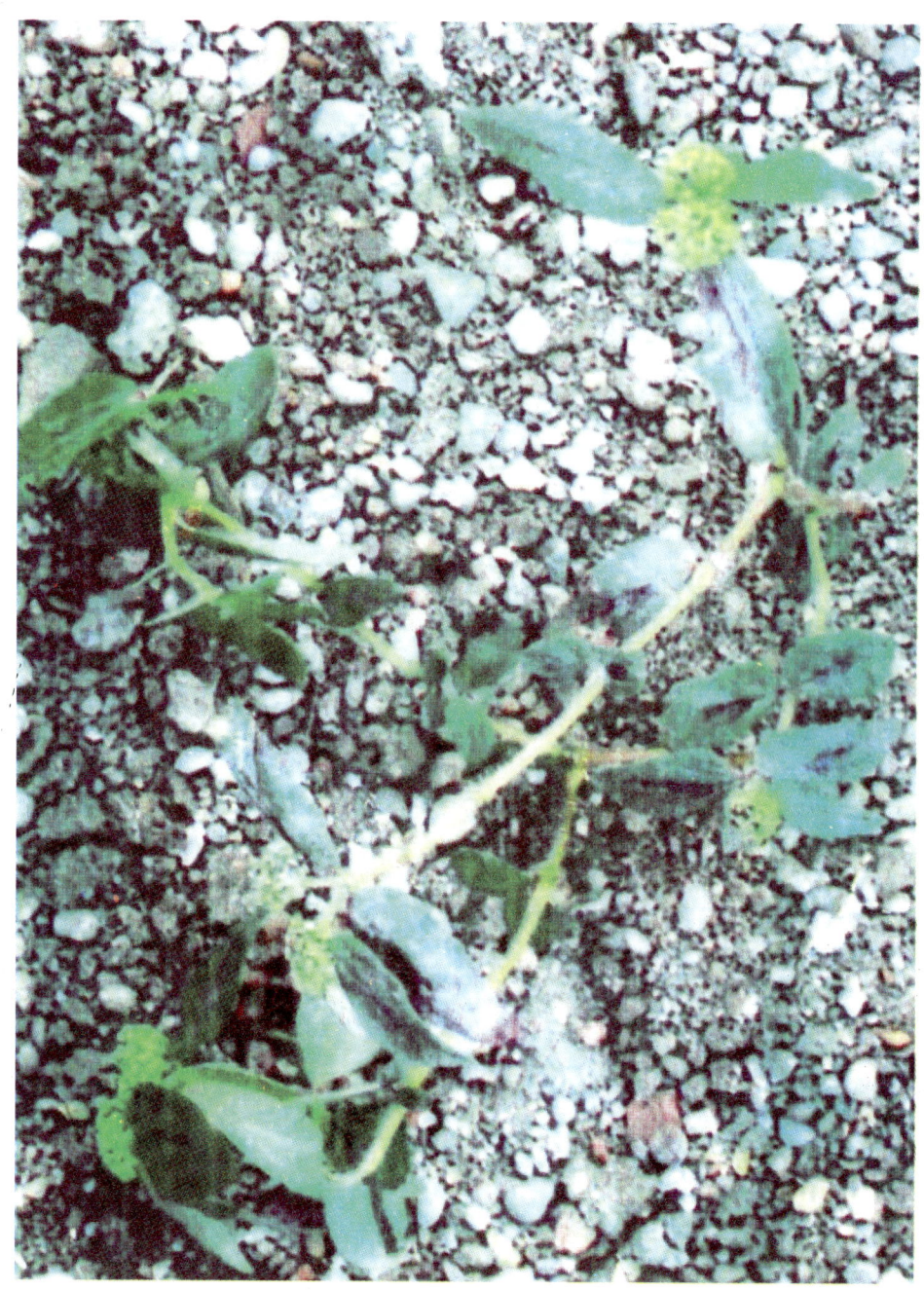

PLATE

63

Euphorbia hirta Linn

EUPHORBIACEAE

Common Names

Eng	:	Australian asthma herb
Hin	:	Dudhi
San	:	Pusitoa
Ben	:	Burakeru
Tam	:	Ammampatcharisi
Mal	:	Nelapalai

Parts Used

Whole plant

Constituents

Steroids, polyphenols, flavonoids

Uses

Diuretic, molluscicidals, antidiarrhoeal, analgesic and anti-inflammatory

Classification	
Kingdom	Plantae – Plants
Subkingdom	Tracheobionta – Vascular plants
Superdivision	Spermatophyta – Seed plants
Division	Magnoliophyta – Flowering plants
Class	Magnoliopsida – Dicotyledons
Subclass	Rosidae –
Order	Euphorbiales –
Family	Euphorbiaceae – Spurge family
Genus	Euphorbia L – sandmat

Euphorbia neriifolia Linn

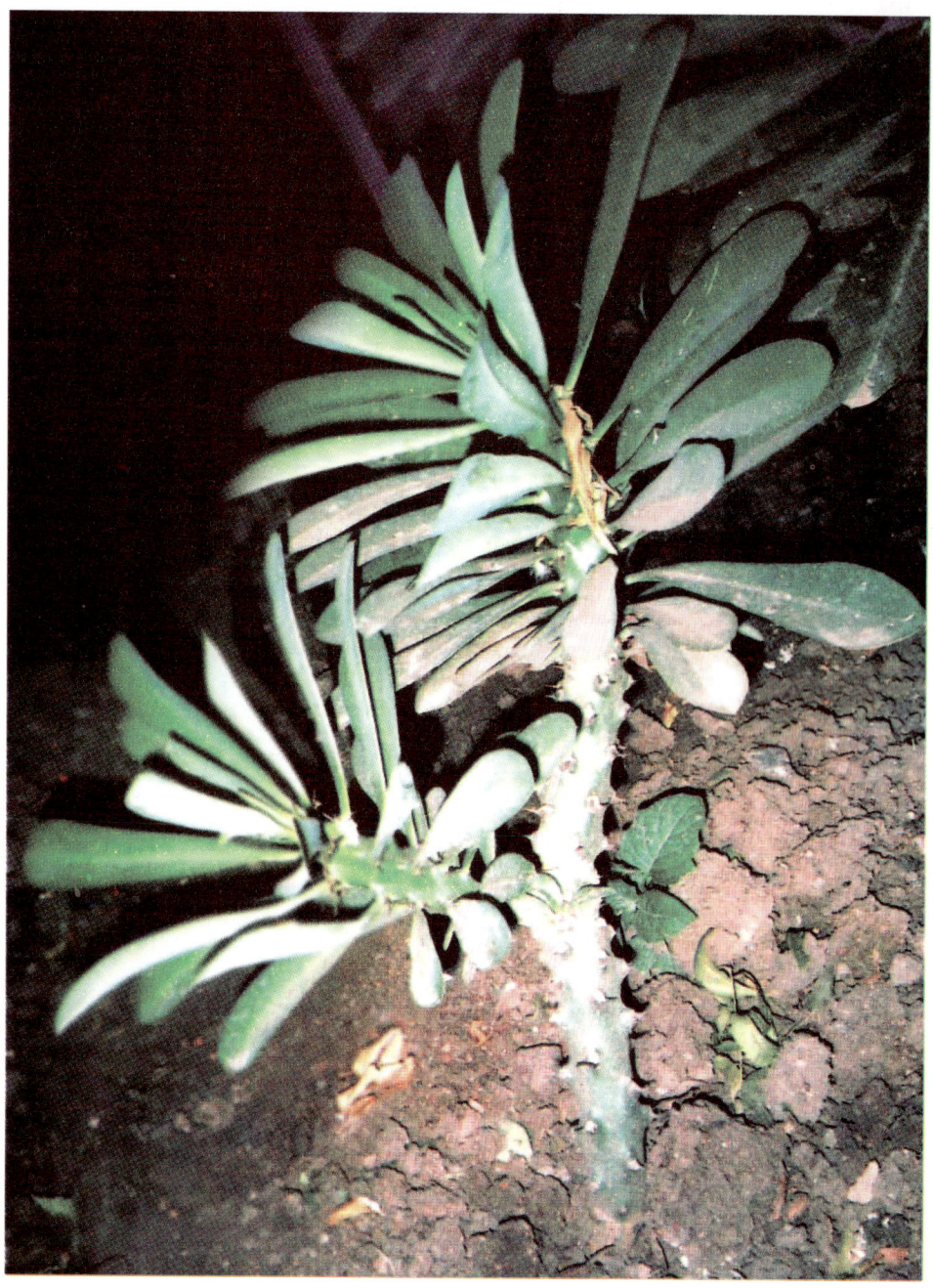

PLATE

64

Euphorbia neriifolia Linn

EUPHORBIACEAE

Common Names

Eng	:	Common milk hedge
Hin	:	Sehund
San	:	vajra
Ben	:	Mansasij
Tam	:	Ilaikalli
Mal	:	Ilaikalli

Parts Used

Juice and root

Constituents

Steroids, flavonoids, resins, gum

Uses

Latex is used as wormicidal, expectorant and purgative. Root is antispasmodic.

Classification	
Kingdom	Plantae – Plants
Subkingdom	Tracheobionta – Vascular plants
Superdivision	Spermatophyta – Seed plants
Division	Magnoliophyta – Flowering plants
Class	Magnoliopsida – Dicotyledons
Subclass	Rosidae –
Order	Euphorbiales –
Family	Euphorbiaceae – Spurge family
Genus	Euphorbia L – common milk hedge

Evolvulus alsinoides Wall & Linn

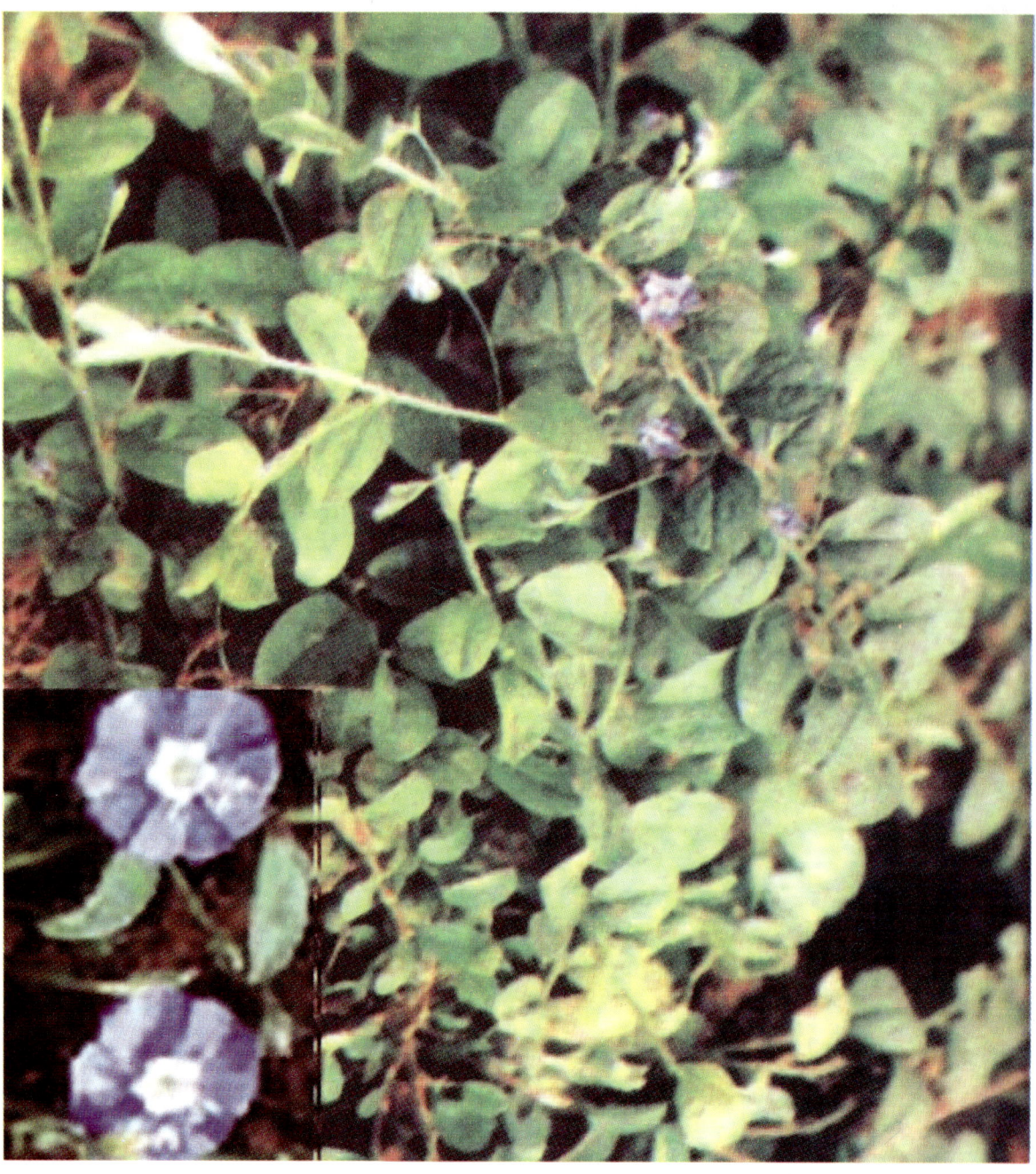

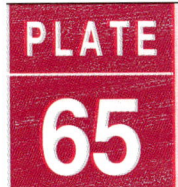

PLATE 65

Evolvulus alsinoides Wall & Linn

CONVOLVULACEAE

Common Names

Eng	:	Slender dwarf morning-glory
Hind	:	Shankhapushpi
Sans	:	Vishnukranta
Tam	:	Vishnukranti
Mal	:	Vishnu karaeli

Parts Used

Whole plant

Constituents

Fat, alkaloid - shankhapushpine

Uses

Nervous debility, loss of memory, also in syphilis, and scrofula. It is used as a brain tonic. The root is used by the santals, for intermittent childhood fever. The leaves are made into cigarettes and smoked in chronic bronchitis and asthma. The plant is useful in internal haemorrhages. The oil promotes the growth of hair. Decoction was given in cases of malarial fever. Evolvulus alsinoides has got antidysenteric and antiseptic properties.

Classification	
Kingdom	Plantae – Plants
Subkingdom	Tracheobionta – Vascular plants
Superdivision	Spermatophyta – Seed plants
Division	Magnoliophyta – Flowering plants
Class	Magnoliopsida – Dicotyledons
Subclass	Asteridae –
Order	Solanales –
Family	Convolvulaceae – Morning-glory family
Genus	Evolvulus L. – dwarf morning-glory

Ferula assafoetida Linn

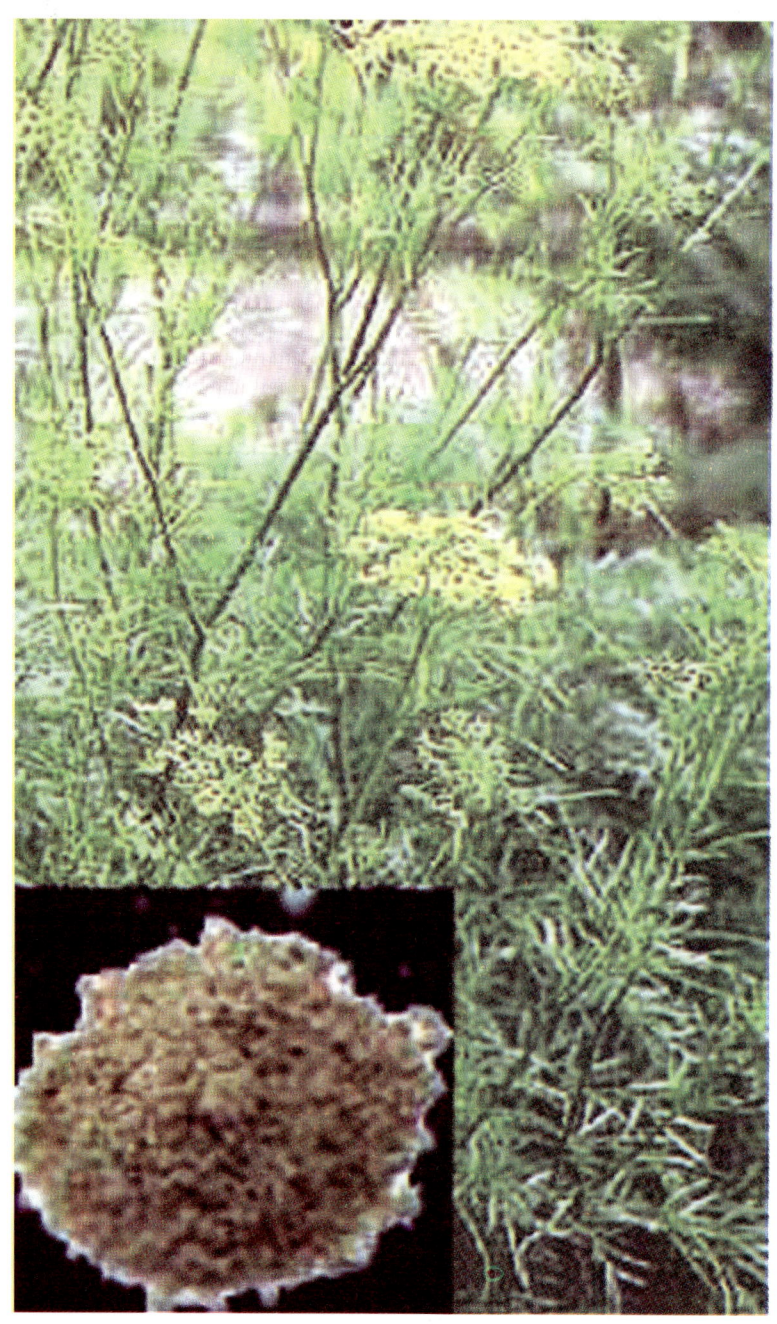

PLATE

66

Ferula assafoetida Linn

UMBELLIFERAE

Common Names

Eng   :   Asafoetida
Hind   :   Hingra
Sans   :   Bhutnasan, Hingu
Ben   :   Hingra
Tam   :   Kayam
Mal   :   Kayam

Parts Used

Gum resin

Constituents

Organic sulphur compound, volatile oil, foetidae, luteolin, luteolin – 7 -0 - β- D glucopyranoside. The gum resins contain coumarins, 5-hydroxyumbelliprenin, assafoetidin, ferocolicin, asacoumarinA and B, farnesiferol A, B, C and disulphide, asadisulphide, and sec-butylpropenyl disulphide.

Uses

Stimulant, carminative, antispasmodic, expectorant, slightly laxative, anthelmintic, diuretic, aphrodisiac, emmemagogue, nerve & pulmonary stimulant.

Classification	
Kingdom	Plantae – Plants
Subkingdom	Tracheobionta – Vascular plants
Superdivision	Spermatophyta – Seed plants
Division	Magnoliophyta – Flowering plants
Class	Magnoliopsida – Dicotyledons
Subclass	Rosidae –
Order	Apiales –
Family	Apiaceae – Carrot family
Genus	Ferula L. – ferula

Ficus bengalensis Linn

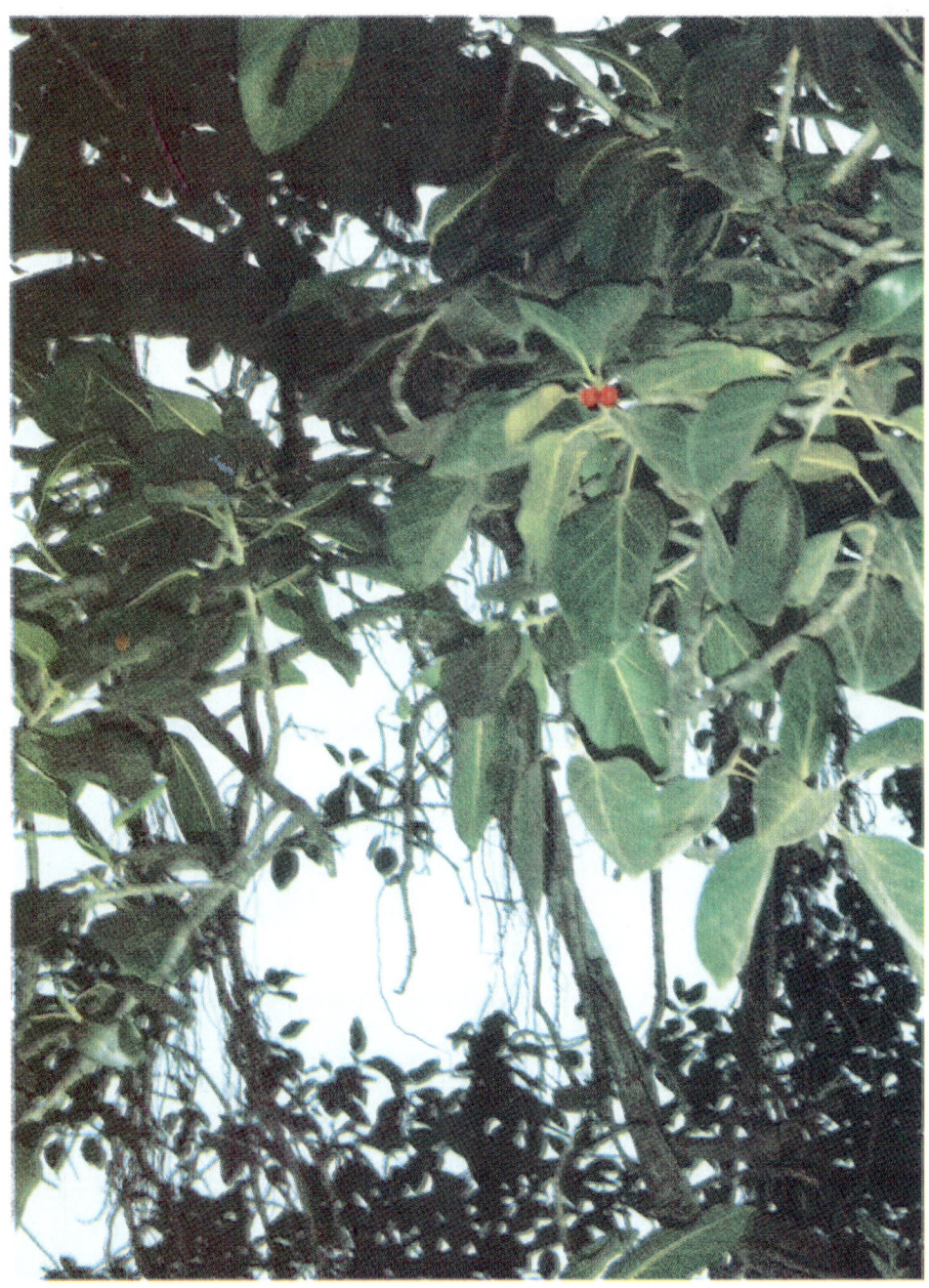

PLATE

67

Ficus bengalensis Linn

URTICACEAE

Common Names

Eng	:	Banyan Tree
Hind	:	Vada, Ber
Sans	:	Vata
Ben	:	Bar, Bargat
Tam	:	Vada, Alam, Ara
Mal	:	Paeral, Vatam

Parts Used

Latex, bark, fruits, leaves, roots and root bark, buds, bark, aerial roots.

Constituents

A triterpine, friedelin and 8-sitosterol were isolated from the leaves. The tigilic acid ester of a -taraxasterol was isolated from the heartwood. The flavonols of the leaves were identified as quercetin-3- galactoside and rutin. Tannins, waxes, fruit contain oil, albuminoid, carbohydrates.

Uses

Aqueous extract of aerial root is given in the treatment of diabetes, tonic, astringent, cooling, and diuretic. Bark is tonic, astringent, cooling and hypoglycemic. The fruits are cooling and tonic.

Classification	
Kingdom	Plantae – Plants
Subkingdom	Tracheobionta – Vascular plants
Superdivision	Spermatophyta – Seed plants
Division	Magnoliophyta – Flowering plants
Class	Magnoliopsida – Dicotyledons
Subclass	Hamamelidae –
Order	Urticales –
Family	Moraceae – Mulberry family
Genus	Ficus L. – Banyan tree

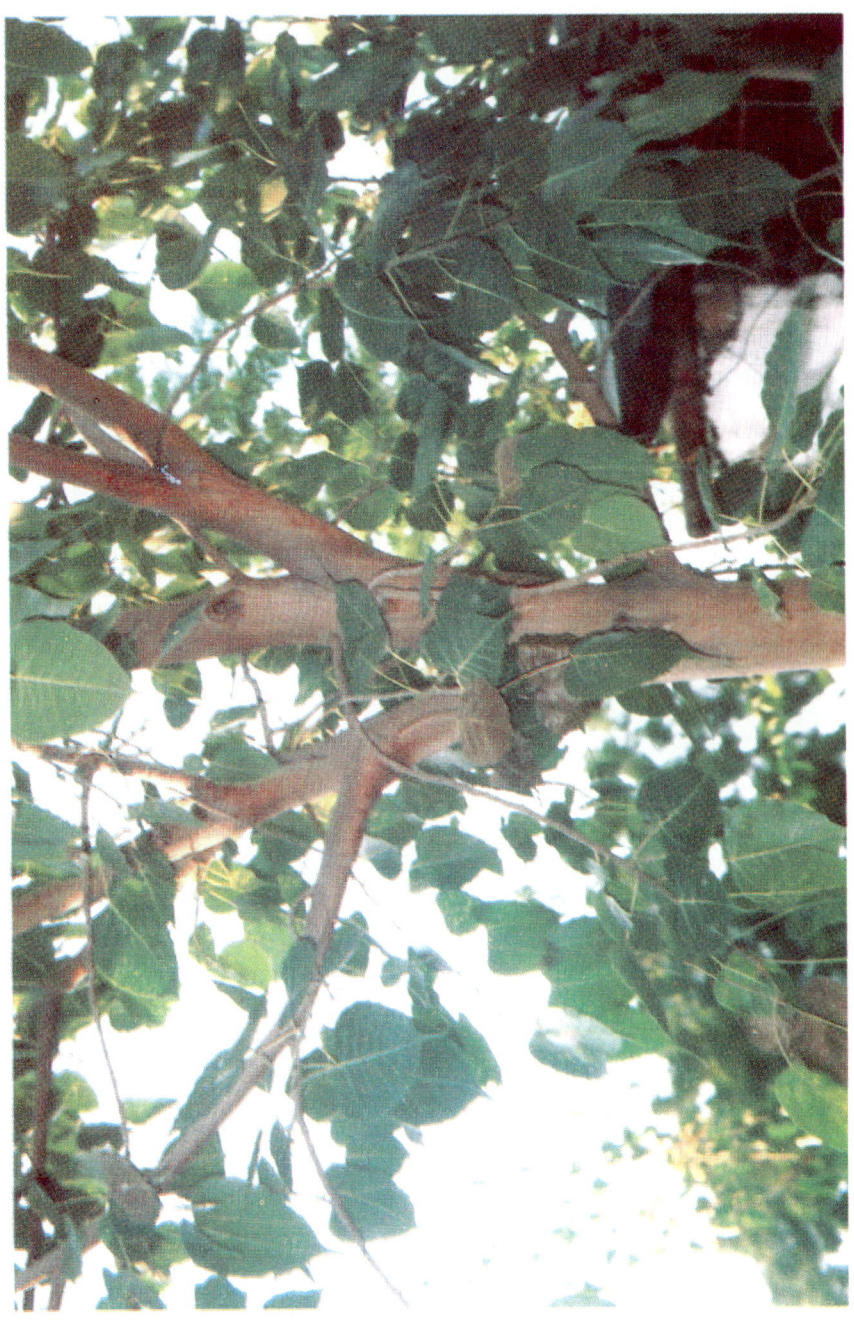

PLATE

68

Ficus glomerata Roxb

MORACEAE

Common Names

Eng	:	Cluster- fig
Hind	:	Gular, Paroa
Sans	:	Udambara
Ben	:	Jajndumar
Tam	:	Atti
Mal	:	Atti

Parts Used

Bark, root, leaves, fruits

Constituents

Tannins, wax, lignin.

Uses

Ripe fruit is eaten raw and roasted fruit is taken along with milk as a tonic. Lignin the main constituent prevents the serum cholesterol level, astringent, carminative stomachic, vermicide.

Classification	
Kingdom	Plantae – Plants
Subkingdom	Tracheobionta – Vascular plants
Superdivision	Spermatophyta – Seed plants
Division	Magnoliophyta – Flowering plants
Class	Magnoliopsida – Dicotyledons
Subclass	Hamamelidae –
Order	Urticales –
Family	Moraceae – Mulberry family
Genus	Ficus L. – fig

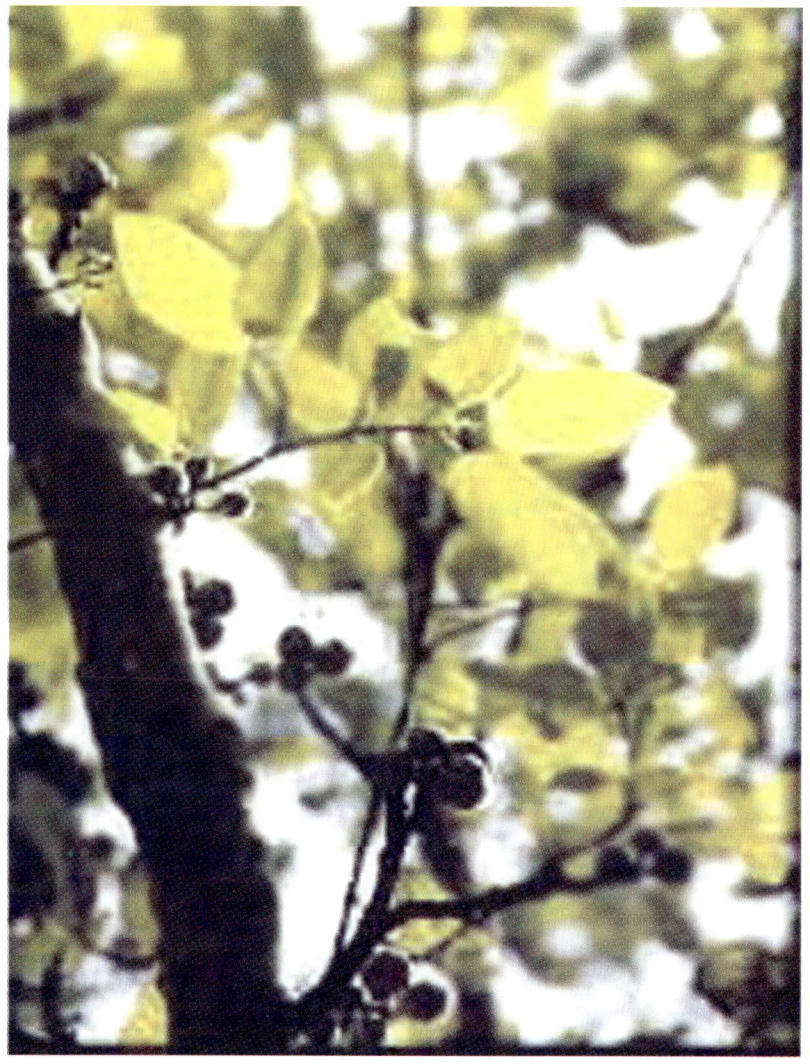

PLATE

69

Ficus religiosa Linn

MORACEAE

Common Names

Eng	:	Sacred fig
Hind	:	Pipal
Sans	:	Pippala
Ben	:	Asud
Tam	:	Arasha maram
Mal	:	Areyal

Parts Used

Barks, roots, leaves, seeds

Constituents

Bark contains tannins, sitosterol, stigmasterol, lanosterol, caffeic acid, wax, fruits contain proteins,

Uses

Seeds are cooling, refrigerant, laxative, leaves are purgative, barks are hypoglycemic, used in the treatment of cold.

Classification	
Kingdom	Plantae – Plants
Subkingdom	Tracheobionta – Vascular plants
Superdivision	Spermatophyta – Seed plants
Division	Magnoliophyta – Flowering plants
Class	Magnoliopsida – Dicotyledons
Subclass	Hamamelidae –
Order	Urticales –
Family	Moraceae – Mulberry family
Genus	Ficus L. – fig

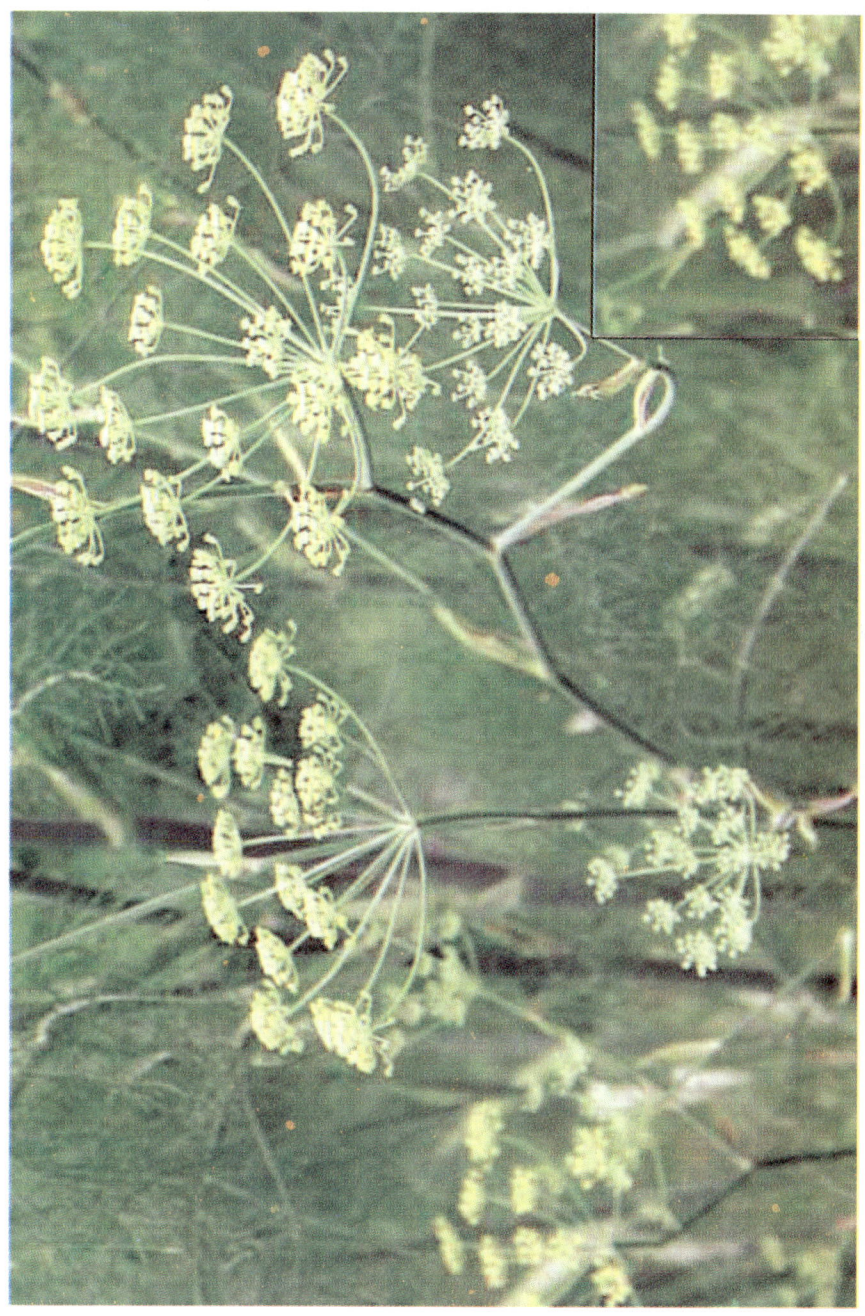

PLATE
70

Foeniculum vulgare Miller

UMBELLIFERAE

Common Names

Eng	:	Indian sweet fennel
Hind	:	Badi Saunf
Sans	:	Madhurika
Ben	:	Panmouri
Tam	:	Shombu
Mal	:	Shombu

Parts Used

Fruits

Constituents

Volatile oil, protein, fixed oil, ketone, fenchone, phenolic ether, anethole, limonene, methyl chavicol, anisic aldehyde.

Uses

The fruits are used in flatulence, fever, intestinal colic, burning sensation, constipation. It is also used as toothpaste for the prevention of dental caries, periodonal diseases, The hot infusion of fruit is useful in amenorrhoe. The fennel extract have been reported for its antimicrobial, estrogenic activity, carminative aromatic, stimulant, expectorant, flavoring agent.

Classification	
Kingdom	Plantae – Plants
Subkingdom	Tracheobionta – Vascular plants
Superdivision	Spermatophyta – Seed plants
Division	Magnoliophyta – Flowering plants
Class	Magnoliopsida – Dicotyledons
Subclass	Rosidae –
Order	Apiales –
Family	Apiaceae – Carrot family
Genus	Foeniculum P. Mill. – fennel

Gaultheria procumbens L.

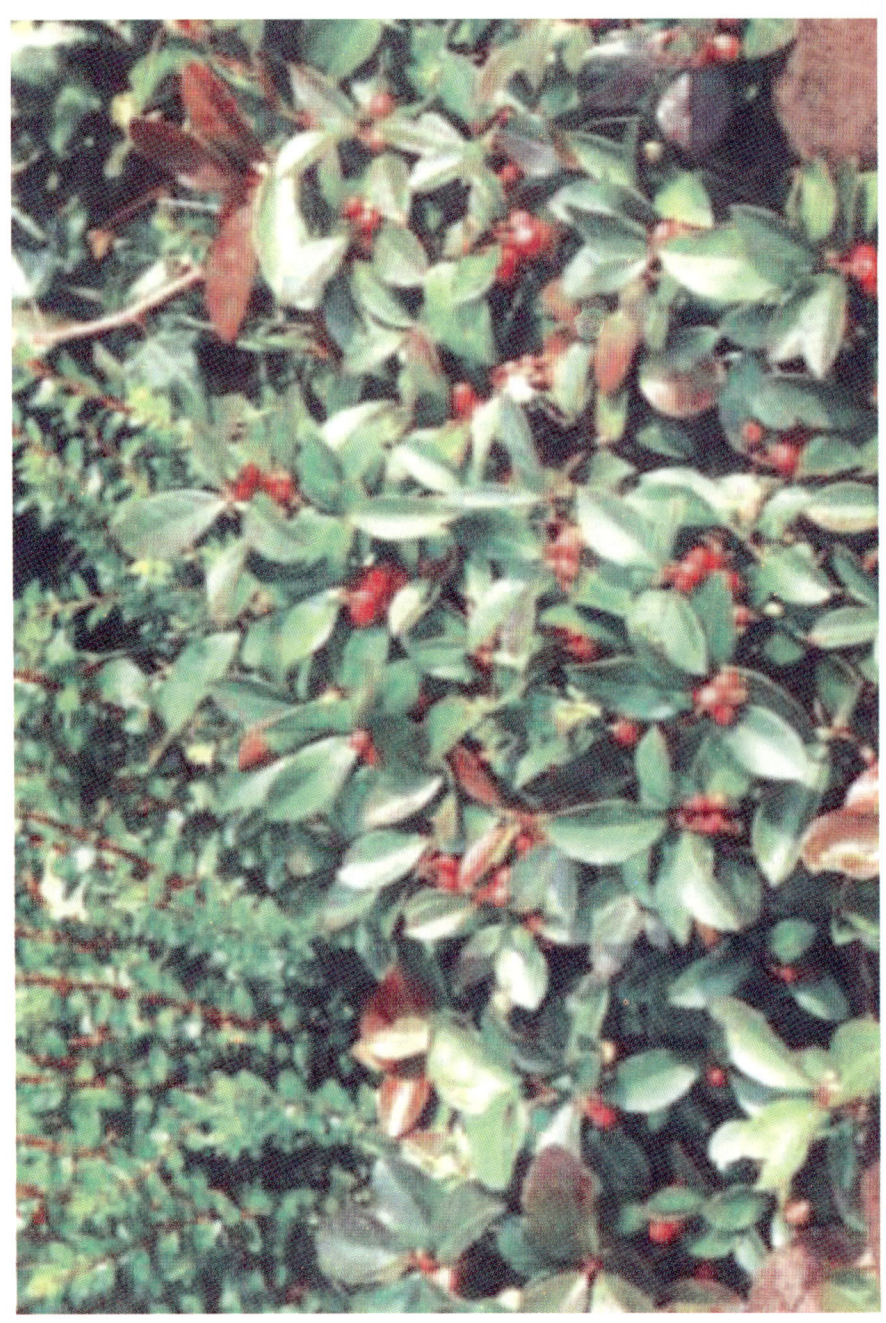

PLATE

71

Gaultheria procumbens L.

ERICACEAE

Common Names

Eng   :   Betula oil

Parts Used

Leaves

Constituents

Oil contain methyl salicylate, formed by hydrolysis of a glycoside gaultheri in presence of water by natural enzyme gaultherase

Uses

Counter irritant, treatment of rheumatism, vermicide, flavouring agent

Classification	
Kingdom	Plantae – Plants
Subkingdom	Tracheobionta – Vascular plants
Superdivision	Spermatophyta – Seed plants
Division	Magnoliophyta – Flowering plants
Class	Magnoliopsida – Dicotyledons
Subclass	Dilleniidae –
Order	Ericales –
Family	Ericaceae – Heath family
Genus	Gaultheria L. – snowberry

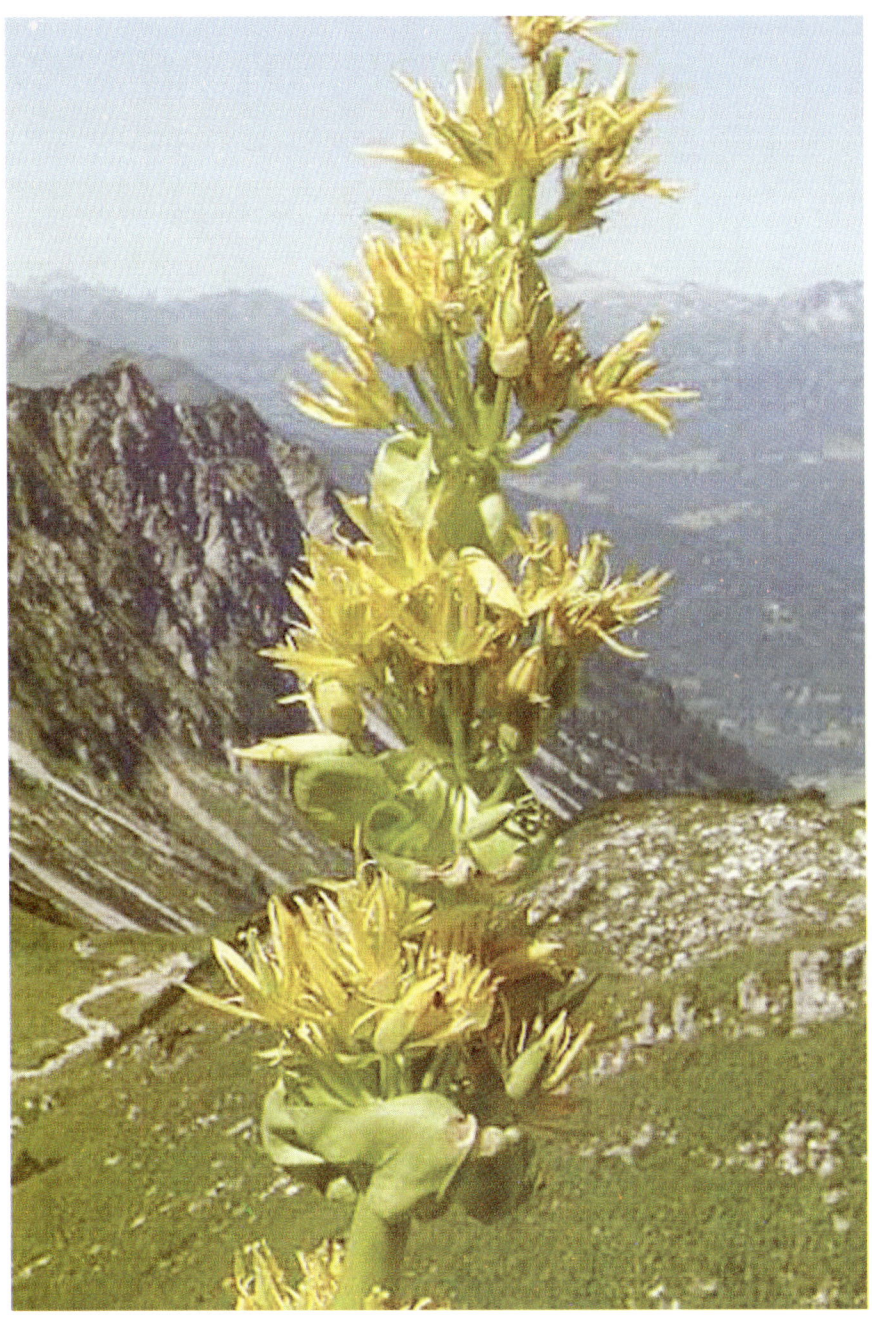

PLATE

72

Gentiana lutea L.

GENTIANACEAE

Common Names

Eng   :   Yellow gentian

Parts used

Roots and Rhizomes

Constituents

Biter glycoside mainly gentiopicrin, gentiogenin, glucose, amarogenitin, amaroswerin, gentioside, gentisin

Uses

It is used as bitter tonic to stimulate the gastric secretion and hence improve the appetite.

Classification	
Kingdom	Plantae – Plants
Subkingdom	Tracheobionta – Vascular plants
Superdivision	Spermatophyta – Seed plants
Division	Magnoliophyta – Flowering plants
Class	Magnoliopsida – Dicotyledons
Subclass	Asteridae –
Order	Gentianales –
Family	Gentianaceae – Gentian family
Genus	Gentiana L. – gentian

Ginkgo biloba L.

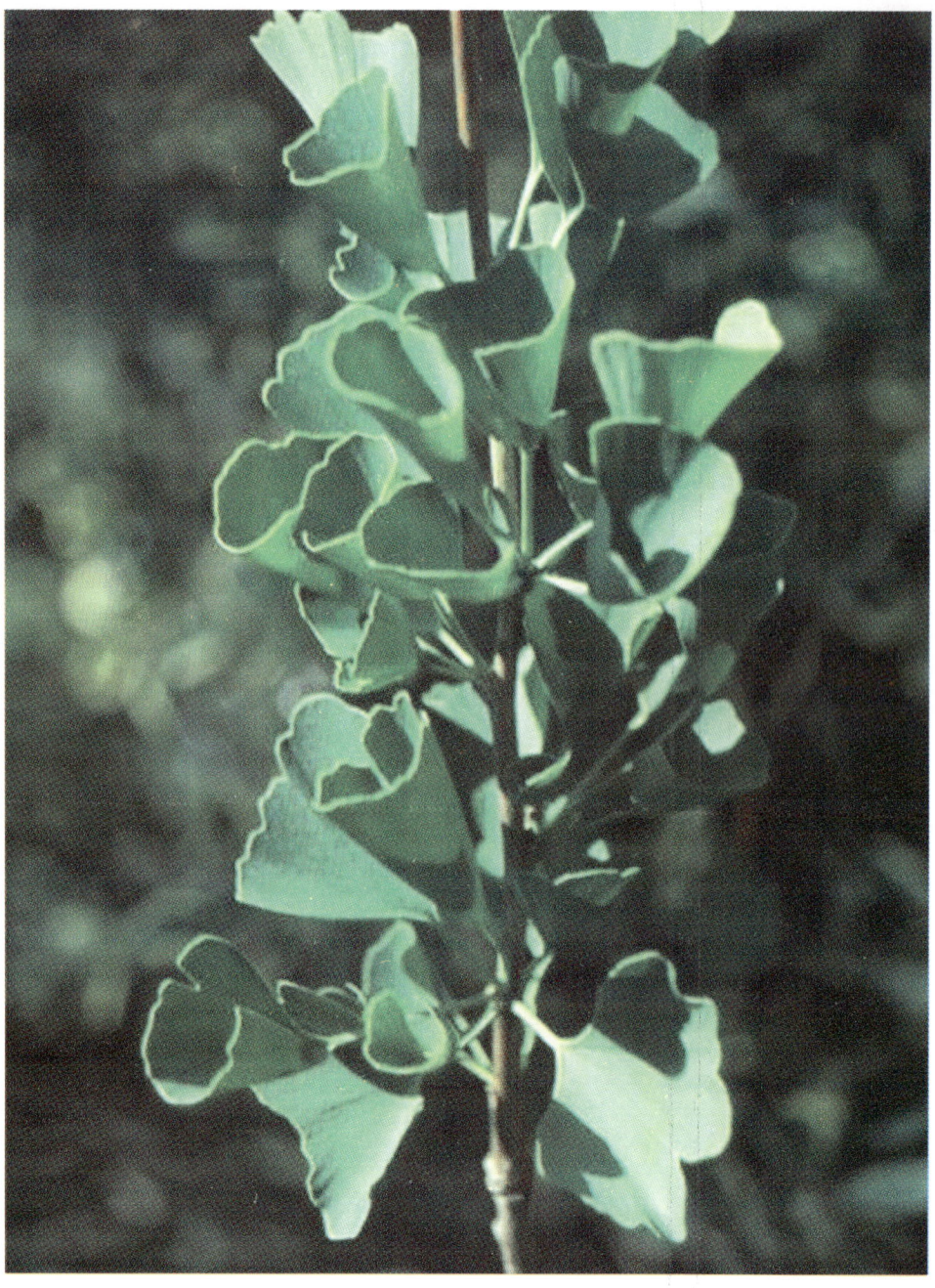

PLATE
73

Ginkgo biloba L.

GINKGOACEAE

Common Name

    Eng   :   maiden hair tree

Parts Used

Leaves

Constituents

The active ingridents are flavonol glycoside, which mainly include flavonol, mono- di- and triglycosides of kaempferol, quercetin and isorhamnetin, biflavones present are ginkgetin, isoginkgetin, bilobetin which occur in the form of coumaric ester of glucorhamnosides.

Uses

In the treatment of metabolic and vascular disorders, asthma, memory impairment.

Classification	
Kingdom	Plantae – Plants
Subkingdom	Tracheobionta – Vascular plants
Superdivision	Spermatophyta – Seed plants
Division	Ginkgophyta – Ginkgo
Class	Ginkgoopsida –
Order	Ginkgoales –
Family	Ginkgoaceae – Ginkgo family
Genus	Ginkgo L. – ginkgo

Glycyrrhiza glabra Linn

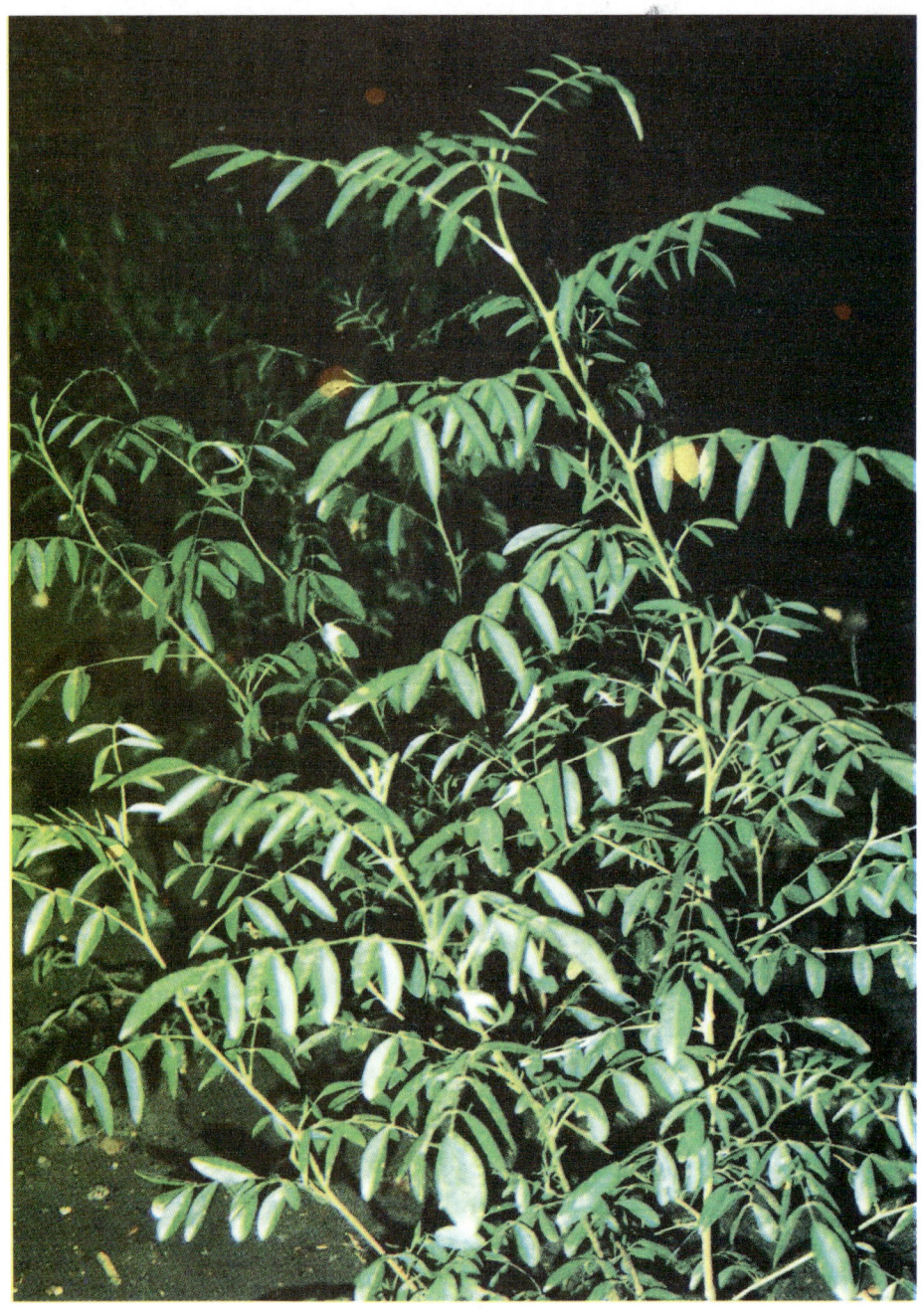

PLATE

74

Glycyrrhiza glabra Linn

PAPILIONACEAE

Common Names

Eng	:	Sweet wood, Liquorice
Hind	:	Mithilakdi, Mulathee
Sans	:	Yashti mudhu, Madhuka
Ben	:	Jashti madhu
Tam	:	Ati Maduram, Athimathurappat

Parts Used

Peeled roots

Constituents

It consist of many volatile constituents like pentanol, hexanol, linalool oxide A, B, tetramethyl pyrazine, terpinen-4-ol, β- terpinol, geraniol and acids like propionic acid, benzoic acid, ethyl linolenate, methyl ethyl ketone, butanediol, feufuraldehyde, furfuryl formate, trimethylpyrazine, maltol and many other compounds like glycyrrhizin, asparagin, sugar starch, acid resin, gum, mucilage, tannin, glycyrrhizic, acid are reported.

Uses

It is used in the treatment of asthma, acute and chronic bronchitis, chronic cough, prevention of urinary tract infection and also as tonic, cooling, demulcent, expectorant, diuretic, emmenagogue, gentle laxative, anti ulcer.

Classification	
Kingdom	Plantae – Plants
Subkingdom	Tracheobionta – Vascular plants
Superdivision	Spermatophyta – Seed plants
Division	Magnoliophyta – Flowering plants
Class	Magnoliopsida – Dicotyledons
Subclass	Rosidae –
Order	Fabales –
Family	Fabaceae – Pea family
Genus	Glycyrrhiza L. – licorice

Gossypium herbaceum Linn

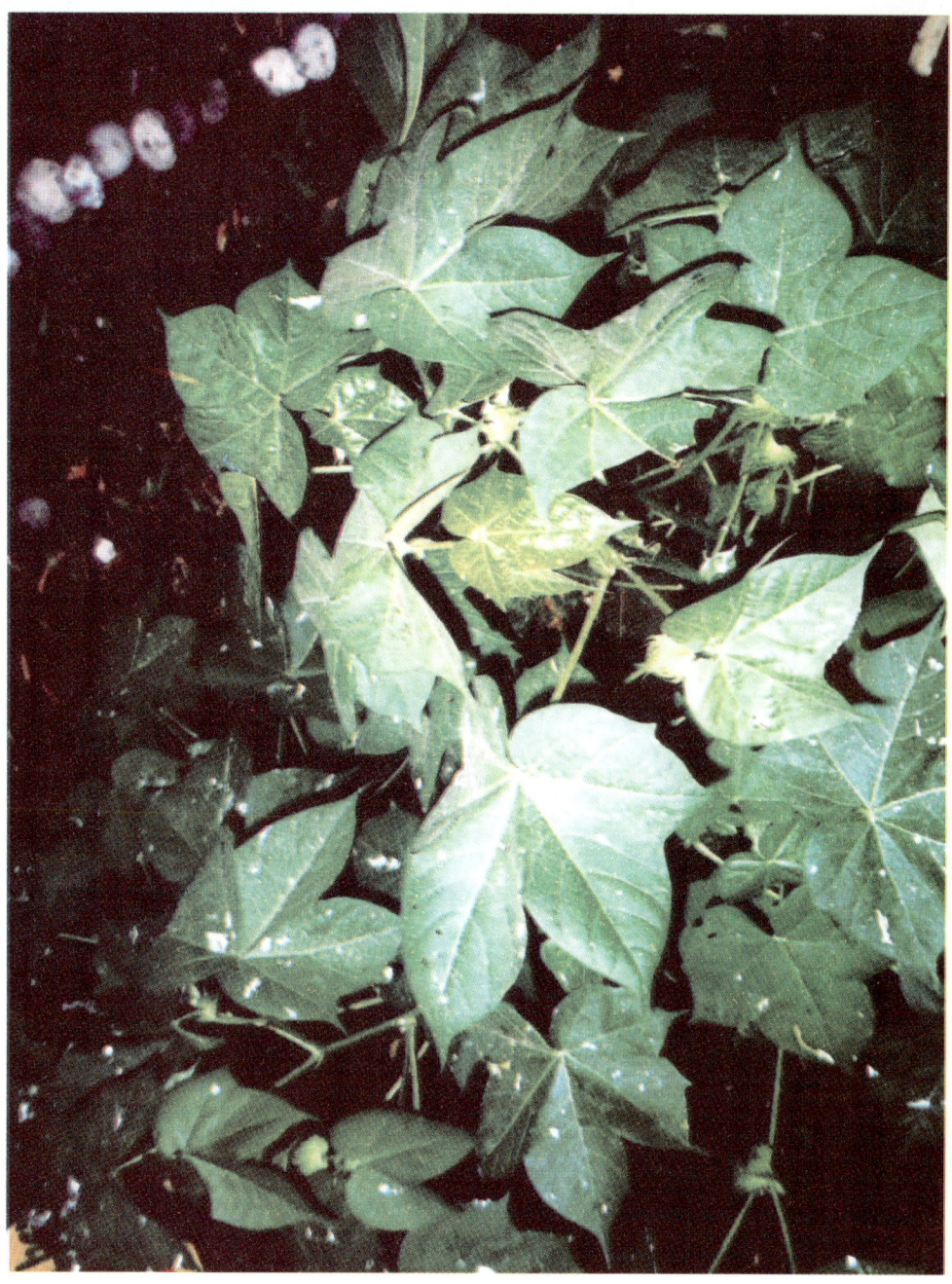

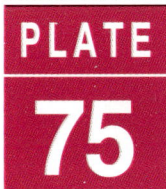

PLATE

75

Gossypium herbaceum Linn

MALVACEAE

Common Names

Eng	:	Cotton
Hind	:	Kupas
Sans	:	Anagnika
Ben	:	Kapas, Tula
Tam	:	Paruti
Mal	:	Pangi

Parts Used

Seeds

Constituents

Triglycerides of fatty acids mainly palmitic, oleic and linoleic acids

Uses

Pharmaceutical aid for the preparation of cosmetics, hydrogenated fats, emollients. It is also used as edible oils for cooking or preparation of margarine. It is also employed as pediculosis, laxative, acaricide.

Classification	
Kingdom	Plantae – Plants
Subkingdom	Tracheobionta – Vascular plants
Superdivision	Spermatophyta – Seed plants
Division	Magnoliophyta – Flowering plants
Class	Magnoliopsida – Dicotyledons
Subclass	Dilleniidae –
Order	Malvales –
Family	Malvaceae – Mallow family
Genus	Gossypium L. – cotton

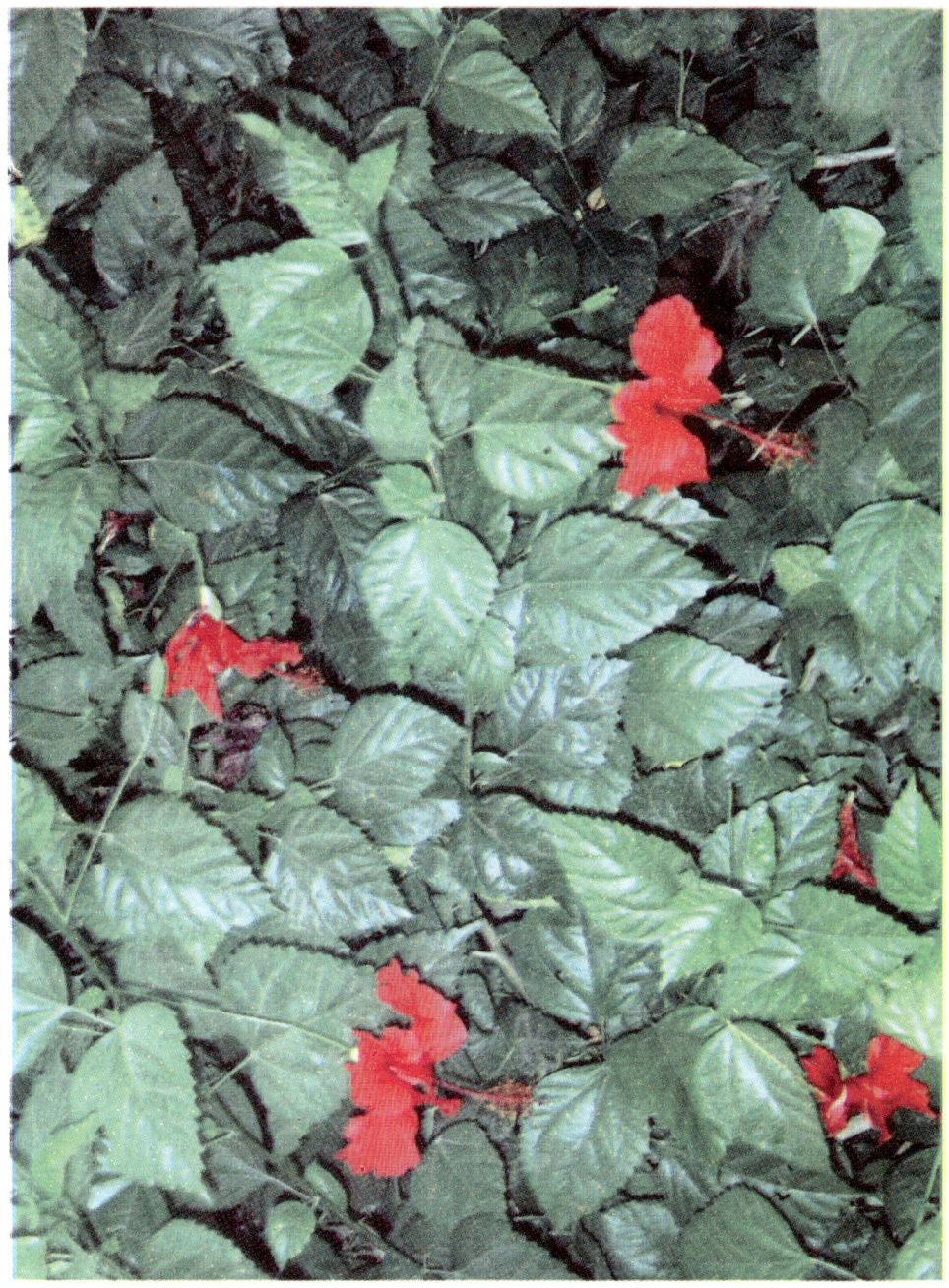

PLATE 76

Hibiscus rosasinensis Linn

MALVACEAE

Common Names

Eng	:	China rose, shoe flower plant
Hind	:	Jasund, Gudhal
Sans	:	Japa
Ben	:	Jaba
Tam	:	Shamberaltar
Mal	:	Champuratti

Parts Used

Roots, Flowers, Seeds

Constituents

The anthocyanins from petals are used as colouring agents. The major anthocynidin are 3- sophoroside, the flower nector is rich in amino acids mainly aspartic acid and asparagin, quercetin 3 diglucoside, 3-7 diglucoside, cyanidine – 3, 5-diglucoside, cyanide 3-sopheraside – 5 – glucoside are reported .

Uses

Antitumour, anti-complementary activity, anti-inflammatory, refrigerant, emollient, demulcent, aphrodisiac, emmenogogue.

Classification	
Kingdom	Plantae – Plants
Subkingdom	Tracheobionta – Vascular plants
Superdivision	Spermatophyta – Seed plants
Division	Magnoliophyta – Flowering plants
Class	Magnoliopsida – Dicotyledons
Subclass	Dilleniidae –
Order	Malvales –
Family	Malvaceae – Mallow family
Genus	Hibiscus L. – rosemallow

Holarrhena antidysenterica Wall

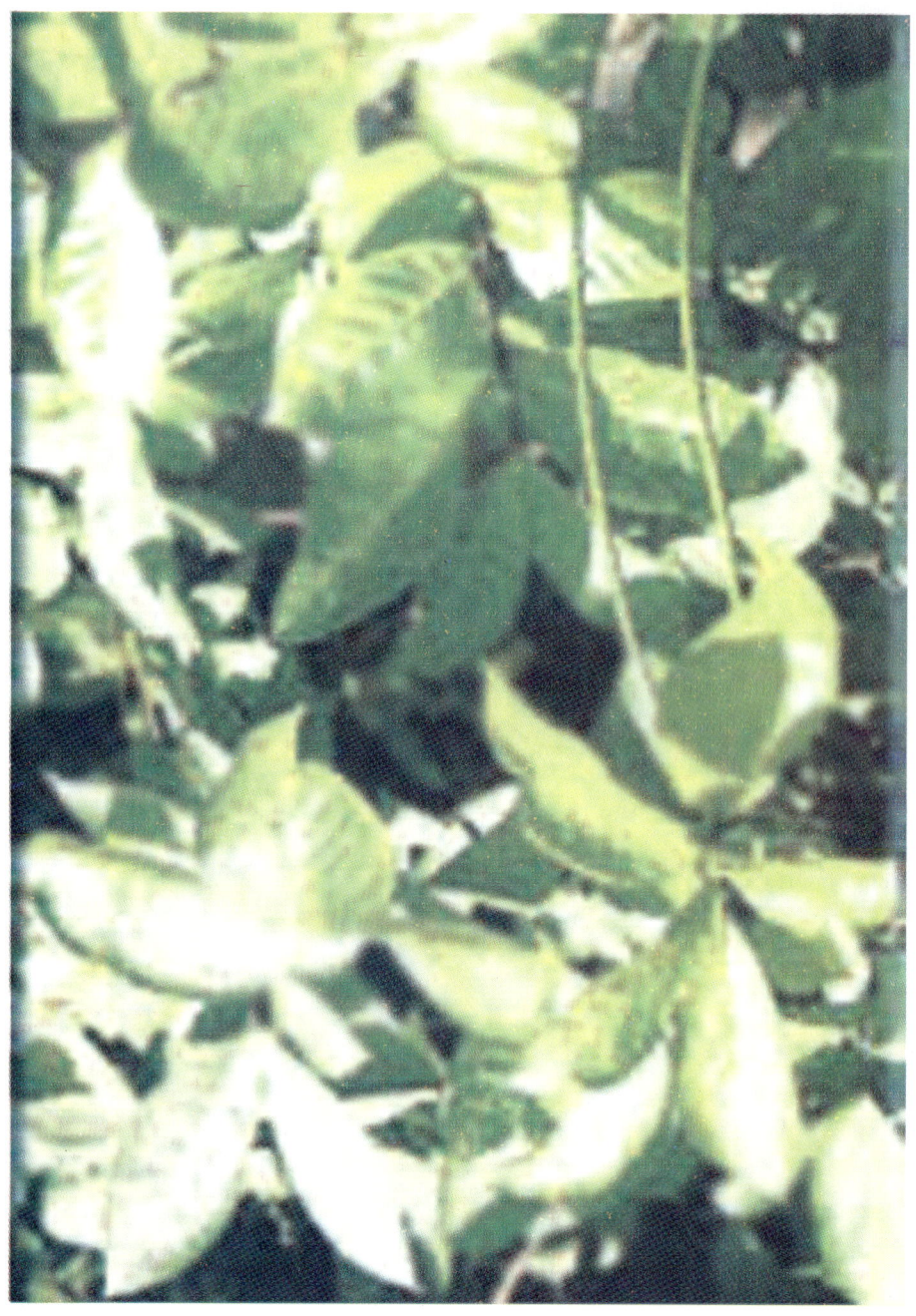

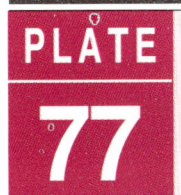

PLATE

77

Holarrhena antidysenterica Wall

APOCYNACEAE

Common Names

Eng	:	Kurchi, Tellicherry
Hind	:	Karchi, Kura
Sans	:	Kutaja, Kalinga
Ben	:	Kurchi, Khureya
Tam	:	Kashappu - vetpalarishi

Parts Used

Backs, Seeds, Leaves

Constituents

Non-oxygenerated alkaloid, wrightine, conessine, karchisine, holarrlenine.

Uses

Stomachic, astringent, antidysenteric, febrifuge, anthelmintic, carminative, antiperiodic.

Classification	
Kingdom	Plantae – Plants
Subkingdom	Tracheobionta – Vascular plants
Superdivision	Spermatophyta – Seed plants
Division	Magnoliophyta – Flowering plants
Class	Magnoliopsida – Dicotyledons
Subclass	Asteridae –
Order	Gentianales –
Family	Apocynaceae – DogBene family
Genus	Holarrhena R. Br. – holarrhena

Ipomoea batatas Poir

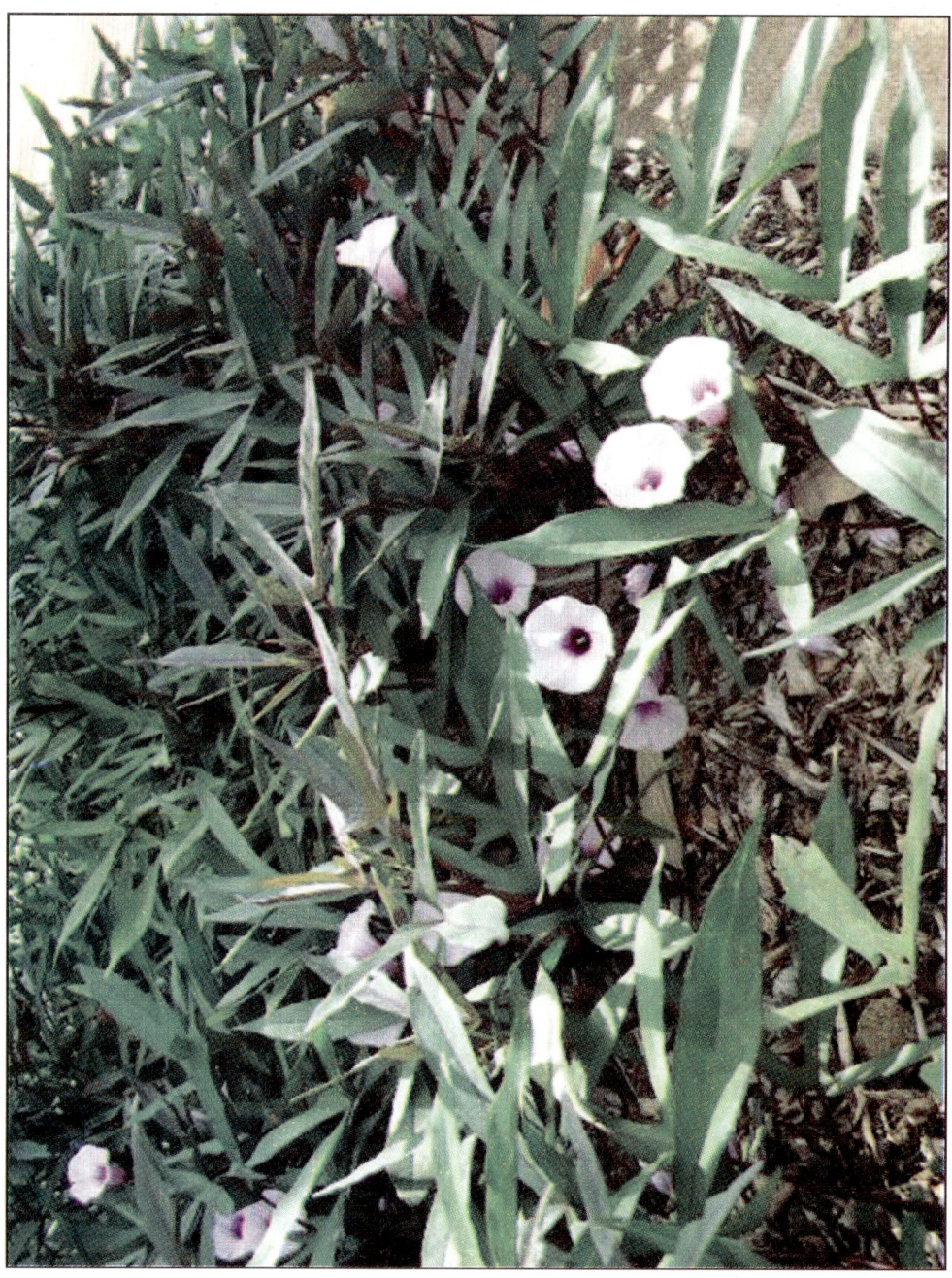

PLATE
78

Ipomoea batatas Poir

CONVOLVULACEAE

Common Names

Eng	:	Sweet potato
Ben	:	Kalmi sak
Tam	:	Sarkarivalli

Parts Used

Roots, leaves

Constituents

Carbohydrates, glycosides, resins, proteins.

Uses

Nutritive, pastes of leaves in scorpion sting.

Classification	
Kingdom	Plantae – Plants
Subkingdom	Tracheobionta – Vascular plants
Superdivision	Spermatophyta – Seed plants
Division	Magnoliophyta – Flowering plants
Class	Magnoliopsida – Dicotyledons
Subclass	Asteridae –
Order	Solanales –
Family	Convolvulaceae –
Genus	Ipomoea L. – Sweet potato

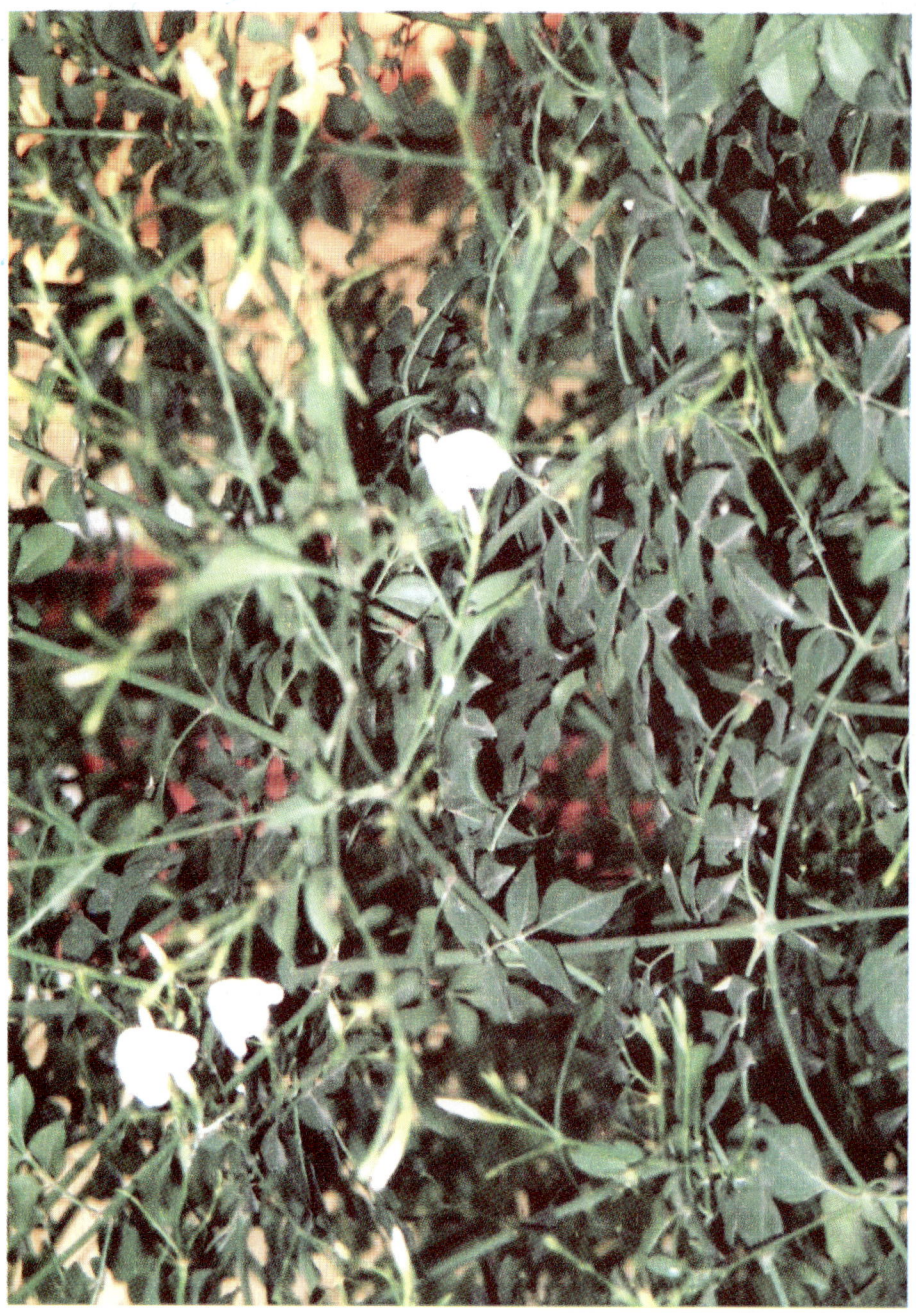

PLATE 79

Jasminum grandiflorum Linn

OLEACEAE

Common Names

Eng	:	Spanish Jasmine
Hin	:	Jati
San	:	Jati
Ben	:	Chameli
Tam	:	Malli
Mal	:	Pichhakam

Parts Used

Whole Plants

Constituents

Leaves and flowers contain resin, salicylic acid, the main odorous components present are benzyl acetate, benzyl benzoate, phytol, jasmone, methyljasmonate, linalool, geranyl linalool, isophytol.

Uses

Astringent, anthelmintic, deobstruent, diuretic, emmenagogue, headache, aphrodisiac, mouth ulcerations.

Classification	
Kingdom	Plantae – Plants
Subkingdom	Tracheobionta – Vascular plants
Superdivision	Spermatophyta – Seed plants
Division	Magnoliophyta – Flowering plants
Class	Magnoliopsida – Dicotyledons
Subclass	Asteridae –
Order	Scrophulariales –
Family	Oleaceae – Olive family
Genus	Jasminum L. – jasmine

Jatropha curcus Linn

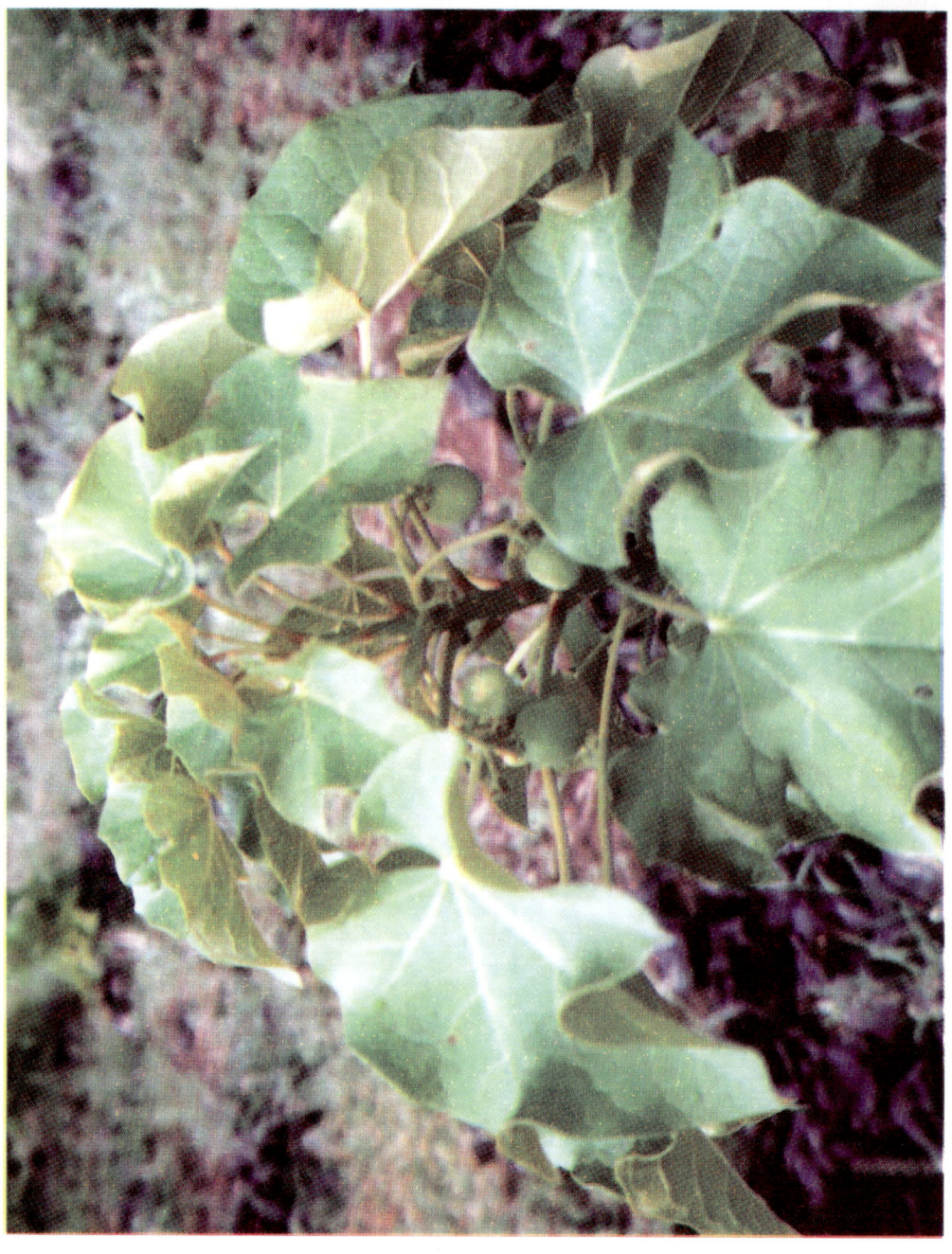

PLATE 80

Jatropha curcus Linn

EUPHORBIACEAE

Common Names

Eng	:	Angular leaved physic nut
Hin	:	Jangli erandi
San	:	Parveta-eranda
Ben	:	Bonbheranda
Tel	:	Pepalam
Tam	:	Kattamanakku
Mal	:	Katamanak

Parts Used

Seeds, leaves and juice.

Constituents

Proteins, sterols, enzymes, sugar, starch, etc.

Uses

Seed oil is used as purgative, antiseptic and depurative. Leaves are lactagogue. Stem juice is used in ulcers and wounds.

Classification	
Kingdom	Plantae – Plants
Subkingdom	Tracheobionta – Vascular plants
Superdivision	Spermatophyta – Seed plants
Division	Magnoliophyta – Flowering plants
Class	Magnoliopsida – Dicotyledons
Subclass	Rosidae –
Order	Euphorbiales –
Family	Euphorbiaceae – Spurge family
Genus	Jatropha L. – nettlespurge

Lantana camara Linn

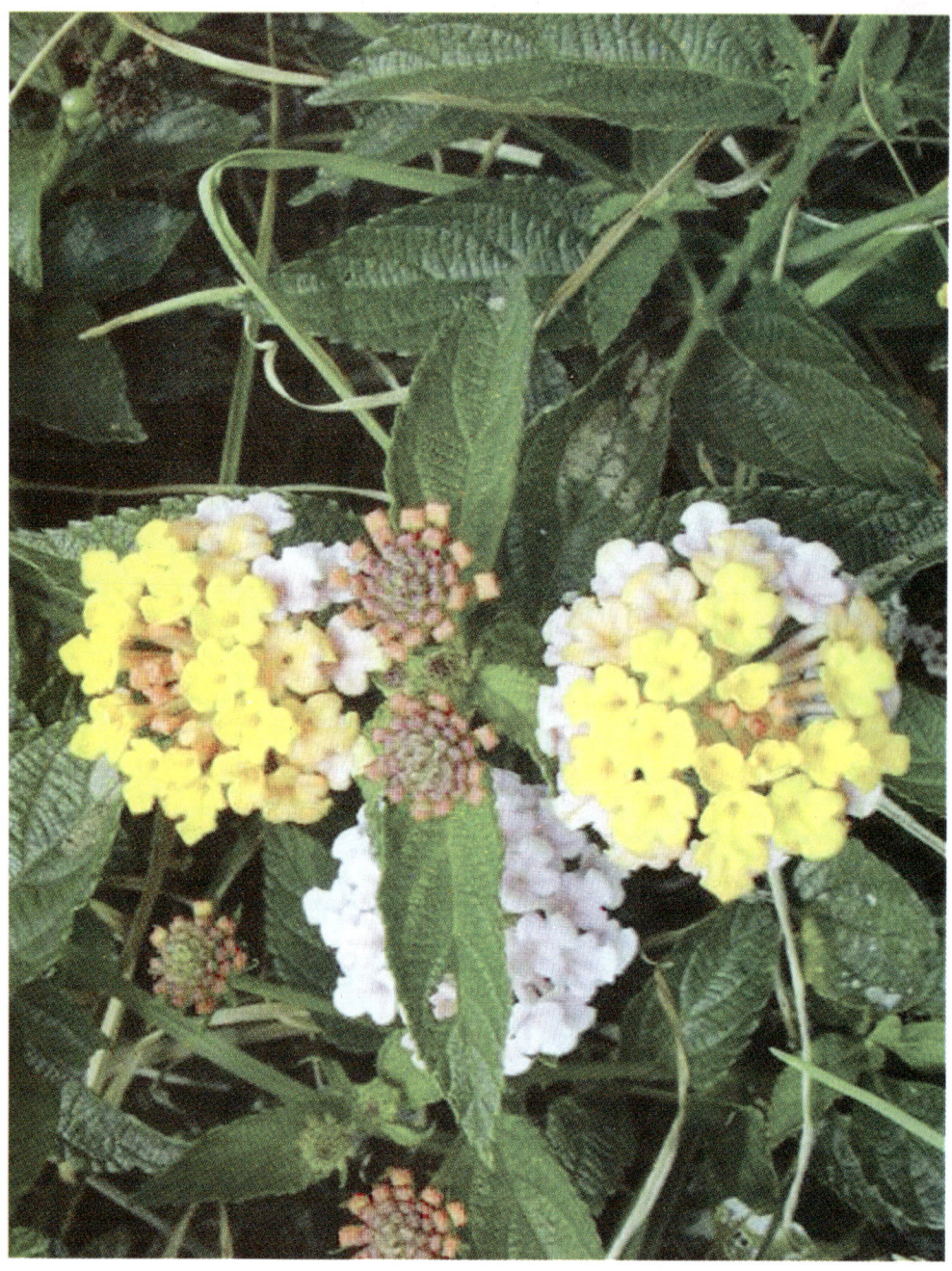

PLATE

81

Lantana camara Linn

VERBENACEAE

Common Names

Eng	:	Lantana, wild sage
Tam	:	Arippu
Mal	:	Arippu
Tel	:	Pulikampa
Kan	:	Nata hu gida

Parts Used

Leaves, flowers

Constituents

Leaves contain essential oils, lantadenes A-D, lantanilic acid, icterogenin, farnesene, caryaphyllene.

Uses

Antifungal, nematicidal, antifeedant.

Classification	
Kingdom	Plantae – Plants
Subkingdom	Tracheobionta – Vascular plants
Superdivision	Spermatophyta – Seed plants
Division	Magnoliophyta – Flowering plants
Class	Magnoliopsida – Dicotyledons
Subclass	Asteridae –
Order	Lamiales –
Family	Verbenaceae – Verbena family
Genus	Lantana L. – lantana

Lawsonia inermis Linn

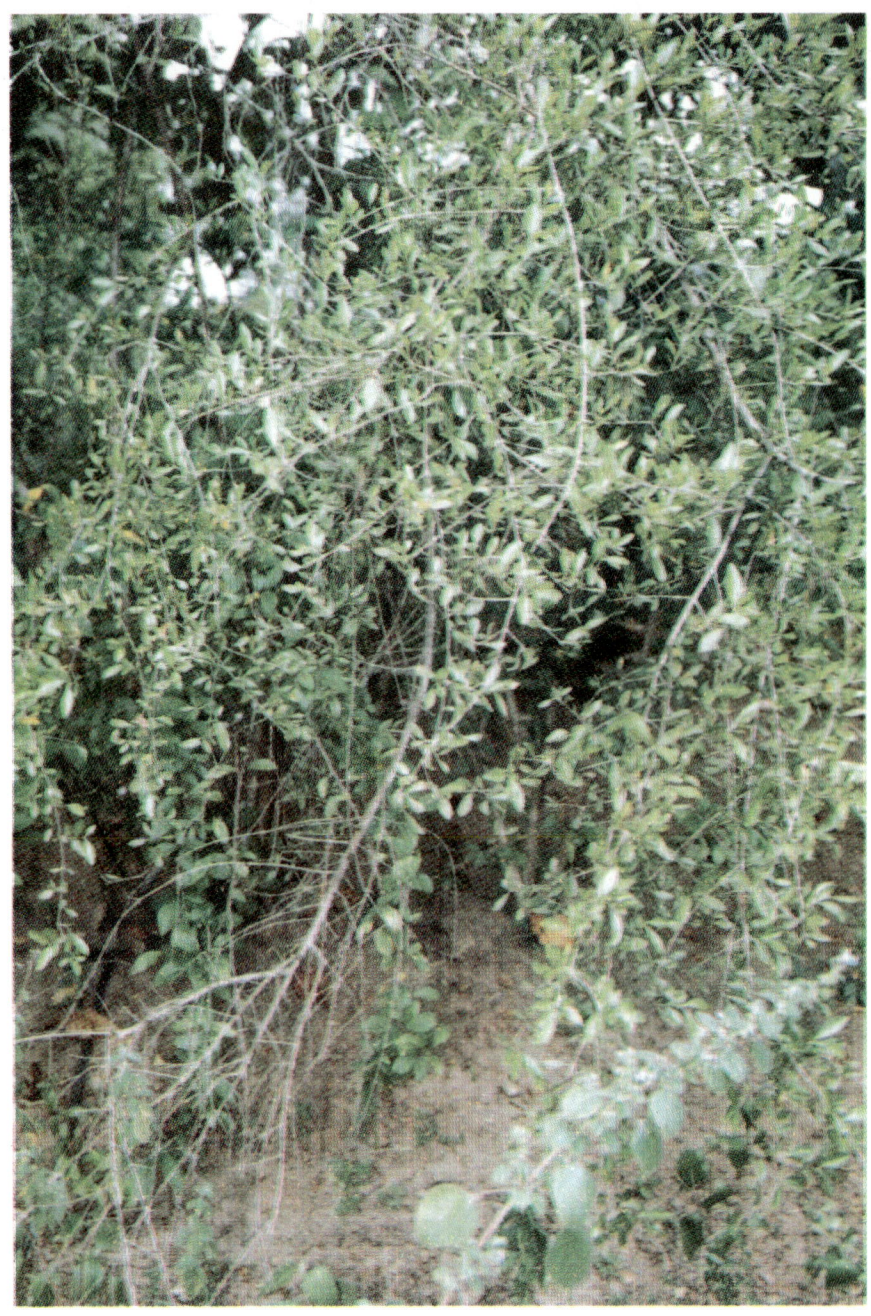

PLATE
82

Lawsonia inermis Linn

LYTHRACEAE

Common Names

Eng	:	Henna, Samphire
Hind	:	Hena, Mehandi
Sans	:	Mendhi, Mendika
Ben	:	Mehendi
Tam	:	Maruthoni
Mal	:	Mailanchi

Parts Used

Leaves, back, flowers, seeds

Constituents

Leaves are rich in minerals like K, Ca, Mg, Na, Fe, Mn, Zn, Cu, phenolic glucoside, lawsoniaside, lalioside. Stem contain isoplumbagin and 3 methyl nonacosan-1-ol, fatty acid composition of oil is palmitic acid, stearic acid, oleic acid and linolinic acid, colouring matter, homo-tannic acid, tannin.

Uses

Anti bacterial, antimicrobial, wound healing, skin lesions, hepatoprotective, antifungal, sedative, astringent.

Classification	
Kingdom	Plantae – Plants
Subkingdom	Tracheobionta – Vascular plants
Superdivision	Spermatophyta – Seed plants
Division	Magnoliophyta – Flowering plants
Class	Magnoliopsida – Dicotyledons
Subclass	Rosidae –
Order	Myrtales –
Family	Lythraceae – Loosestrife family
Genus	Lawsonia L. – lawsonia

Mangifera indica Linn

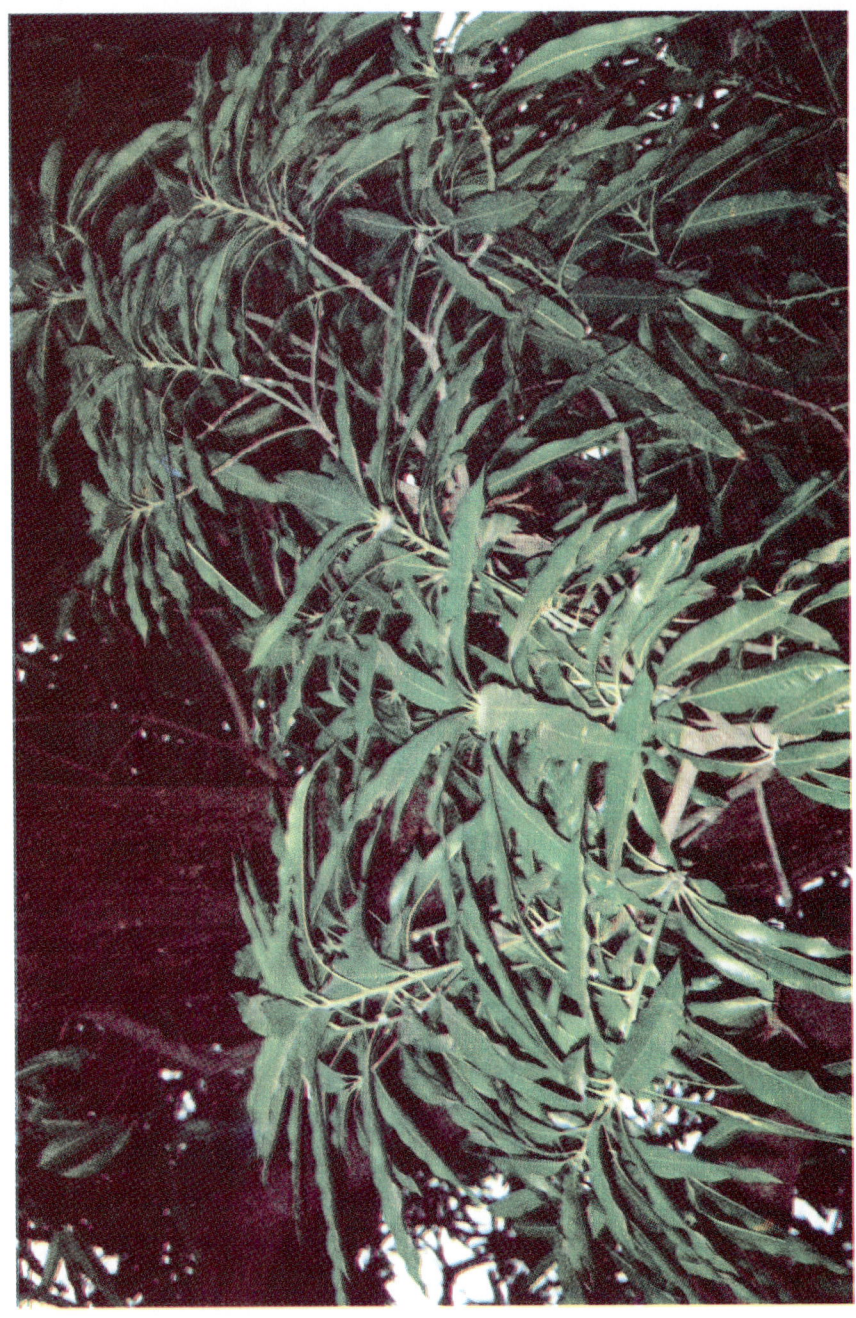

PLATE

83

Mangifera indica Linn

ANACARDIACEAE

Common Names

Eng	:	Mango
Hin	:	Am
San	:	Amva
Ben	:	Am
Tam	:	Mampalam
Mal	:	Mavu

Parts Used

Fruits, kernals, leaves, flowers and bark

Constituents

Tannins, gallic acid, fats, sugar, rich in vitamin C.

Uses

The fruit is laxative, diuretic, diaphoretic, astringent, refrigerant, the unripe fruit is astringent, stomachic, antiscorbutic, kernals are anthelmintic.

Classification	
Kingdom	Plantae – Plants
Subkingdom	Tracheobionta – Vascular plants
Superdivision	Spermatophyta – Seed plants
Division	Magnoliophyta – Flowering plants
Class	Magnoliopsida – Dicotyledons
Subclass	Rosidae –
Order	Sapindales –
Family	Anacardiaceae – Sumac family
Genus	Mangifera L. – mango

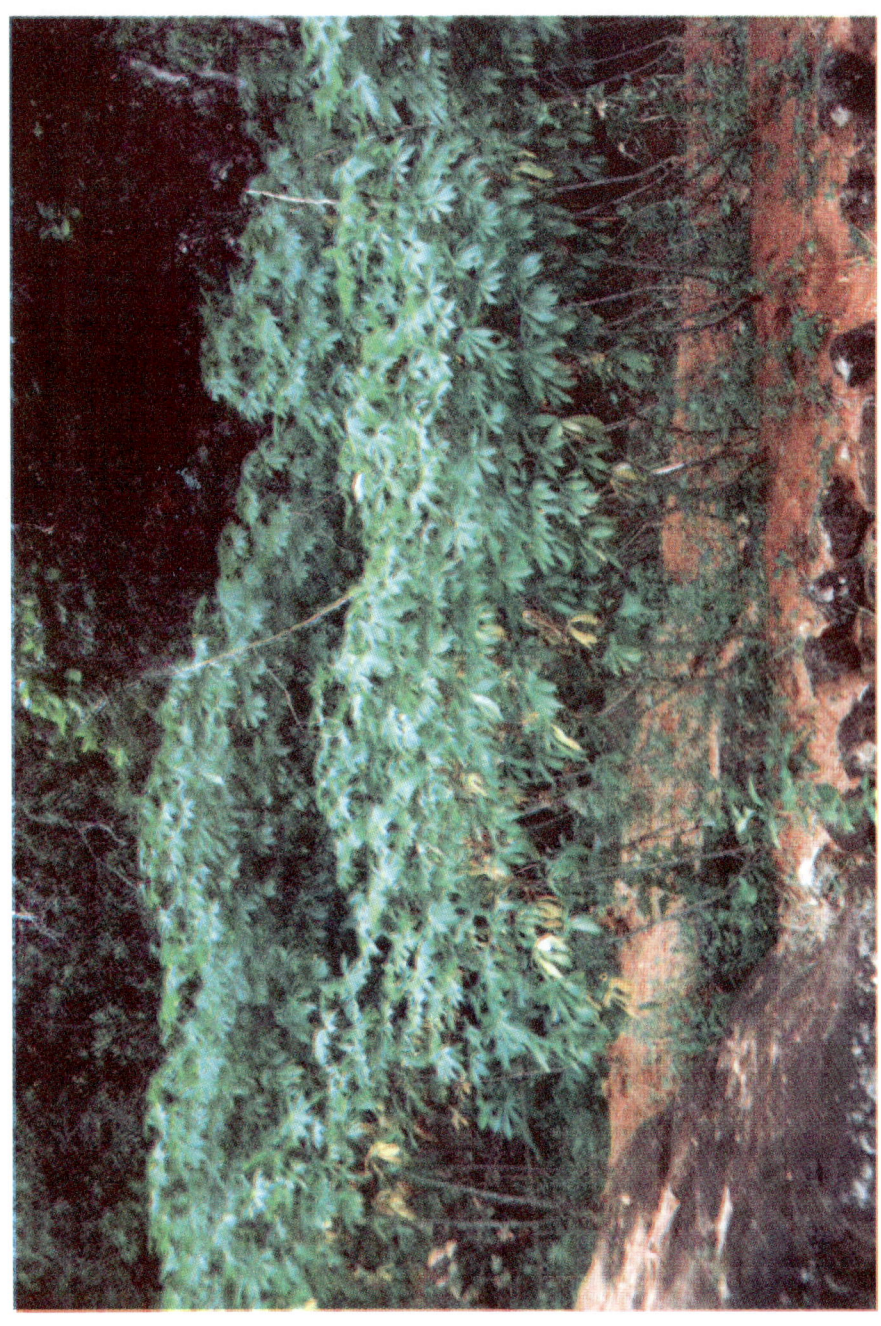

PLATE
84

Manihot esculentum Pohl

EUPHORBIACEAE

Common Names

Eng	:	Tapioca
Hin	:	Sakarkanda
Tam	:	Maravalli
Mal	:	Marichini

Parts used

Tubers

Constituents

Tubers Contain β carotene lutein carotenoids includes α-, γ-, æ -carotenes & β cryptoxanthum. It is a good source of provetanen, bitterness is due to cyanoglycoside, leaf proteins has high tannin and high level of chymotrypsin.

Use

Nutritive

Classification	
Kingdom	Plantae – Plants
Subkingdom	Tracheobionta – Vascular plants
Superdivision	Spermatophyta – Seed plants
Division	Magnoliophyta – Flowering plants
Class	Magnoliopsida – Dicotyledons
Subclass	Rosidae –
Order	Euphorbiales –
Family	Euphorbiaceae – Spurge family
Genus	Manihot P. Mill. – manihot

Mentha arvensis Linn

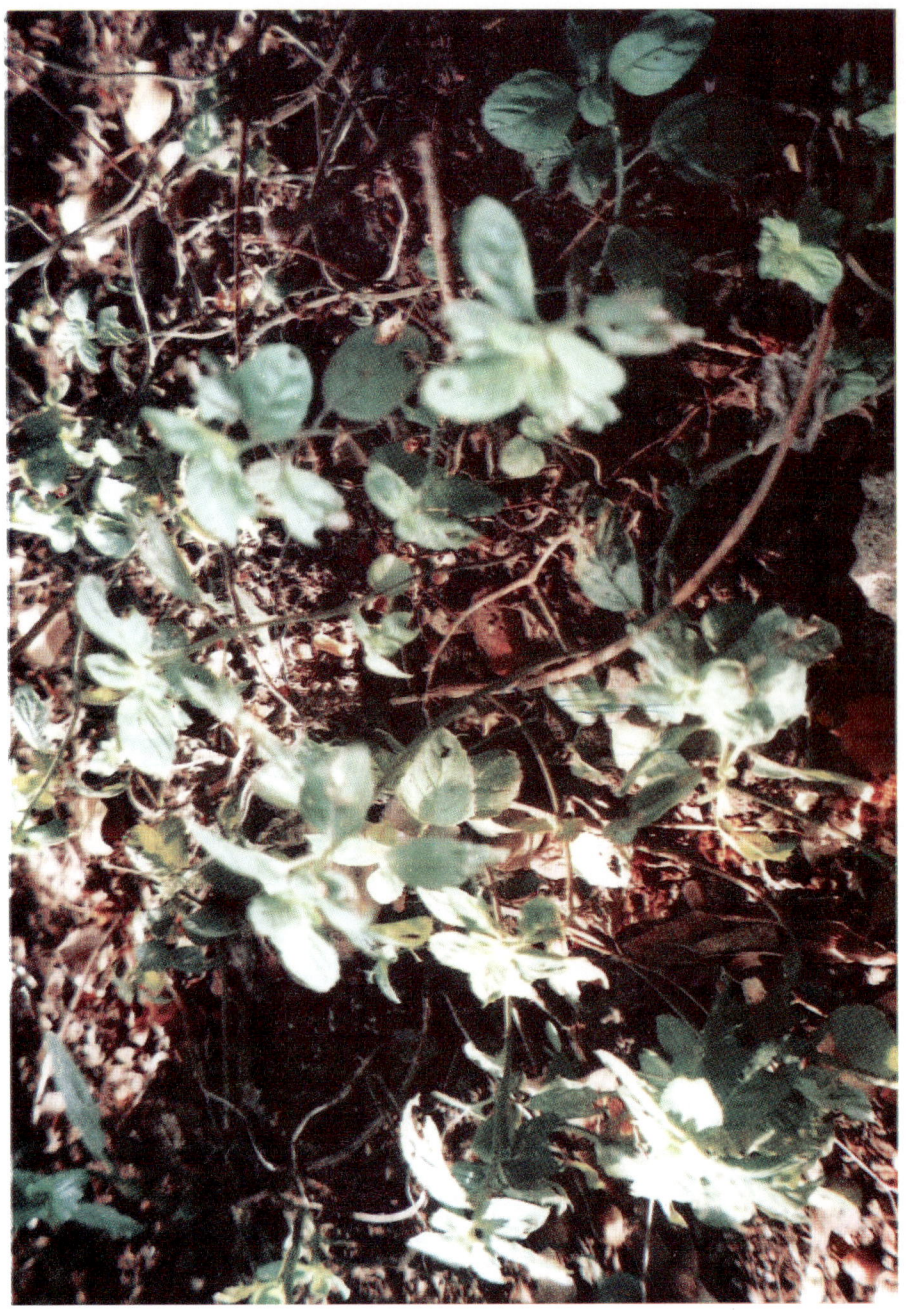

PLATE
85

Mentha arvensis Linn

LABIATAE

Common Names

Eng	:	Japanese mint
Hind	:	Pudinah
Ben	:	Pudinah
Tam	:	Pudinah
Mal	:	Puttiyana

Parts Used

Whole plant

Constituents

Volatile oil- menthone, menthol, isomenthone, methyl acetate, neomenthol, piperitone, isomenthol, pulegone.

Uses

Aromatic, carminative, stimulant, antispasmodic, antiseptic, stomachic, rheumatic pain, indigestion, spleen disease, asthma, jaundice and emmenogogue.

Classification	
Kingdom	Plantae – Plants
Subkingdom	Tracheobionta – Vascular plants
Superdivision	Spermatophyta – Seed plants
Division	Magnoliophyta – Flowering plants
Class	Magnoliopsida – Dicotyledons
Subclass	Asteridae –
Order	Lamiales –
Family	Lamiaceae – Mint family
Genus	Mentha L. –mint

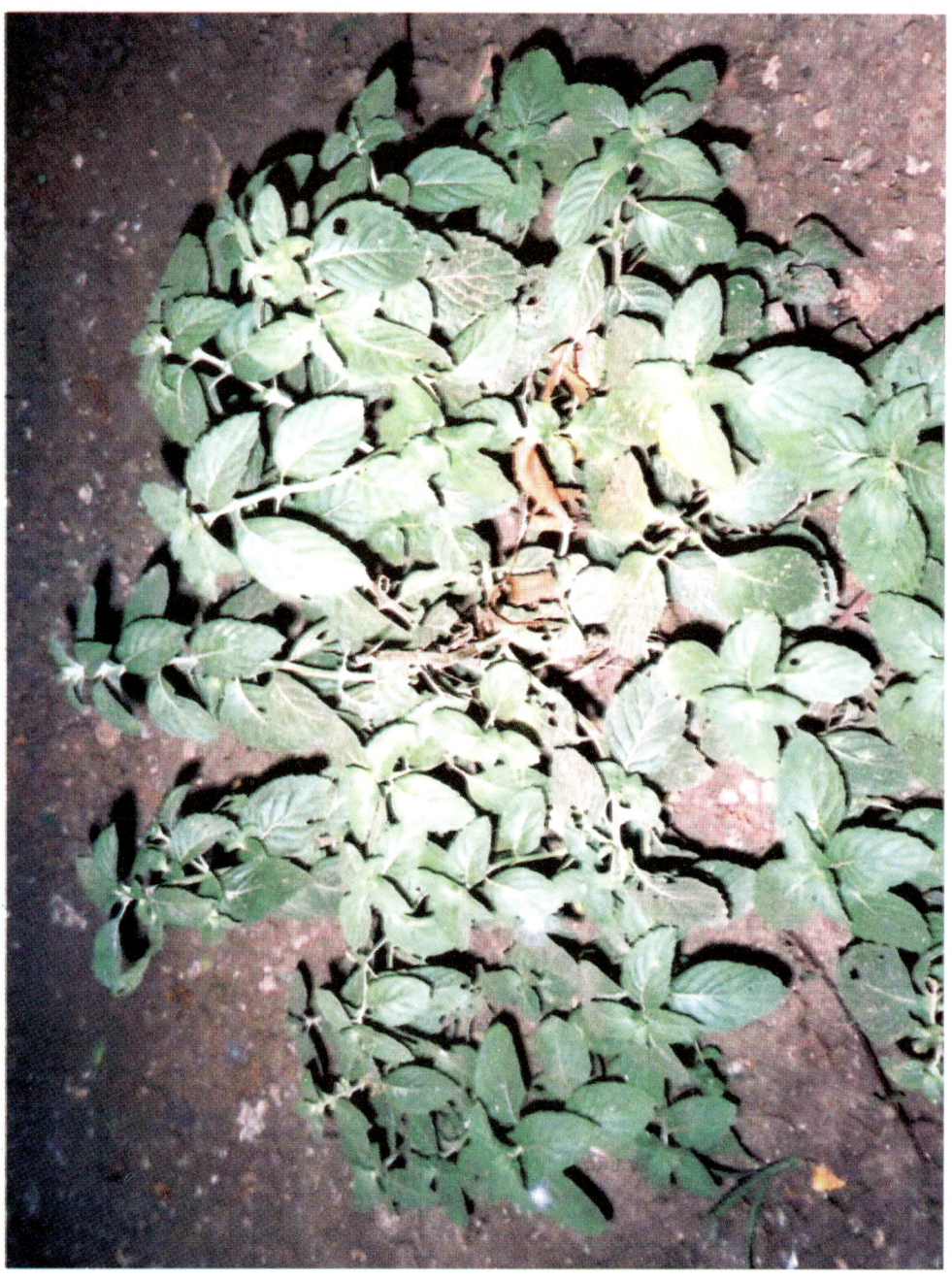

PLATE
86

Mentha piperita Linn

LABIATAE

Common Names

Eng	:	Peppermint
Hind	:	Gamathi pudinah
Ben	:	Pudinah
Tam	:	Pudinah
Mal	:	Puttiyana

Parts Used

Leaves and flowering tops.

Constituents

Volatile oil- menthone, menthol, isomenthone, methyl acetate, neomenthol, piperitone, isomenthol, pulegone.

Uses

Expectorant, emmenagogue, useful in diseases of liver, spleen, asthma, it is also refrigerant stomachic, diuretic, stimulant, antispasmodic, antiimplantation, antibacterial, anti fungal, cardiotonic, etc.

Classification	
Kingdom	Plantae – Plants
Subkingdom	Tracheobionta – Vascular plants
Superdivision	Spermatophyta – Seed plants
Division	Magnoliophyta – Flowering plants
Class	Magnoliopsida – Dicotyledons
Subclass	Asteridae –
Order	Lamiales –
Family	Lamiaceae – Mint family
Genus	Mentha L. – Peppermint

Mentha spicata Linn

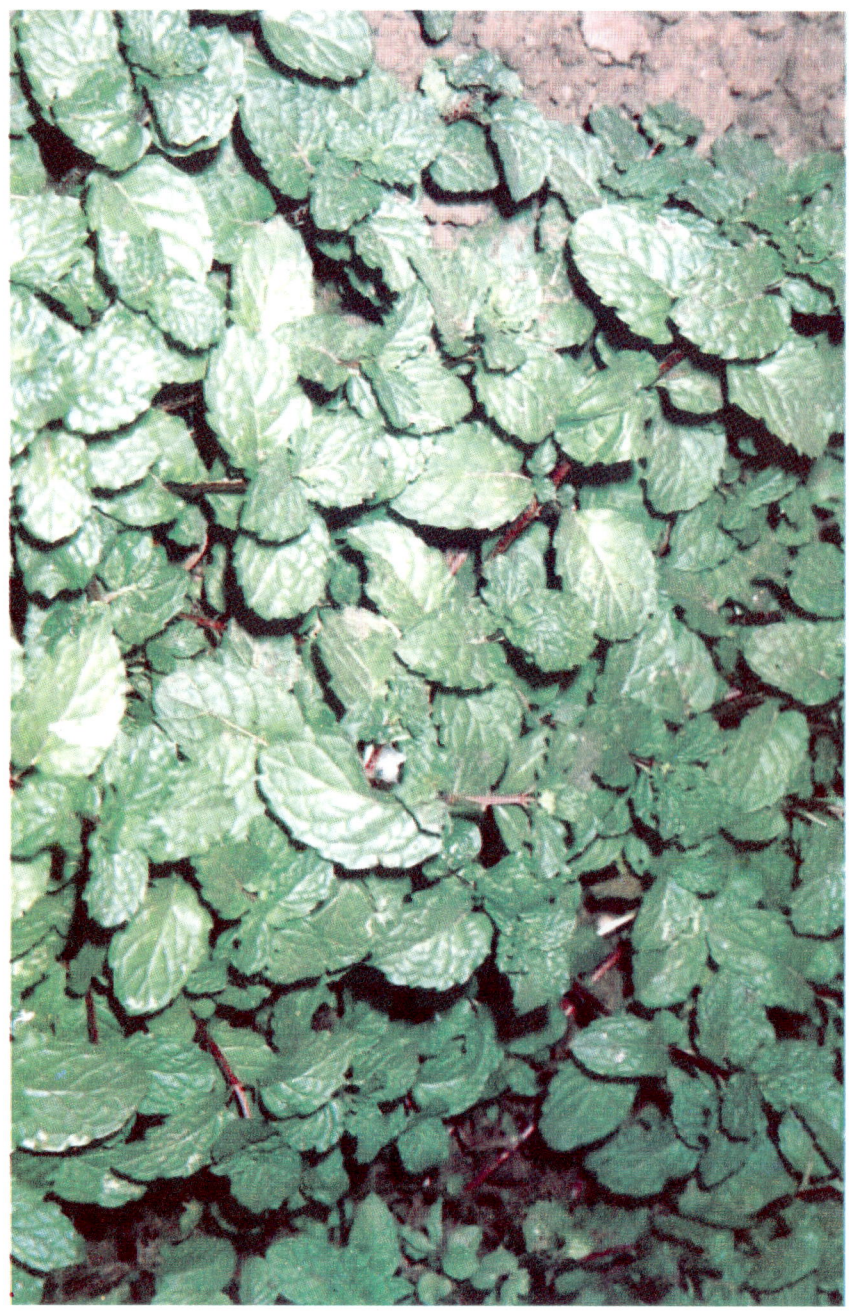

PLATE

87

Mentha spicata Linn

LABIATAE

Common Names

Eng	:	Spearmint
Hind	:	Pudinah
Ben	:	Pudinah
Tam	:	Pudinah
Mal	:	Puttiyana

Parts Used

Leaves and flowering tops.

Constituents

Volatile oil- carvone, linolool, pinene, cineol and phellendrene, resins and tannins.

Uses

Carminative, flavouring agent and digestant.

Classification	
Kingdom	Plantae – Plants
Subkingdom	Tracheobionta – Vascular plants
Superdivision	Spermatophyta – Seed plants
Division	Magnoliophyta – Flowering plants
Class	Magnoliopsida – Dicotyledons
Subclass	Asteridae –
Order	Lamiales –
Family	Lamiaceae – Mint family
Genus	Mentha L. – Spearmint

Mimosa pudica Linn

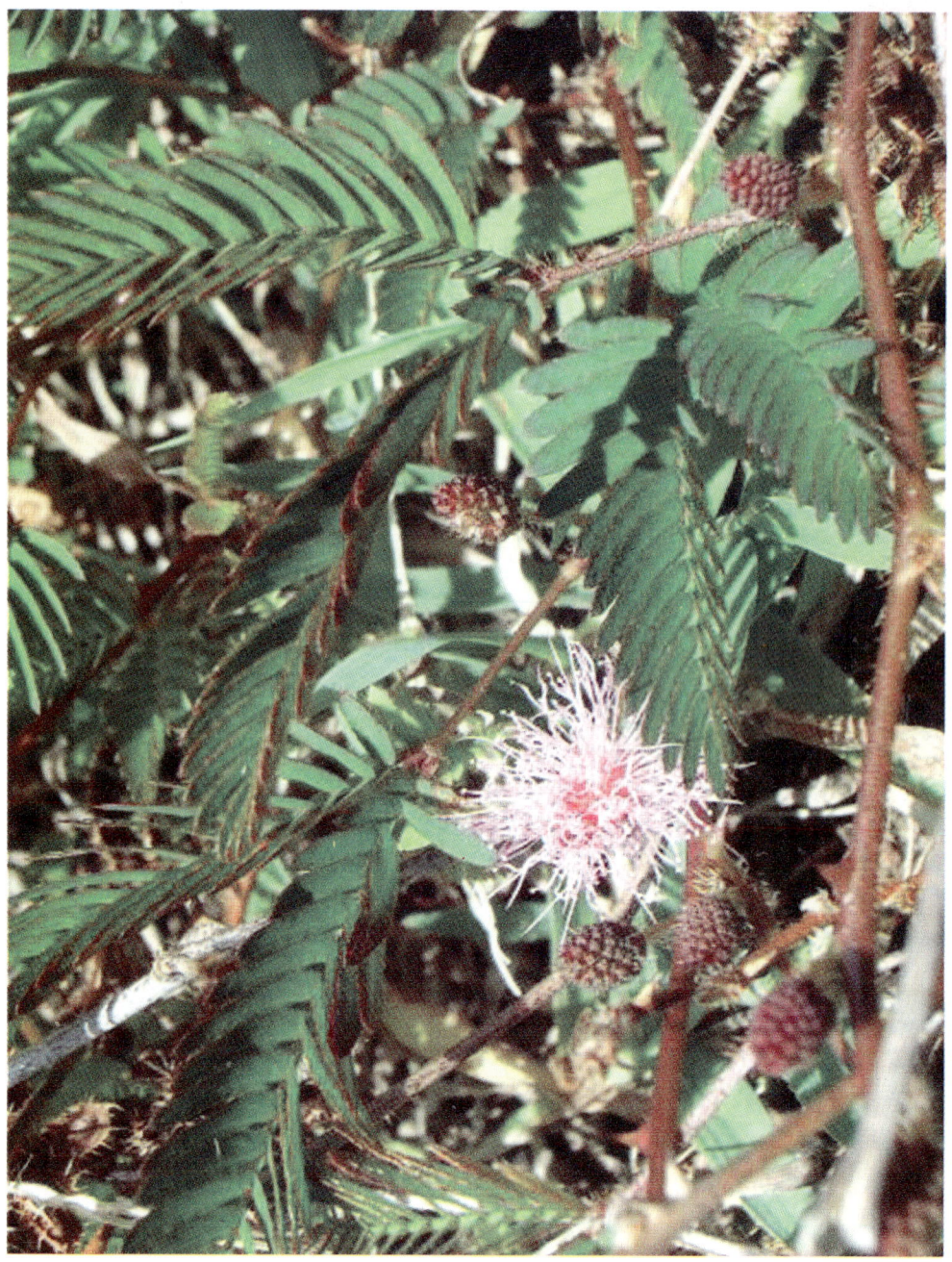

PLATE
88

Mimosa pudica Linn

MIMOSACEAE

Common Names

Eng	:	Sensitive plant, humble plant
Hind	:	Lajalu
Sans	:	Lajjalu
Ben	:	Lajak
Tam	:	Tottalvadi
Mal	:	Thottavadi

Parts Used

Roots & leaves

Constituents

Tannin mimosine, turqorins, phytohormone, tubulin, aerial part contain C glycosyl flavone, 2″ O-rhamnosylorientin, 2″ O- rhamnosylisoorientin, The seed contain moisture, crude protein, pentosan, water soluble gum, seed extract contain saponins.

Uses

Itching, scabic patches, diarrhea, fever, headache, hemorrhage, stomachache, vomiting, carminative, root is aphrodisiac, juice is antiseptic, alternative and blood purifiers.

Classification	
Kingdom	Plantae – Plants
Subkingdom	Tracheobionta – Vascular plants
Superdivision	Spermatophyta – Seed plants
Division	Magnoliophyta – Flowering plants
Class	Magnoliopsida – Dicotyledons
Subclass	Rosidae –
Order	Fabales –
Family	Fabaceae – Pea family
Genus	Mimosa L. – sensitive plant

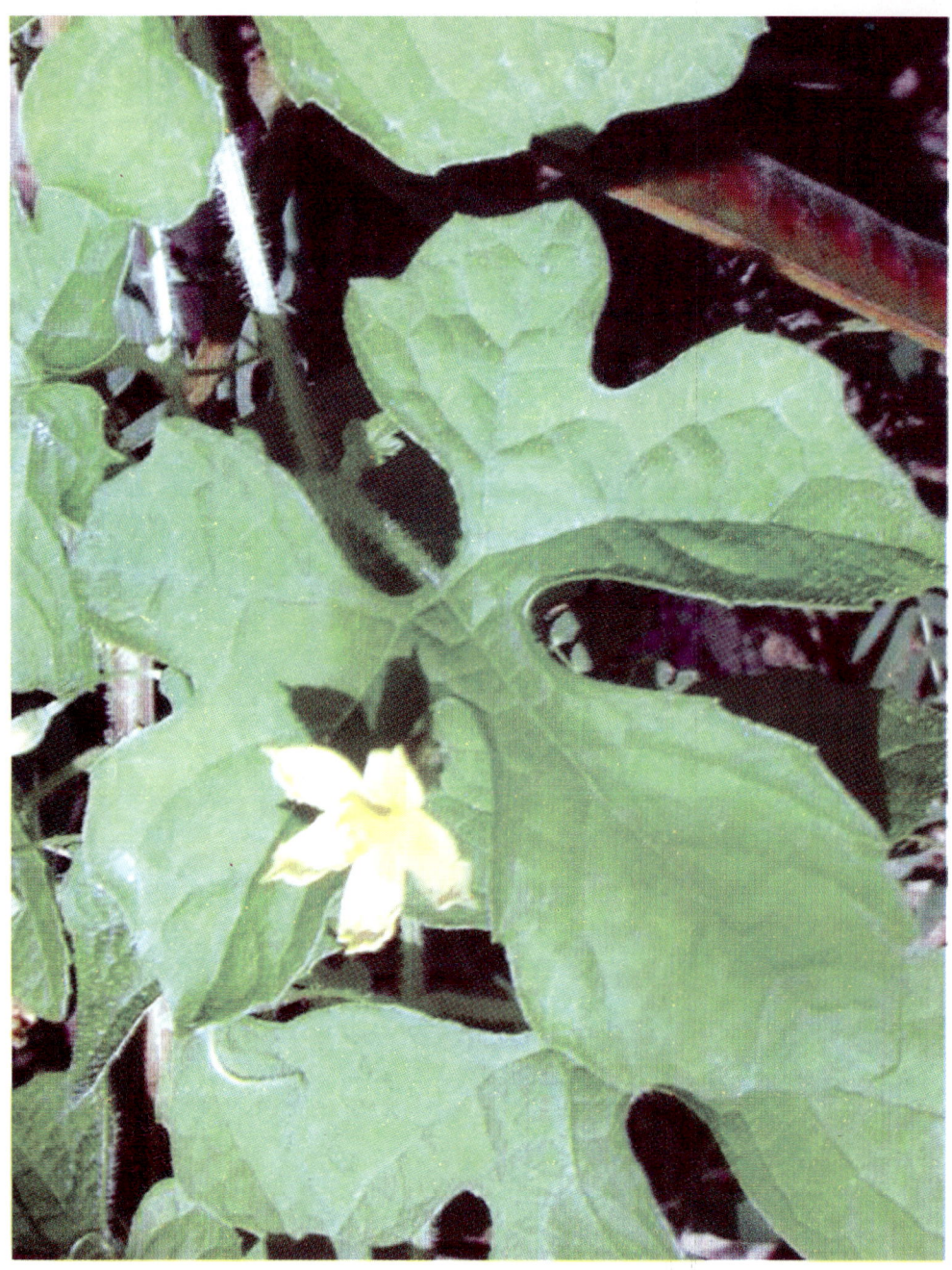

PLATE

89

Momordica charantia Linn

CUCURBITACEAE

Common Names

Eng	:	Bitter gourd
Hind	:	Karela
Sans	:	Karavella
Ben	:	Uchchhe, Karala
Tam	:	Pava
Mal	:	Pavakka- chedi

Parts Used

Fruits, seeds, leaves

Constituents

Glucoside, albuminoids, the predominant fatty acid are á- eleostearic acid in nonpolar lipid, linolenic acid in glycolipids, and palmitic acid in phospholipids. Volatile components of the fruit and veins are identified as myrtenol, cis-3- hexenol, benzyl alcohol,1- penten-3- Ol, acylglycosylsterols, seeds contain glycoproteins.

Uses

Hepatoprotective, seeds and fruits inhibit HIV MAP-30 (momordica anti HIV protein), anti tumour, as tonic, stimulant, emetic, laxative, stomachic. In treatment of gout, rheumatism, blood purifier.

Classification	
Kingdom	Plantae – Plants
Subkingdom	Tracheobionta – Vascular plants
Superdivision	Spermatophyta – Seed plants
Division	Magnoliophyta – Flowering plants
Class	Magnoliopsida – Dicotyledons
Subclass	Dilleniidae –
Order	Violales –
Family	Cucurbitaceae – Cucumber family
Genus	Momordica L. – momordica

Moringa oleifera Lam

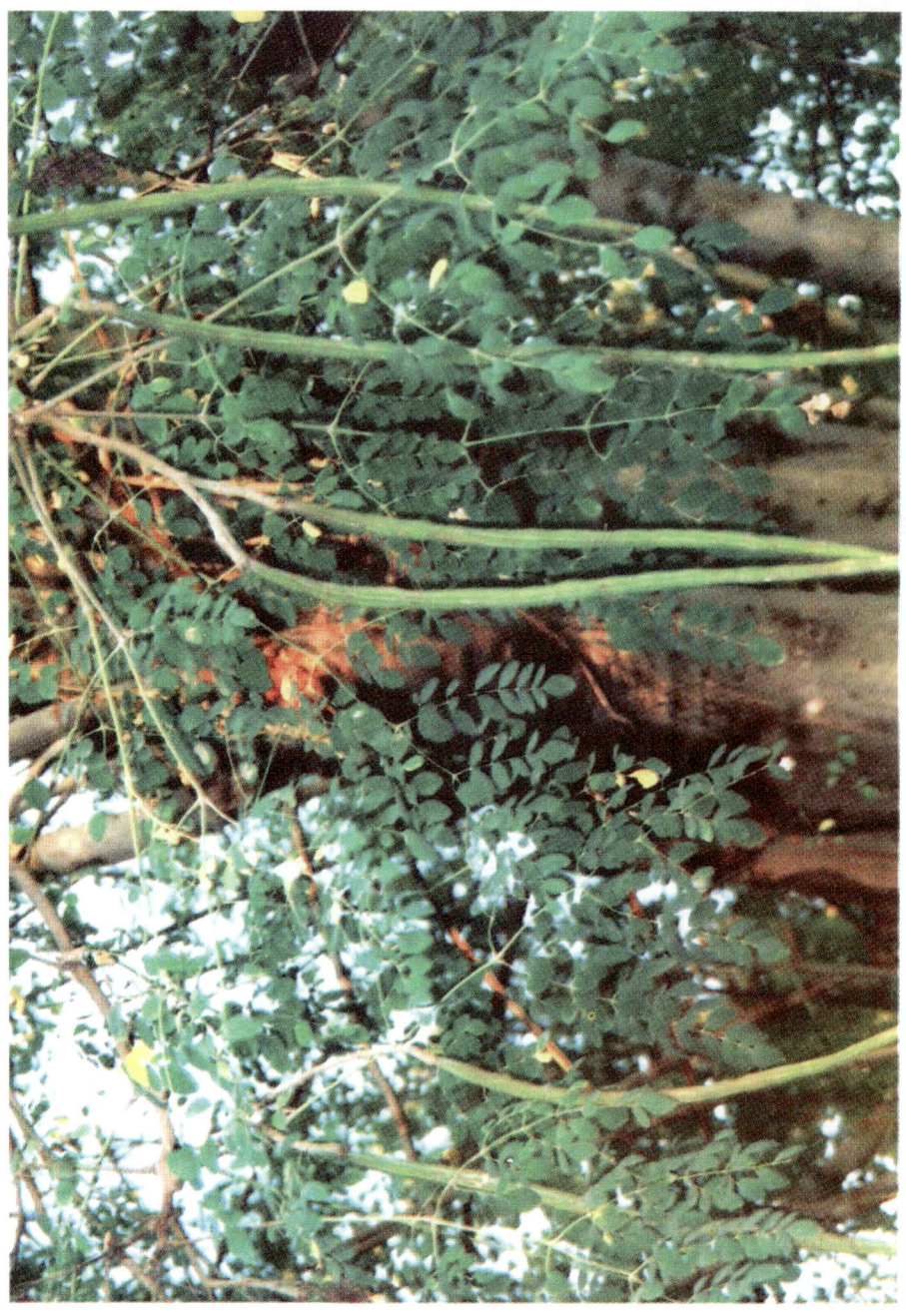

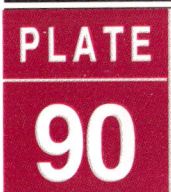

PLATE

90

Moringa oleifera Lam

MORINGACEAE

Common Names

Eng	:	Horse radish
Hind	:	Sahinjan, Soanjha
Sans	:	Sobhanjana
Ben	:	Sojna
Tam	:	Murungai
Mal	:	Murina

Parts Used

Bark, Fruit, Flower, Leaves, Seeds, Gum

Constituents

The pods are rich in vitamins and minerals, it's a good source of α-linolinic acid, mucilage made of galactose, dextrose, xylose, sodium, potasium, calcium, magnisium, salts of glucoronic acid, alkaloids, resin, inorganic acid, gum.

Uses

Antispasmodic, stimulant, expectorant, diuretic, roots are acrid, vesicant, antibiotic, laxative, antibacterial effect against both gram positive and gram negative bacteria,used in upper respiratory tract diseases, and as coagulant.

Classification	
Kingdom	Plantae – Plants
Subkingdom	Tracheobionta – Vascular plants
Superdivision	Spermatophyta – Seed plants
Division	Magnoliophyta – Flowering plants
Class	Magnoliopsida – Dicotyledons
Subclass	Dilleniidae –
Order	Capparales –
Family	Moringaceae – Horse-radish tree family
Genus	Moringa Adans. – moringa

Murraya koenigii Linn

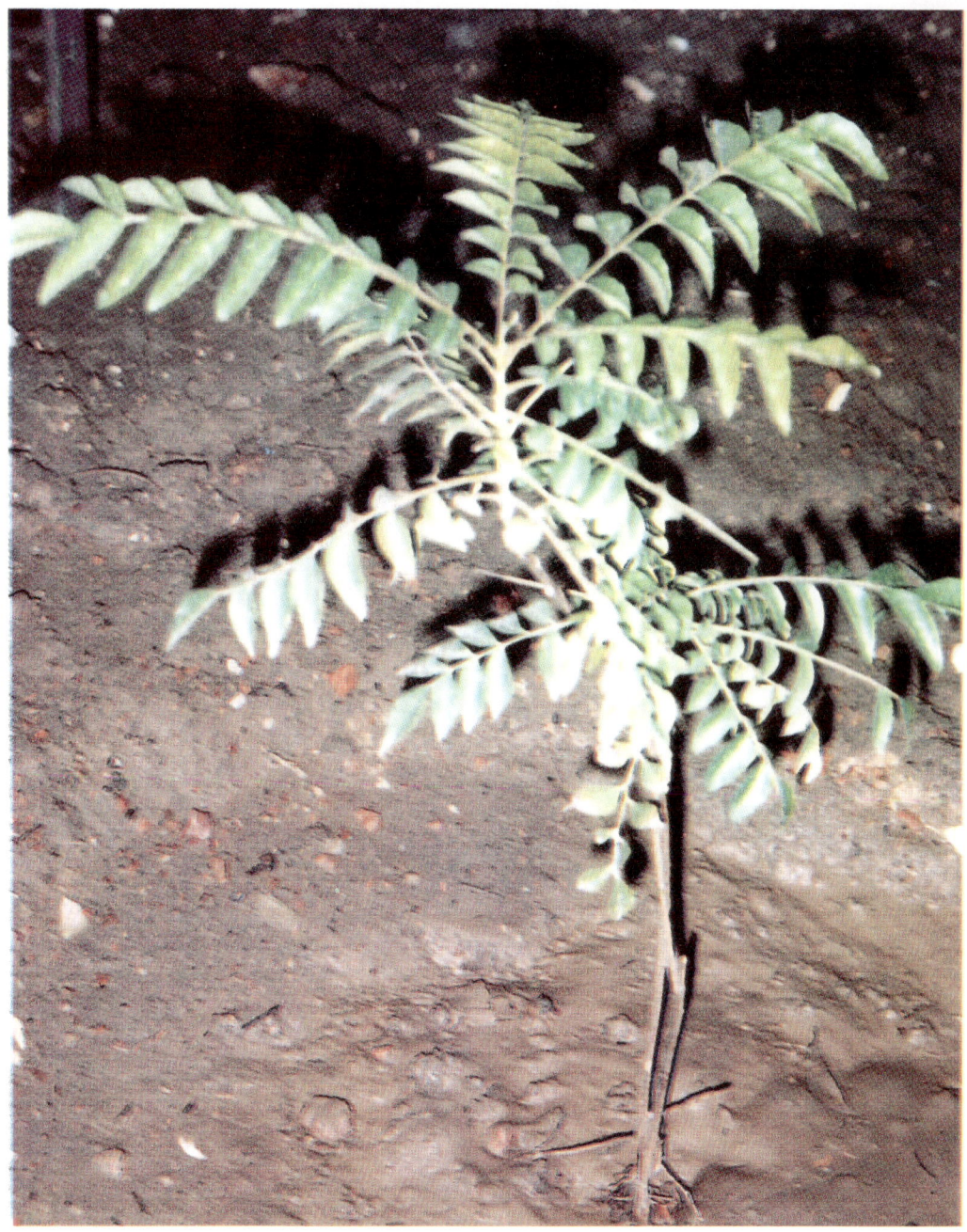

PLATE

91

Murraya koenigii Linn

RUTACEAE

Common Names

Eng	:	Curry leaf
Hind	:	Karipatta
Sans	:	Krishnanimba
Ben	:	Barsunga
Tam	:	Kariveppilai
Mal	:	Karivaeppu

Parts Used

Leaves, barks, roots

Constituents

Volatile oil, resins, crystalline principle glucoside named koenigin, seeds contain oil, stem contain alkaloids – girinimbine, mahanimbine.

Uses

Infusions of root-bark is used in vomiting, decoction of leaves is febrifuge, antioxidant.

Classification	
Kingdom	Plantae – Plants
Subkingdom	Tracheobionta – Vascular plants
Superdivision	Spermatophyta – Seed plants
Division	Magnoliophyta – Flowering plants
Class	Magnoliopsida – Dicotyledons
Subclass	Rosidae –
Order	Sapindales –
Family	Rutaceae – Rue family
Genus	Murraya L. – murraya

Musa paradisica Linn

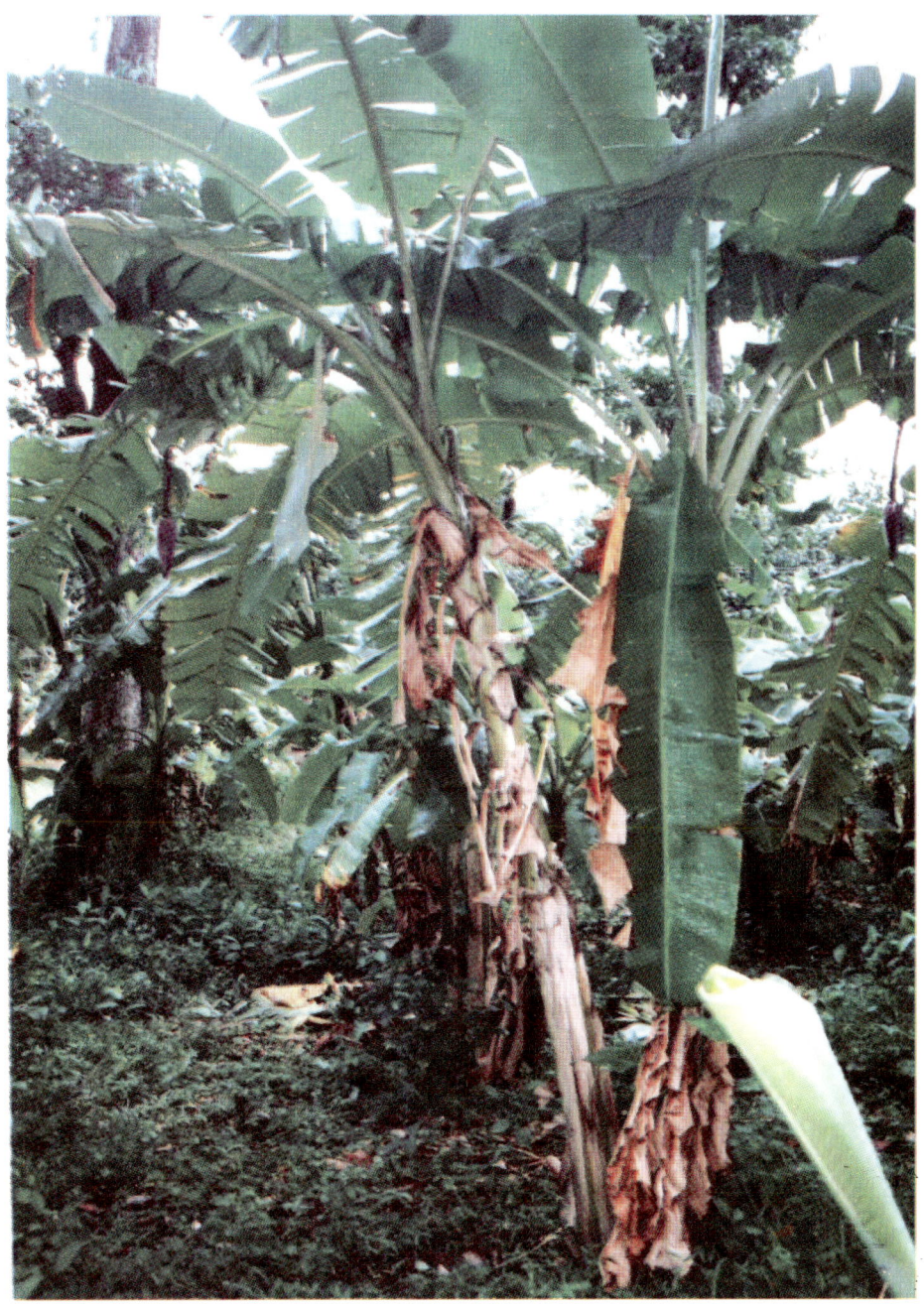

PLATE

92

Musa paradisica Linn

SCITAMINACEAE

Common Names

Eng	:	Banana
Hind	:	Kela
Sans	:	Kadali
Ben	:	Keli
Tam	:	Vazhai
Mal	:	Vazha

Parts Used

Whole plant

Constituents

Tannic acid, gallic acid, vitamin C, B, volatile components, fruits are very rich in chromium, acylsterylglycoside and sitoindoside are isolated from it.

Uses

Laxative, demulcent, emollient, antiulcerogenic.

Classification	
Kingdom	Plantae – Plants
Subkingdom	Tracheobionta – Vascular plants
Superdivision	Spermatophyta – Seed plants
Division	Magnoliophyta – Flowering plants
Class	Liliopsida – Monocotyledons
Subclass	Zingiberidae –
Order	Zingiberales –
Family	Musaceae – Banana family
Genus	Musa L. – banana

Nerium indicum Linn

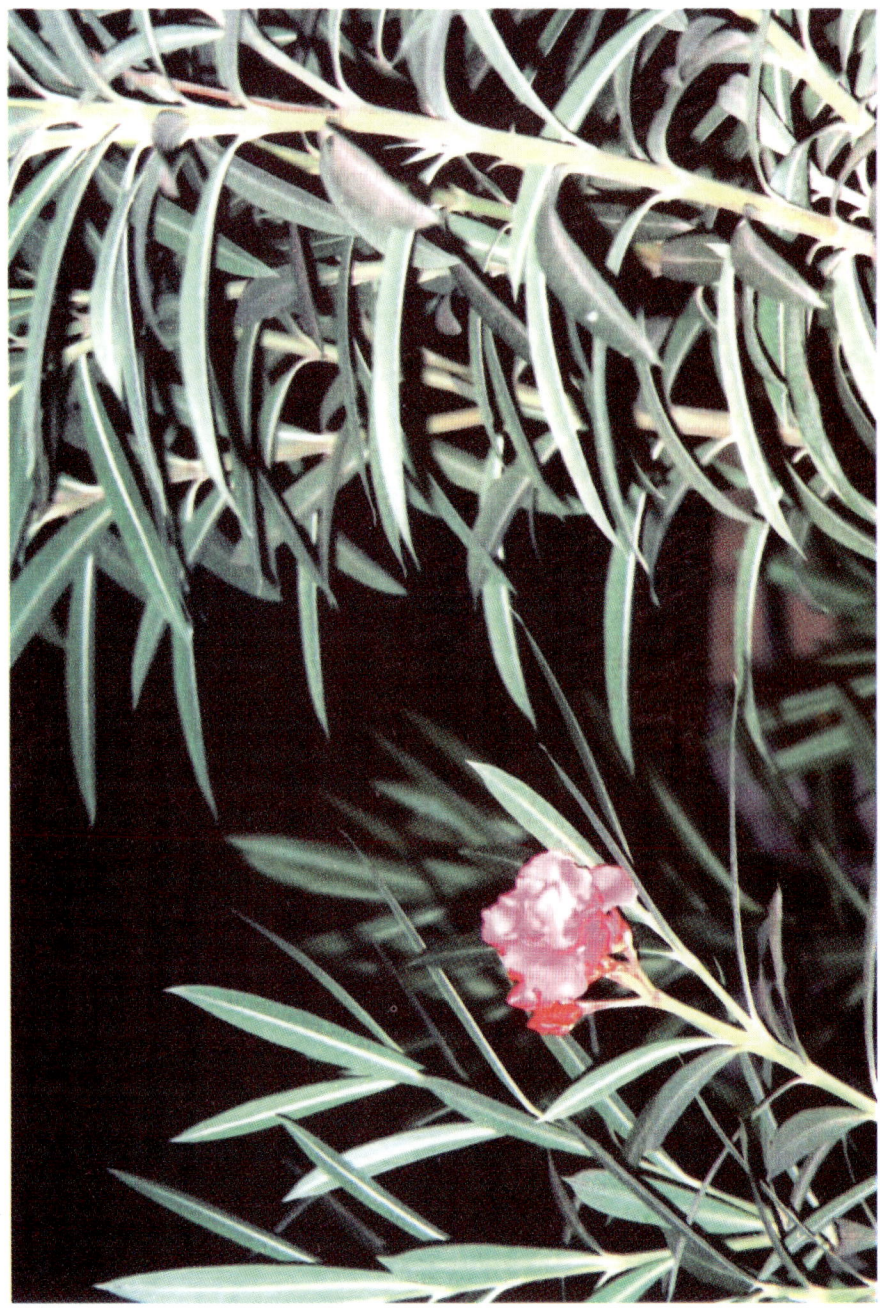

PLATE
93

Nerium indicum Linn

APOCYNACEAE

Common Names

Eng	:	Oleander
Hind	:	Kaner
Sans	:	Raktapushpa
Ben	:	Karavi
Tam	:	Arali
Tel	:	Karaviramu

Parts Used

Seeds, leaves, bark and roots

Constituents

Cardiac glycosides, terpenoids, sterols, tannins, essential oils.

Uses

Leaves are used in cutaneous eruptions. The paste of the root is applied externally in haemorrhoides and ulcerations.

Classification	
Kingdom	Plantae – Plants
Subkingdom	Tracheobionta – Vascular plants
Superdivision	Spermatophyta – Seed plants
Division	Magnoliophyta – Flowering plants
Class	Magnoliopsida – Dicotyledons
Subclass	Asteridae –
Order	Gentianales –
Family	Apocynaceae – Dogbane family
Genus	Nerium L. – oleander

Nicotiana tabacum Linn

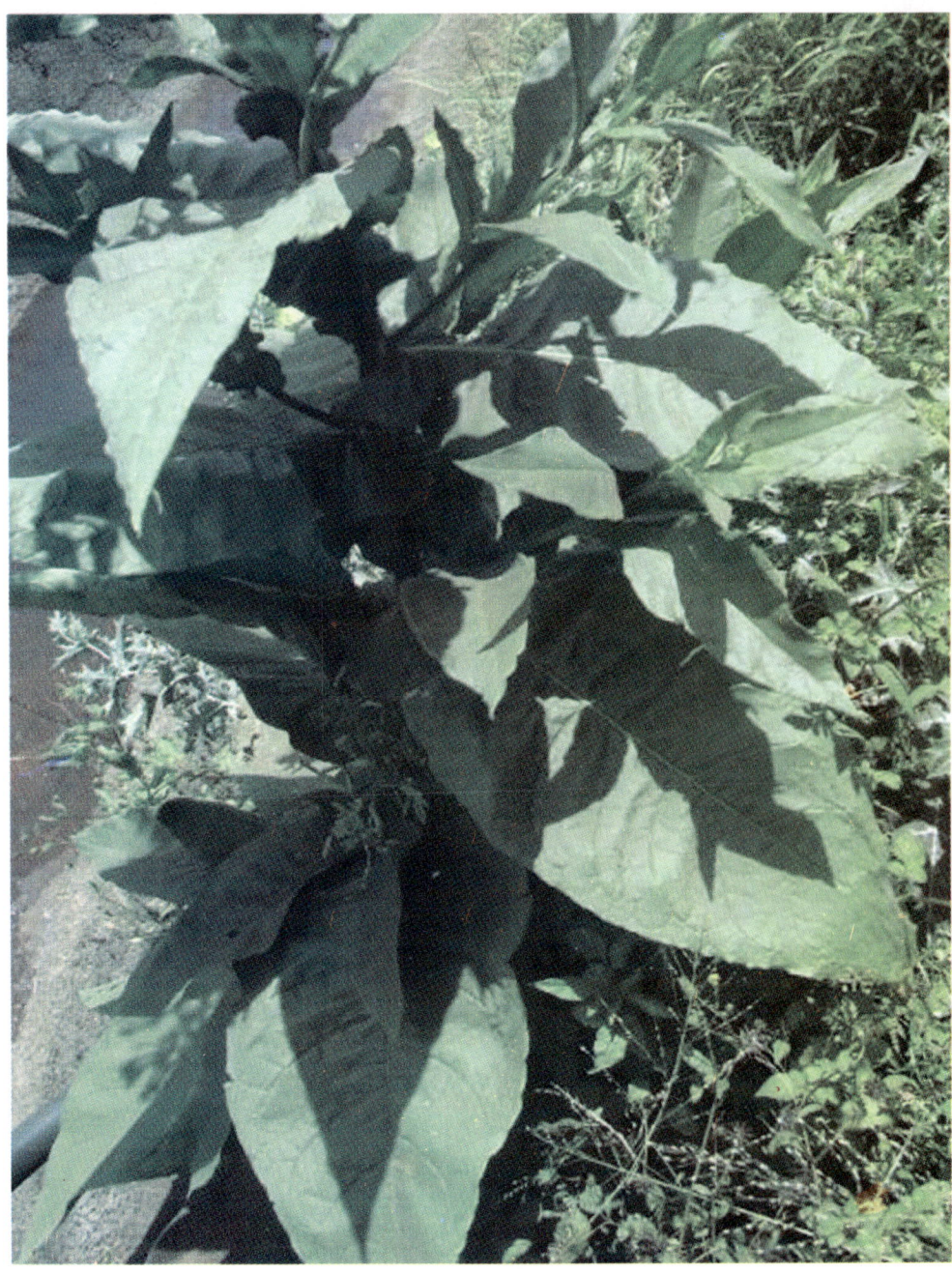

PLATE

94

Nicotiana tabacum Linn

SOLANACEAE

Common Names

Eng	:	Tobacco
Hind	:	Tambaku
Sans	:	Tamrakuta
Ben	:	Tomak
Tam	:	Pogaielai
Mal	:	Pukayil

Parts Used

Dried leaves

Constituents

Leaves contain alkaloid like N-ethylnornicotine, sesquiterpenoids glycoside, 1-β-hydroxy debneyol-12-O-β-D-glucopyranoside, Debneyol and related compounds lactones, coumarin, the trichomes secrete a gum which possesses plant growth inhibitor properties, major cembrenoids in gum are α and β - cembrenoids, other alkaloids like nicotine, anabasine etc.

Uses

Cerebral stimulant, stimulates heart, nervous system, insecticide.

Classification	
Kingdom	Plantae – Plants
Subkingdom	Tracheobionta – Vascular plants
Superdivision	Spermatophyta – Seed plants
Division	Magnoliophyta – Flowering plants
Class	Magnoliopsida – Dicotyledons
Subclass	Asteridae –
Order	Solanales –
Family	Solanaceae – Potato family
Genus	Nicotiana L. – tobacco

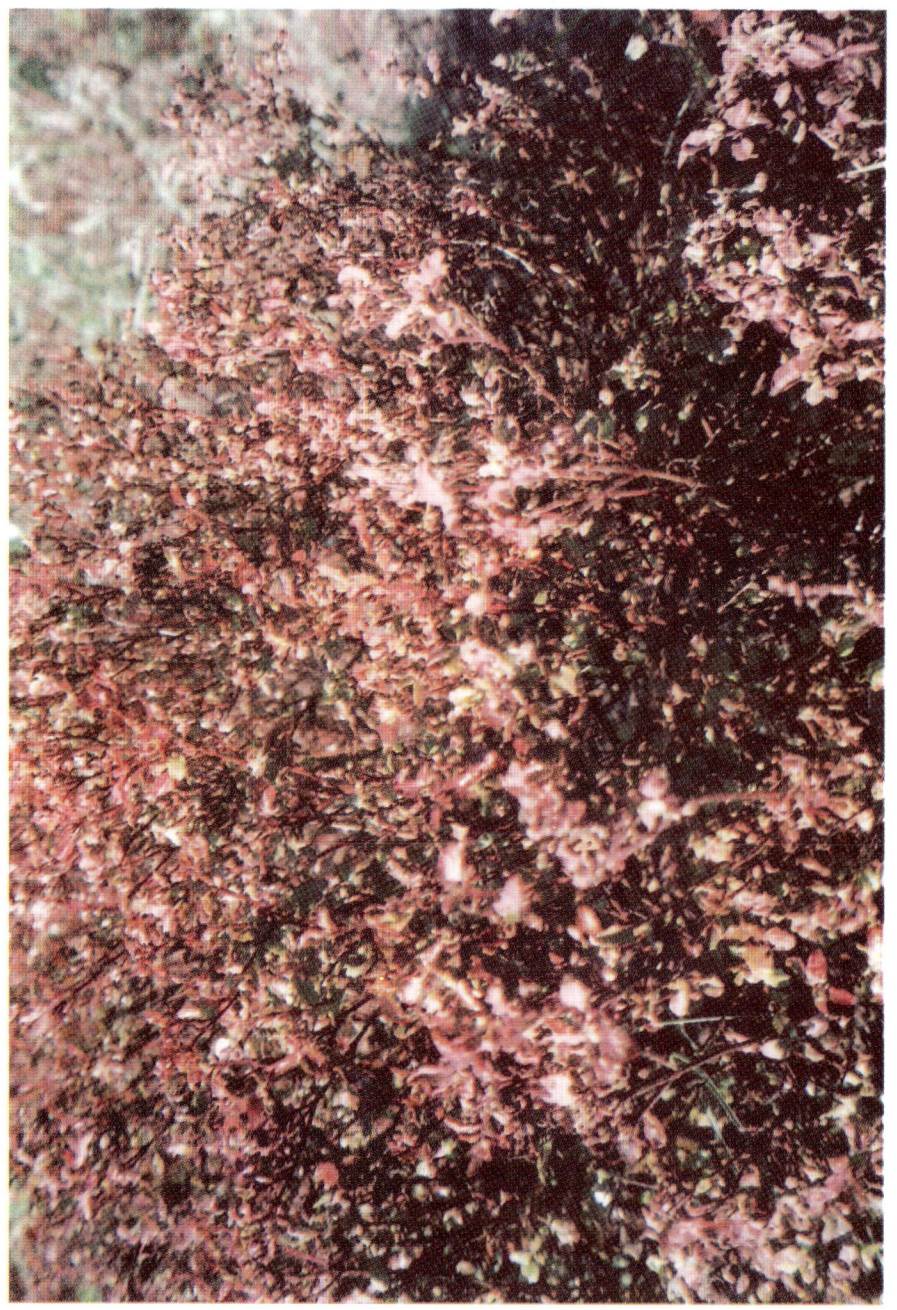

PLATE
95

Ocimum basilicum Linn

LABIATAE

Common Names

Eng	:	Sweet basil
Hind	:	Babui tulasi
Sans	:	Biswa tulasi
Ben	:	Babui tulasi
Tam	:	Thiruniraipachai
Mal	:	Tirunitri

Parts Used

Leaves, seeds, root

Constituents

Essential oil.

Uses

Roots are used for the bowel complaints of children, leaves are anthelmintic and used in scorpion stings, seeds in gonorrhoea, diarrhoea and chronic dysentry.

Classification	
Kingdom	Plantae – Plants
Subkingdom	Tracheobionta – Vascular plants
Superdivision	Spermatophyta – Seed plants
Division	Magnoliophyta – Flowering plants
Class	Magnoliopsida – Dicotyledons
Subclass	Asteridae –
Order	Lamiales –
Family	Lamiaceae – Mint family
Genus	Ocimum L. – Sweet basil

Ocimum sanctum Linn

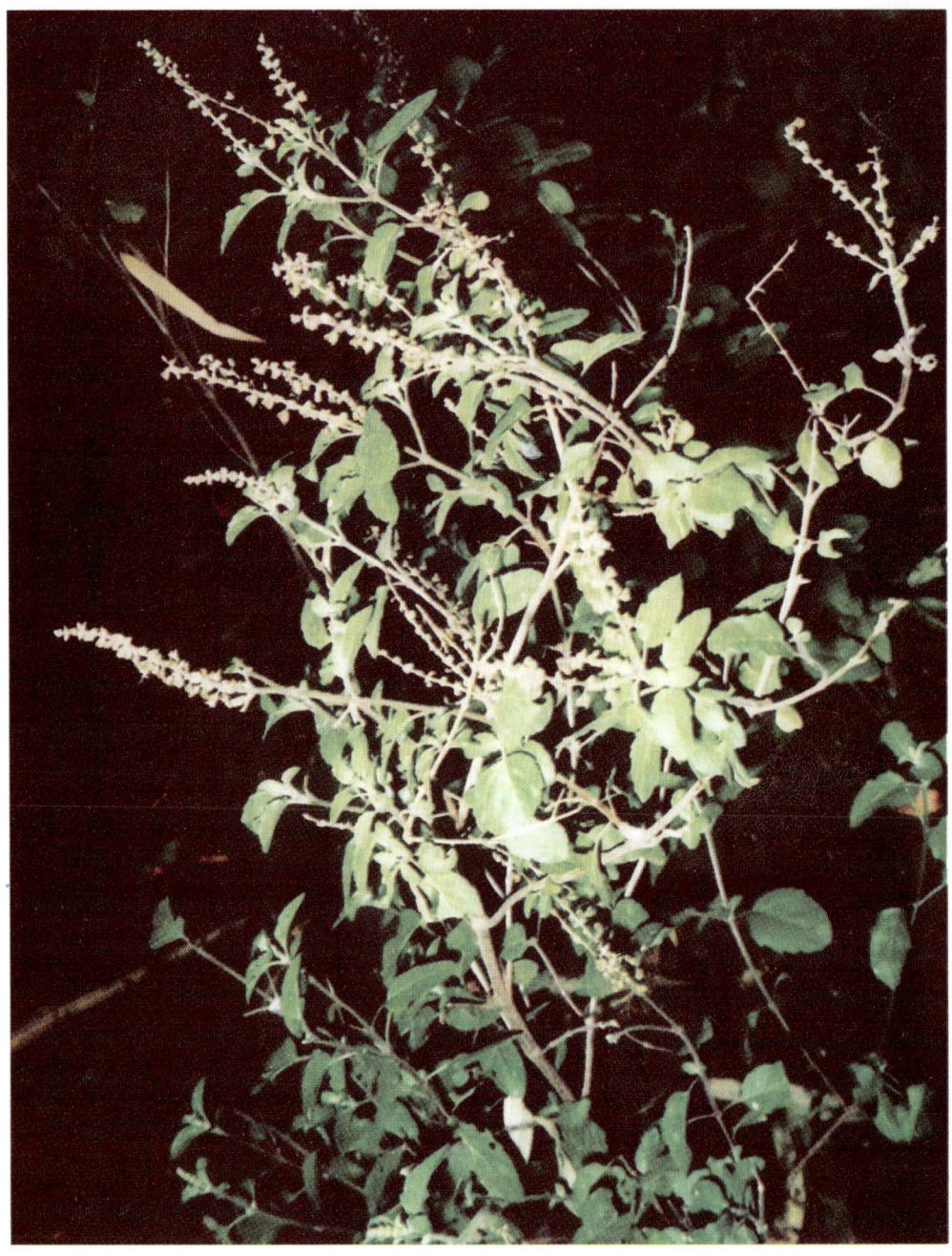

PLATE
96

Ocimum sanctum Linn

LABIATAE

Common Names

Eng	:	Holy basil
Hind	:	Kala Tilasi
Sans	:	Vishnu Priya
Ben	:	Krishna Tulasi
Tam	:	Shiva Tulasi
Mal	:	Shiva Tulasi

Parts Used

Leaves, seeds, root

Constituents

Essential oil.

Uses

Demulcent, expectorant, anti periodic, febrifuge, mucilaginous, demulcent, stomachic, anti-cararrhal, aromatic.

Classification	
Kingdom	Plantae – Plants
Subkingdom	Tracheobionta – Vascular plants
Superdivision	Spermatophyta – Seed plants
Division	Magnoliophyta – Flowering plants
Class	Magnoliopsida – Dicotyledons
Subclass	Asteridae –
Order	Lamiales –
Family	Lamiaceae – Mint family
Genus	Ocimum L. – basil

Oryza sativa Linn

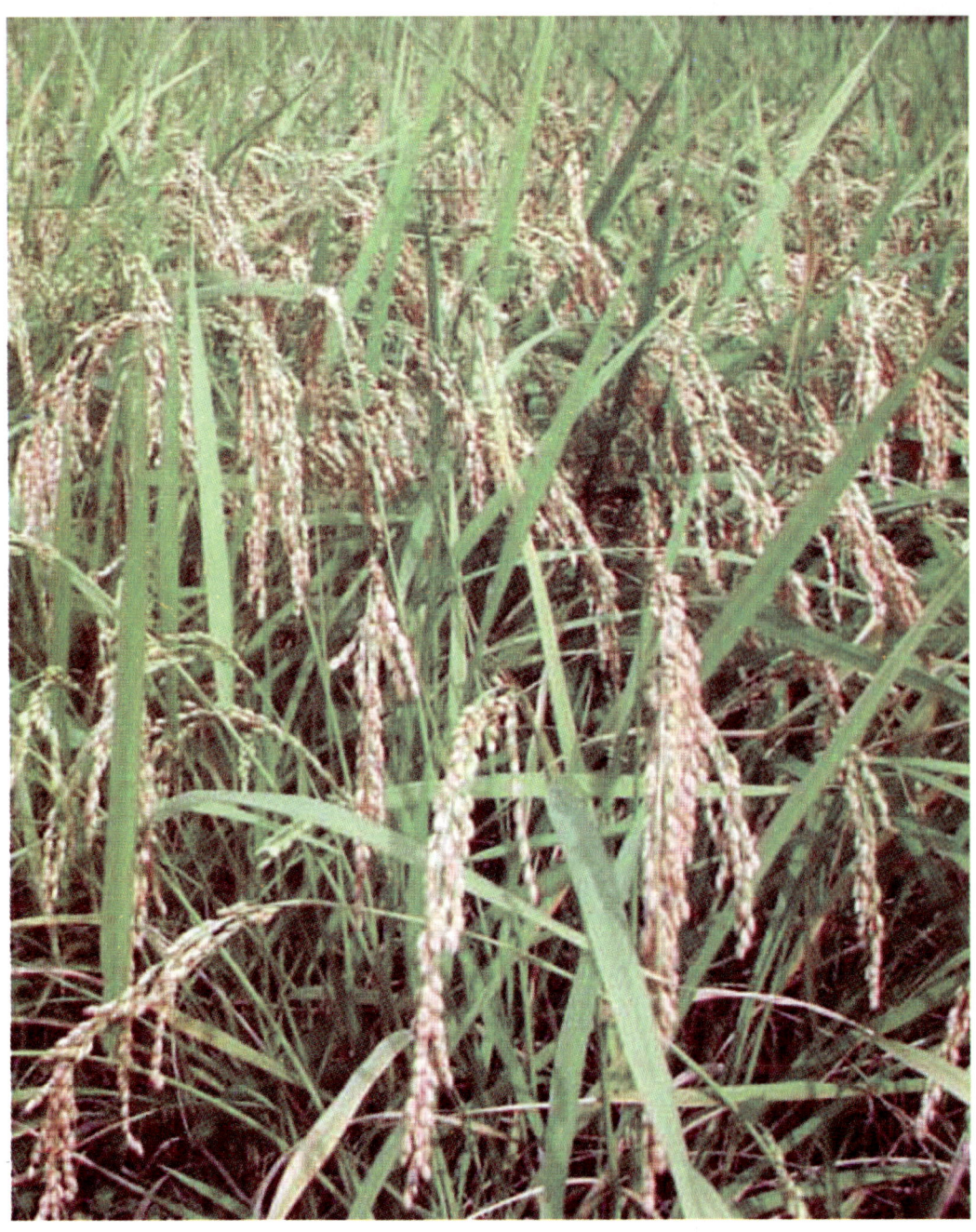

PLATE

97

Oryza sativa Linn

GRAMINAE

Common Names

Eng	:	Rice
Hin	:	Chaval
Sans	:	Vrihi
Ben	:	Dhan
Tam	:	Arshi
Mal	:	Ari

Parts used

Grain

Constituents

Its rich of starch, rice protamins constist of 2 major group of polypeptides, Vit C, β-carotene. The major volatile component of cooked glutinous rice include C_4 - C_8 aldehydes. It also contains protease inhibitors like oryzacystatin, trypsin, chmotrypsin and subtilisin.

Uses

Nutritive, demulcent, protective, antifungal, protein inhibitor.

Classification	
Kingdom	Plantae – Plants
Subkingdom	Tracheobionta – Vascular plants
Superdivision	Spermatophyta – Seed plants
Division	Magnoliophyta – Flowering plants
Class	Liliopsida – Monocotyledons
Subclass	Commelinidae –
Order	Cyperales –
Family	Poaceae – Grass family
Genus	Oryza L. – rice

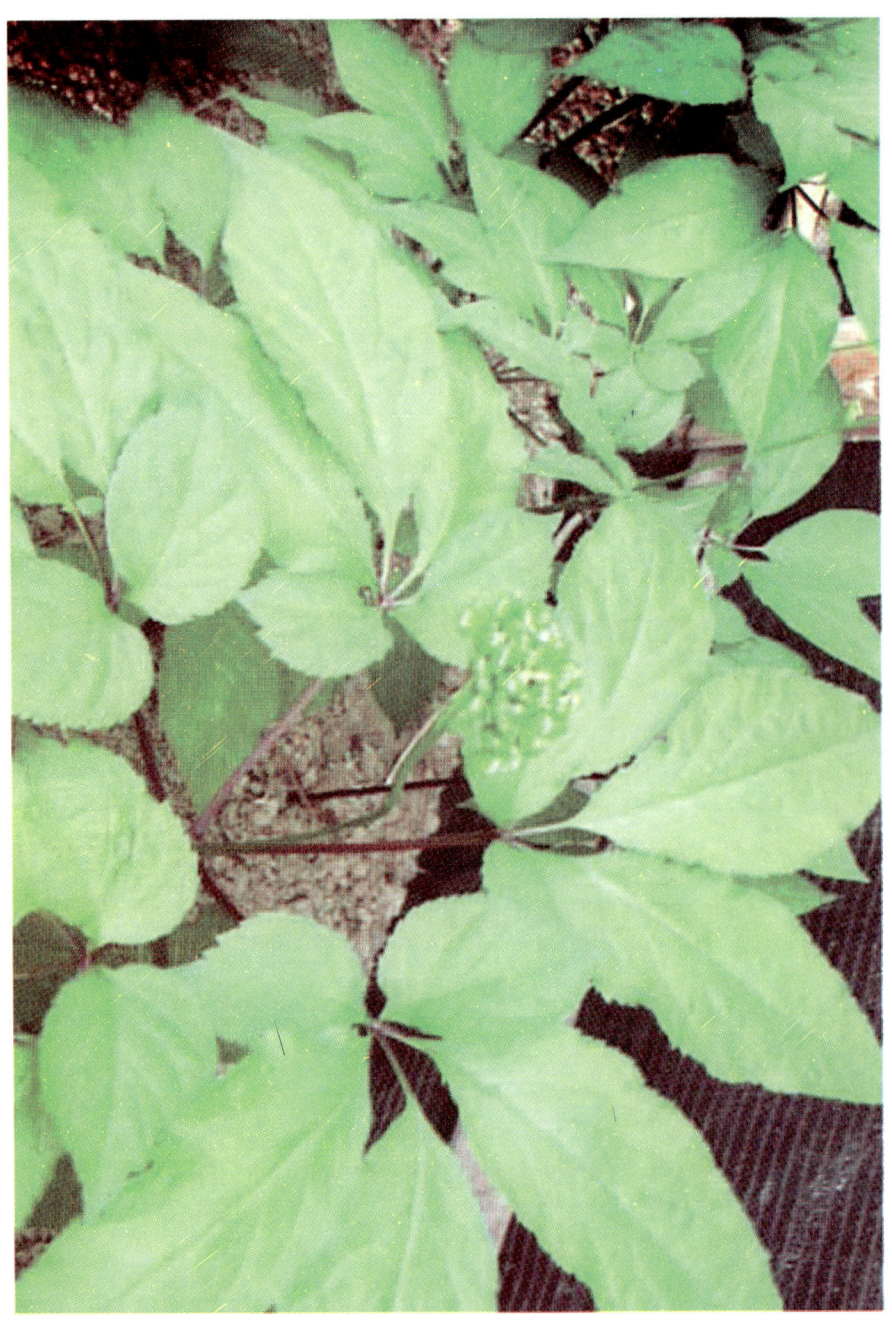

PLATE

98

Panax ginseng C. Meyer

ARALIACEAE

Common Name

Eng   :   Chinese ginseng

Parts used

Roots

Constituents

Ginsenosides, lignans, gomisin, propadecopeptide, pentadecopeptide, sesquiterpenoid, senecrassidiol, aminobutyric acid

Uses

Antiinflamatory, anticancer, antistress

Classification	
Kingdom	Plantae – Plants
Subkingdom	Tracheobionta – Vascular plants
Superdivision	Spermatophyta – Seed plants
Division	Magnoliophyta – Flowering plants
Class	Magnoliopsida – Dicotyledons
Subclass	Rosidae –
Order	Apiales –
Family	Araliaceae – Ginseng family
Genus	Panax L. – ginseng

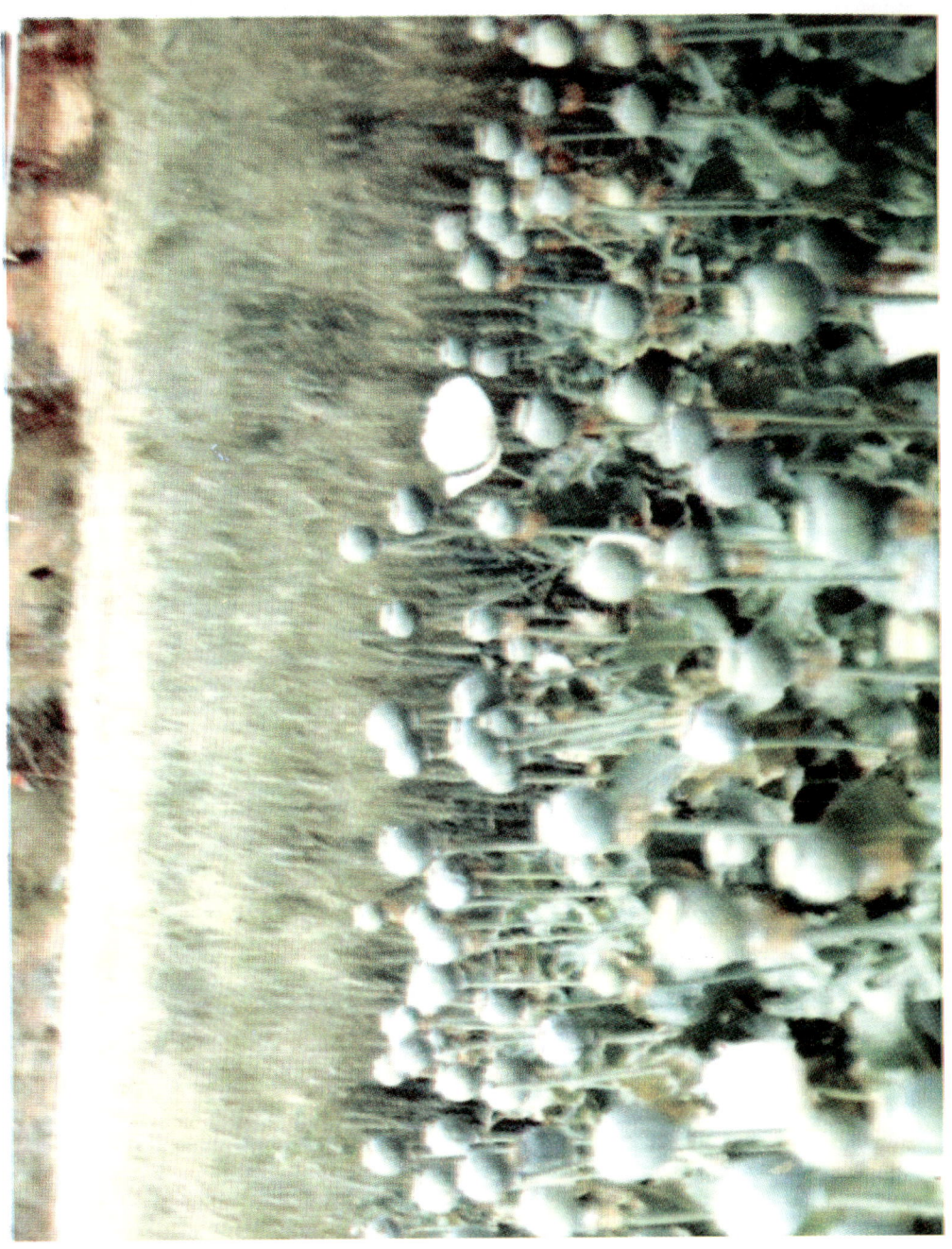

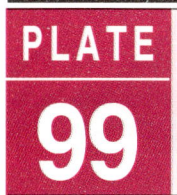

PLATE
99

Papaver somniferum Linn

PAPAVERACEAE

Common Names

Eng	:	Bale-wort
Hind	:	Afin, Afyun
Sans	:	Ahifen, Chosa
Ben	:	Pasto
Tam	:	Abini, Gashagasha
Mal	:	Bungapion

Parts Used

Fruits

Constituents

Alkaloids derived from amino acid phenylalanine, tyrosine, narcotine, narceine, papaverine, morphine, codeine, tetrahydro isoquinoline alkaloid, noscapine, sanguinarine, seeds are good source of water soluble vitamins like thiamine, riboflavin, folic acid, niacin, seed oil contains α tocopherol, β tocopherol, proteins palmitic, steric, oleic, linolenic, linolenic acid.

Uses

Hypnotic, sedative, analgesic, morphine is potent analgesic, codeine relieves irritation, astringent, aphrodisiac, tonic, hypoglycaemic.

Classification	
Kingdom	Plantae – Plants
Subkingdom	Tracheobionta – Vascular plants
Superdivision	Spermatophyta – Seed plants
Division	Magnoliophyta – Flowering plants
Class	Magnoliopsida – Dicotyledons
Subclass	Magnoliidae –
Order	Papaverales –
Family	Papaveraceae – Poppy family
Genus	Papaver L. – poppy

Passiflora edulis Sims

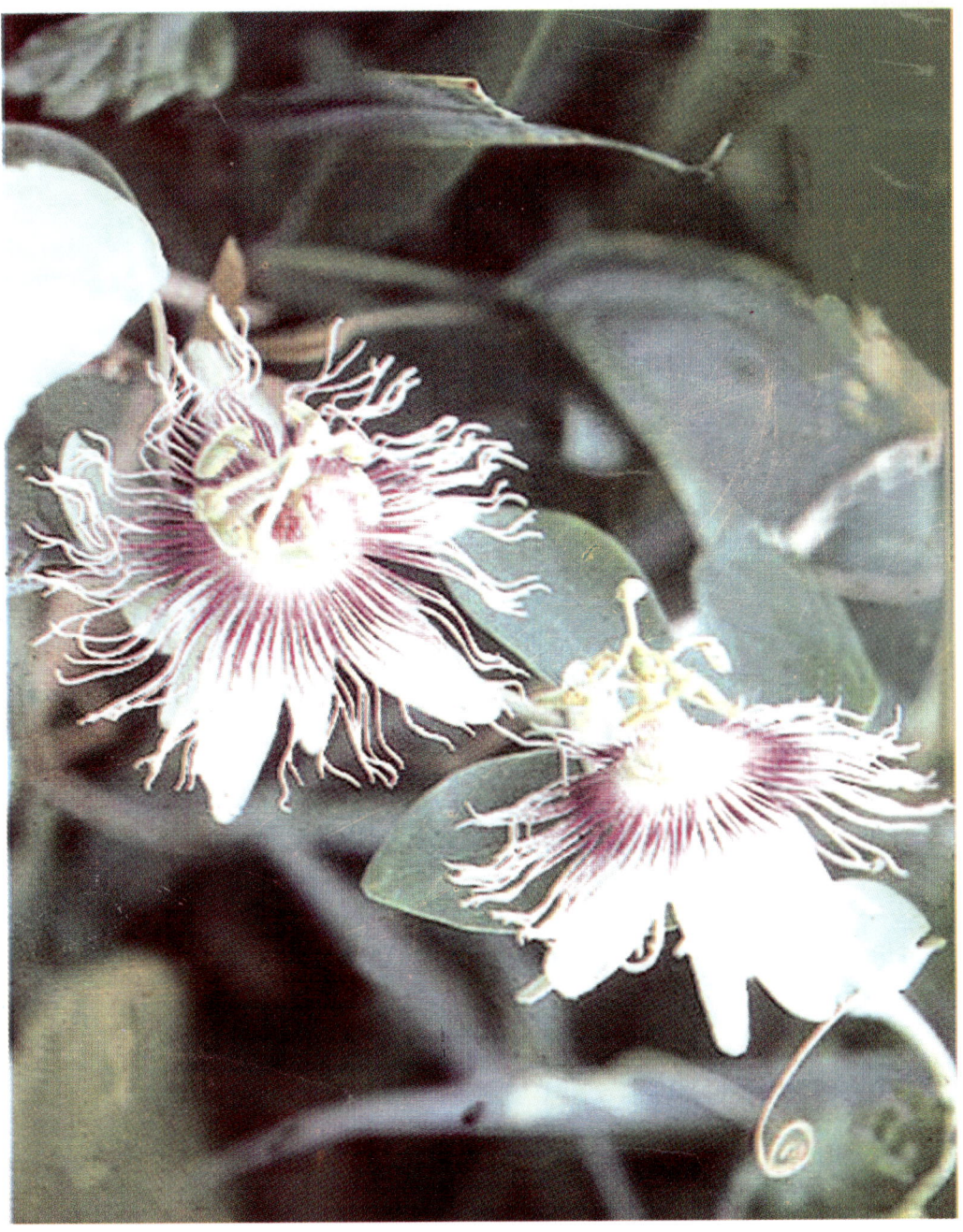

PLATE
100

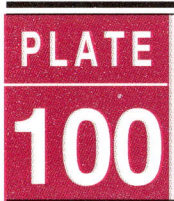

Passiflora edulis Sims

PASSIFLORARACEAE

Common Names

Eng	:	Purple passion fruit
San	:	Passion pal
Ben	:	Mukkopeera
Urdu	:	Kordapacham

Parts Used

Fruits, leaves

Constituents

Several volatile components, terpenoids, alkaloids, flavonoids, saponins, proteins.

Uses

Antifeedant, antidiabetic, anti edema, tranquillizer, diuretic.

Classification	
Kingdom	Plantae – Plants
Subkingdom	Tracheobionta – Vascular plants
Superdivision	Spermatophyta – Seed plants
Division	Magnoliophyta – Flowering plants
Class	Magnoliopsida – Dicotyledons
Subclass	Dilleniidae –
Order	Violales –
Family	Passifloraceae – Passion-flower family
Genus	Passiflora L. – passionflower

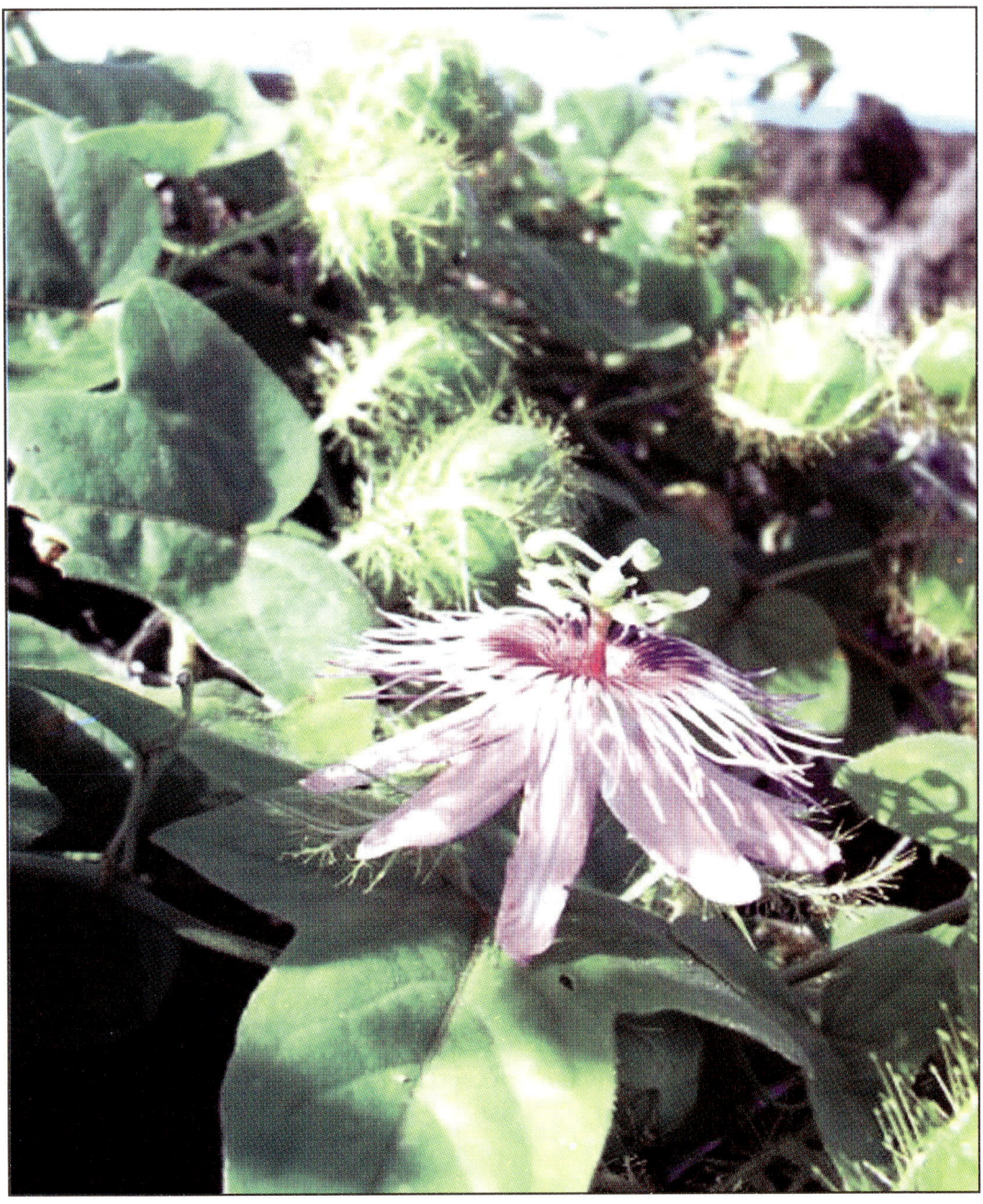

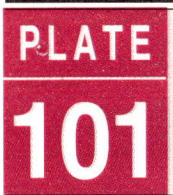

PLATE 101

Passiflora foetida Linn

PASSIFLORARACEAE

Common Names

Eng	:	Purple passion fruit
San	:	Mukkopeera
Tam	:	Mupparisavalli

Parts Used

Fruits, leaves

Constituents

Several volatile components, terpenoids, alkaloids, flavonoids, saponins, proteins.

Uses

Fruit is emetic, decoction is used in biliousness and asthma. Leaves are used in giddiness and head ache.

Classification	
Kingdom	Plantae – Plants
Subkingdom	Tracheobionta – Vascular plants
Superdivision	Spermatophyta – Seed plants
Division	Magnoliophyta – Flowering plants
Class	Magnoliopsida – Dicotyledons
Subclass	Dilleniidae –
Order	Violales –
Family	Passifloraceae – Passion-flower family
Genus	Passiflora L. – passionflower

Passiflora mollisima Bailey

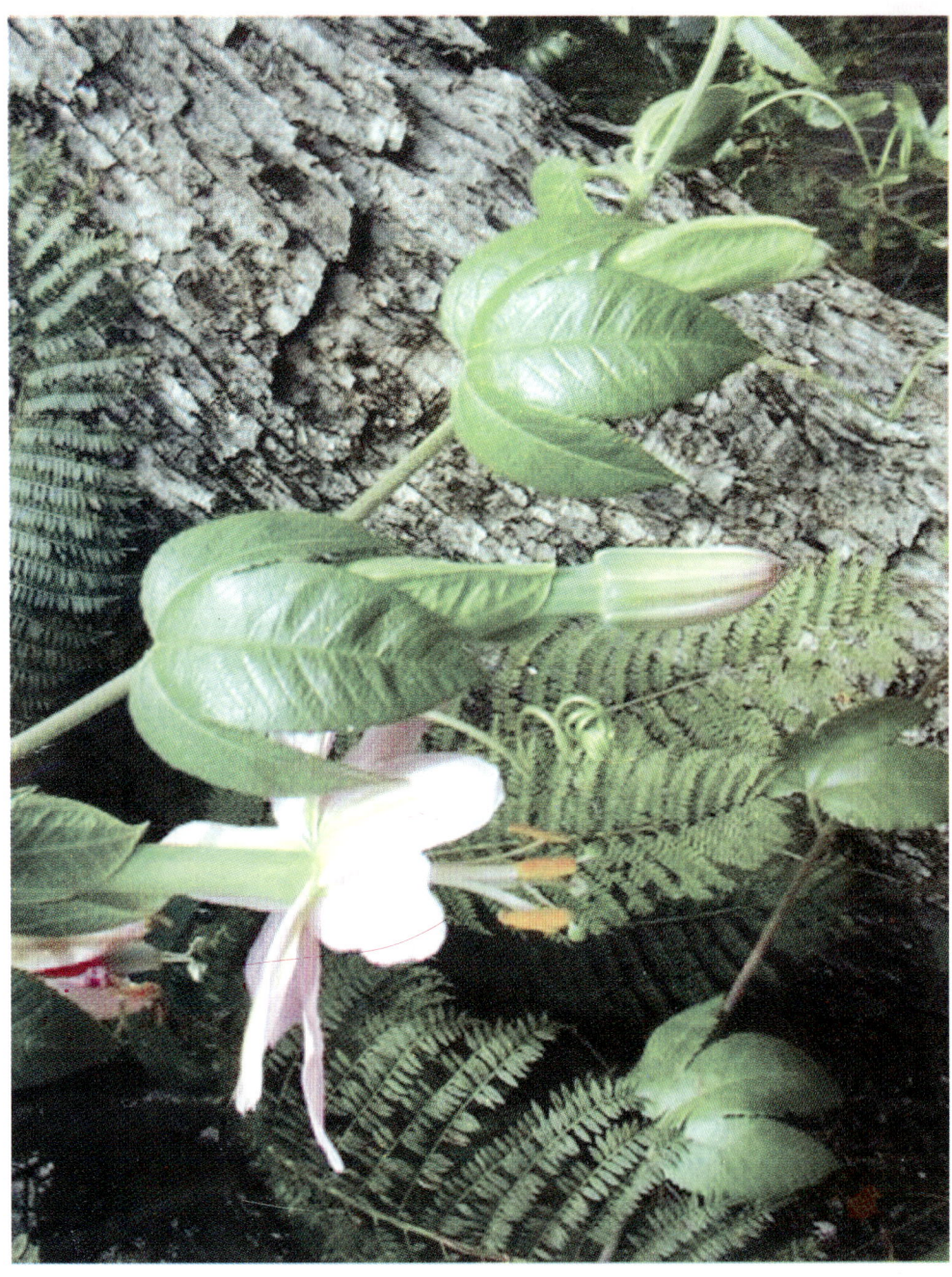

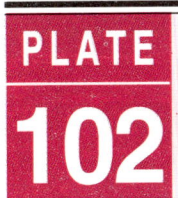

PLATE

102

Passiflora mollisima Bailey

PASSIFLORARACEAE

Common Names

   Eng   :   Banana passion fruit

Parts Used

Fruits, leaves

Constituents

Phenyl proponoids, benzenoid compounds, alkaloids, flavonoids, triterpenoids, saponins.

Uses

Antifungal, antibacterial, antifeedant, antidiabetic.

Classification	
Kingdom	Plantae – Plants
Subkingdom	Tracheobionta – Vascular plants
Superdivision	Spermatophyta – Seed plants
Division	Magnoliophyta – Flowering plants
Class	Magnoliopsida – Dicotyledons
Subclass	Dilleniidae –
Order	Violales –
Family	Passifloraceae – Passion-flower family
Genus	Passiflora L. – passionflower

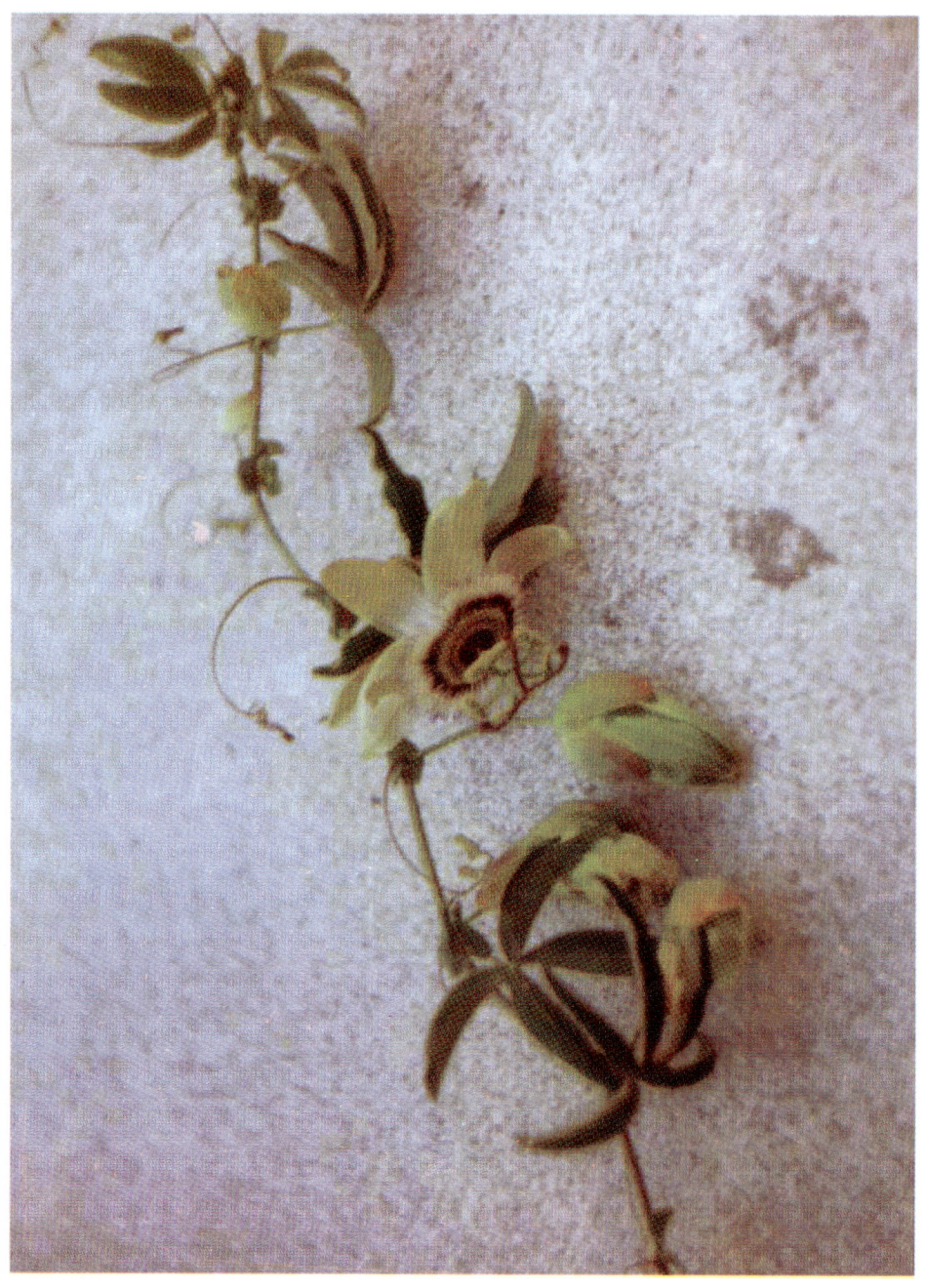

PLATE
103
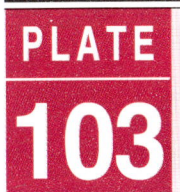

Passiflora quadrangularis Linn

PASSIFLORARACEAE

Common Names

Eng : Giant granadilla

Parts Used

Fruits, leaves

Constituents

Alkaloids, glycosides, flavonoids, tannins, steroids, triterpenoids, saponins.

Uses

Anti algal, antihypertensive, antibacterial, antidiabetic

Classification	
Kingdom	Plantae – Plants
Subkingdom	Tracheobionta – Vascular plants
Superdivision	Spermatophyta – Seed plants
Division	Magnoliophyta – Flowering plants
Class	Magnoliopsida – Dicotyledons
Subclass	Dilleniidae –
Order	Violales –
Family	Passifloraceae – Passion-flower family
Genus	Passiflora L. – passionflower

Phyllanthus emblica Linn

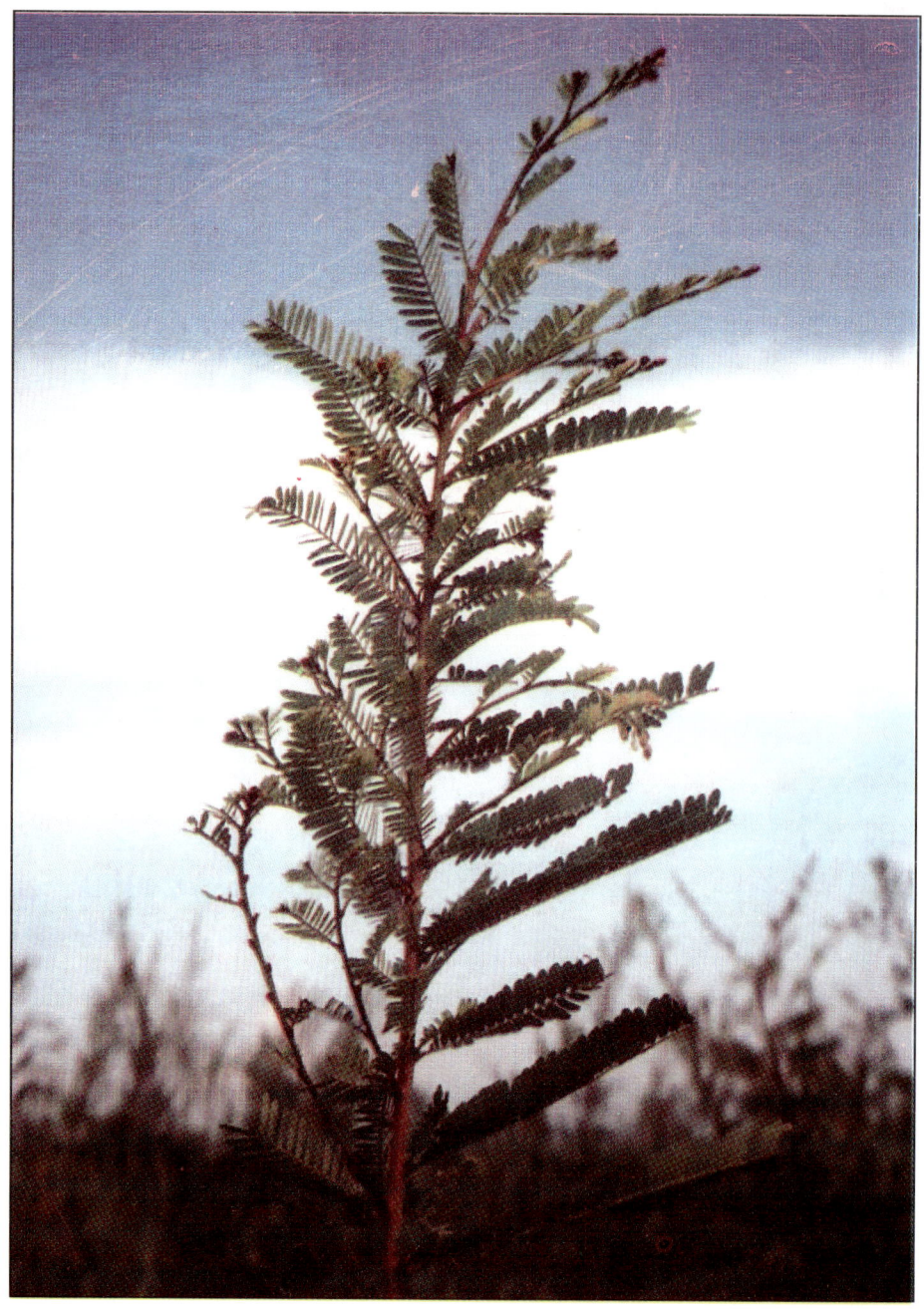

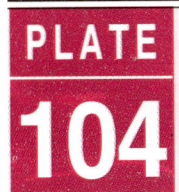

PLATE
104

Phyllanthus emblica Linn

EUPHORBIACEAE

Common Names:

Eng	:	Indian Goose Berry
Hind	:	Amla
Sans	:	Dhatri phala
Ben	:	Amalaki
Tam	:	Toppi, Nellikheyu
Mal	:	Nellikai

Parts Used

Dried fruits, seeds, leaves, root, bark & flowers.

Constituents

Embelin

Uses

Fruit is refrigerant, diuretic, laxative, carminative & stomachic, bark & dried fruits are astringent.

Classification	
Kingdom	Plantae – Plants
Subkingdom	Tracheobionta – Vascular plants
Superdivision	Spermatophyta – Seed plants
Division	Magnoliophyta – Flowering plants
Class	Magnoliopsida – Dicotyledons
Subclass	Rosidae –
Order	Euphorbiales –
Family	Euphorbiaceae – Spurge family
Genus	Phyllanthus L. – Indian goose berry

Piper longum Linn

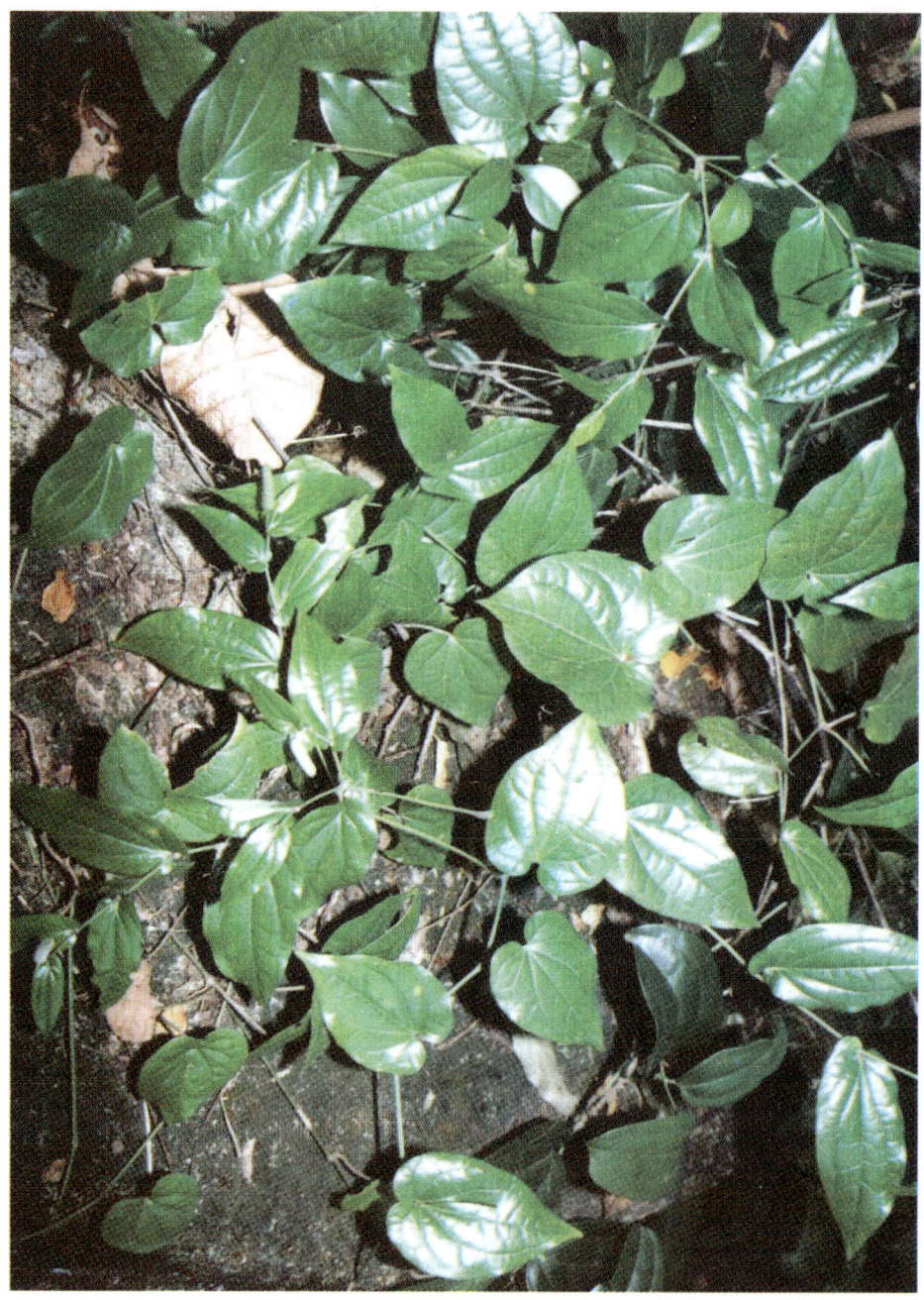

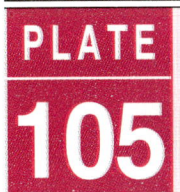

PLATE
105

Piper longum Linn

PIPERACEAE

Common Names

Eng	:	Dried catkins, long pepper
Hind	:	Penpli
Sans	:	Pippali
Ben	:	Pipli
Tam	:	Thippili
Mal	:	Tippli

Parts Used

Immature berries

Constituents

Aristolactums, dioxoaphines, alkaloids like cepharadione A, B, cepharanone B, aristolactum AII, norcepharadione B, piperine, resin, volatile oil.

Uses

Stimulant, carminative, aphrodisiac, liver disorders, lipid peroxidation.

Classification	
Kingdom	Plantae – Plants
Subkingdom	Tracheobionta – Vascular plants
Superdivision	Spermatophyta – Seed plants
Division	Magnoliophyta – Flowering plants
Class	Magnoliopsida – Dicotyledons
Subclass	Magnoliidae –
Order	Piperales –
Family	Piperaceae – Pepper family
Genus	Piper L. – pepper

Piper nigrum Linn

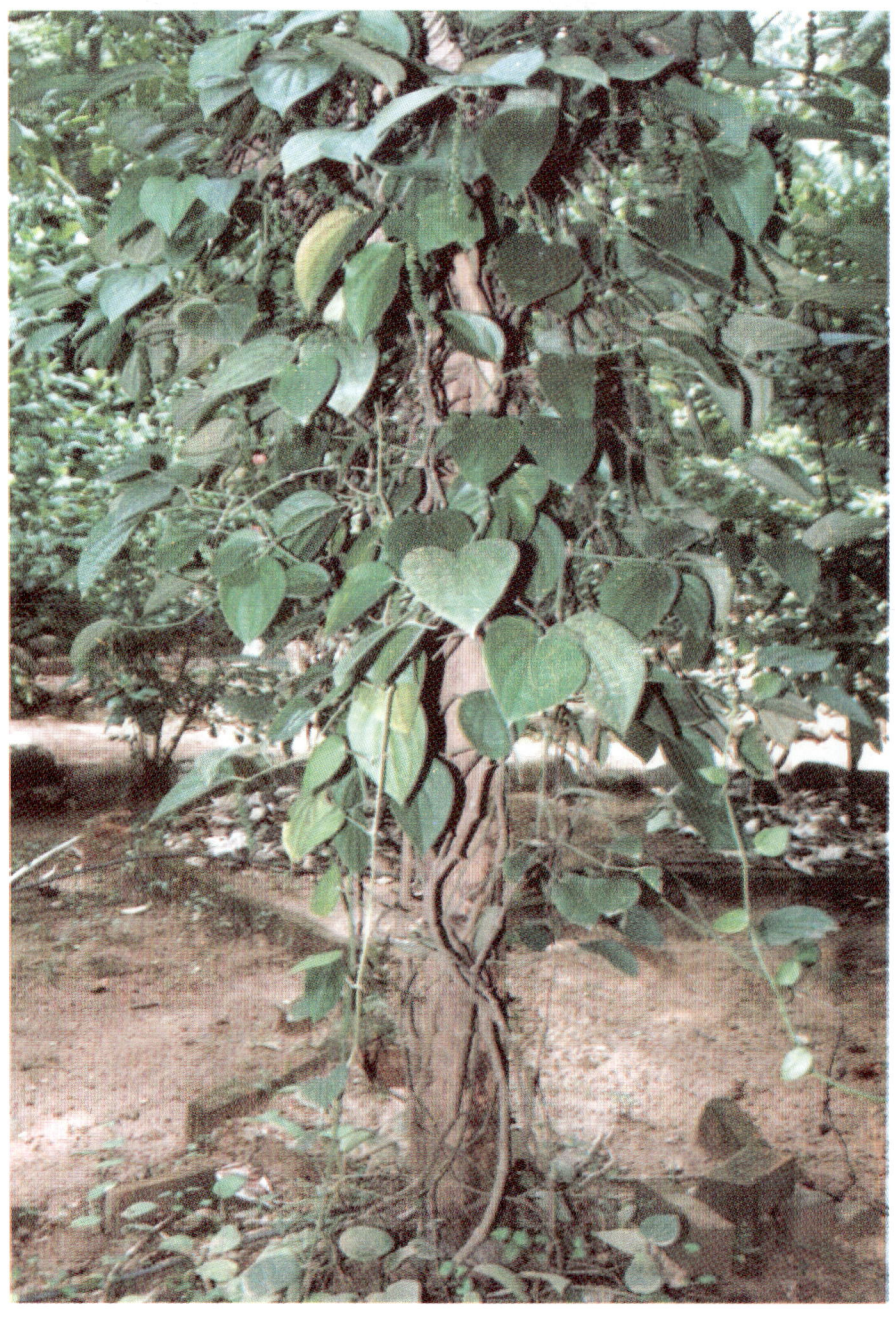

PLATE
106

Piper nigrum Linn

PIPERACEAE

Common Names

Eng	:	Black Pepper
Hind	:	Gulmireh
Sans	:	Maricham
Ben	:	Kalimirich
Tam	:	Milagh
Mal	:	Kuru mulaka, Kurumilagu

Parts Used

Dried unripe fruit

Constituents

Volatile oil, alkaloid, piperine, piperidine, chavicin, safrol, tannic acid, amide of piperamide-C7, pyrrolidine.

Uses

Acrid, pungent, carminative, antiperiodic, stimulant, anti pyretic, anti bacterial, as an anti dote for poisonous bite in cattle, treatment of malaria, nausea, vomiting, excess thirst, cough and inflammatory of penis.

Classification	
Kingdom	Plantae – Plants
Subkingdom	Tracheobionta – Vascular plants
Superdivision	Spermatophyta – Seed plants
Division	Magnoliophyta – Flowering plants
Class	Magnoliopsida – Dicotyledons
Subclass	Magnoliidae –
Order	Piperales –
Family	Piperaceae – Pepper family
Genus	Piper L. – pepper

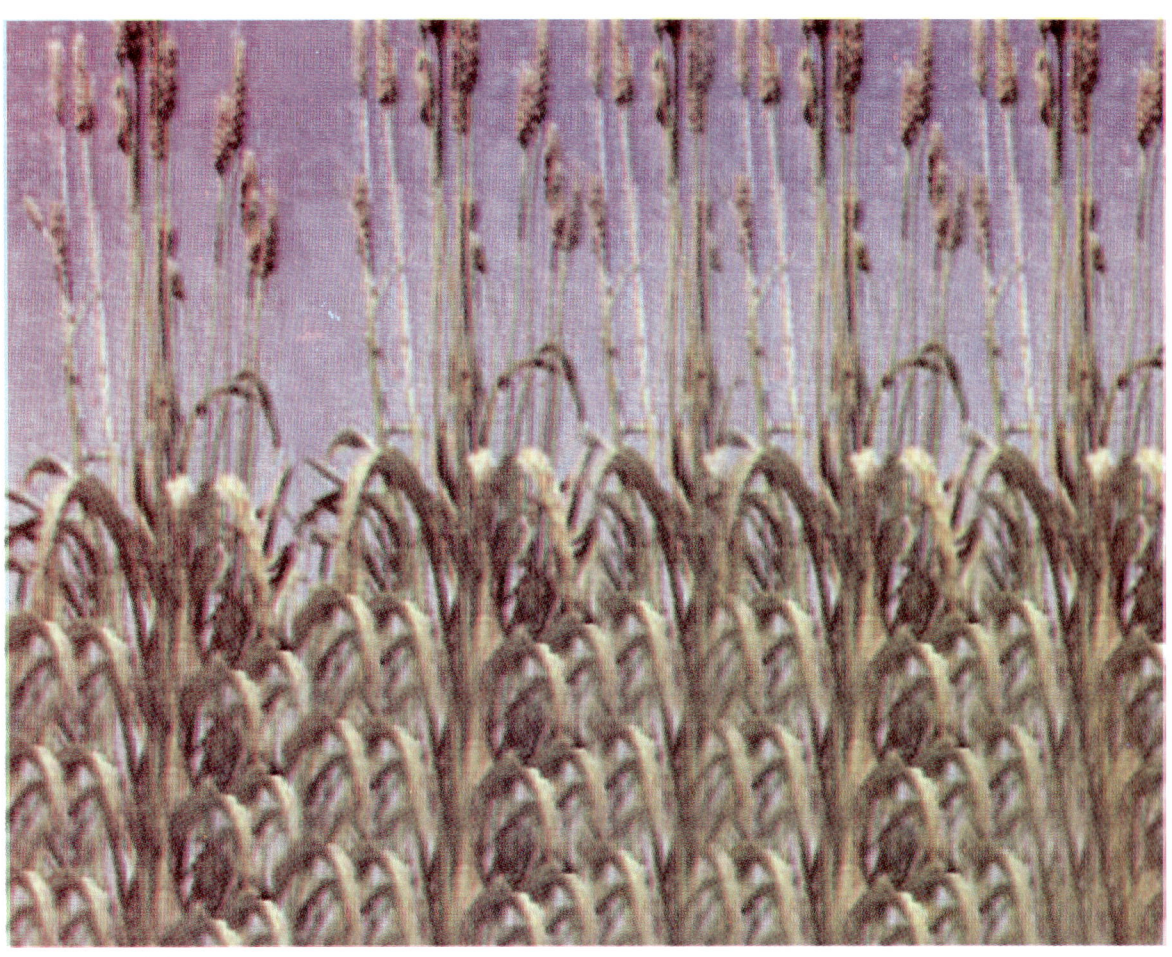

PLATE
107

Plantago ovata Forsk

PLANTAGINACEAE

Common Names

Eng	:	Ispaghula
Hind	:	Issufgul, Isapghul
Sans	:	Snigdhajeera
Ben	:	Isabgul
Tam	:	Ishappukolviri

Parts Used

Seeds

Constituents

Mucilages, fatty oil contains 2-oxygenated fatty acid, (- hydroxy- octadec- 12 enoic acid), 9-oxo octadec – cis – 12- enoic acid.

Uses

Cooling, demulcent, mild astringent, emollient, laxative, diuretic, diarrhoea, dysentery, constipation, lowering blood cholesterol.

Classification	
Kingdom	Plantae – Plants
Subkingdom	Tracheobionta – Vascular plants
Superdivision	Spermatophyta – Seed plants
Division	Magnoliophyta – Flowering plants
Class	Magnoliopsida – Dicotyledons
Subclass	Asteridae –
Order	Plantaginales –
Family	Plantaginaceae – Plantain family
Genus	Plantago L. – plantain

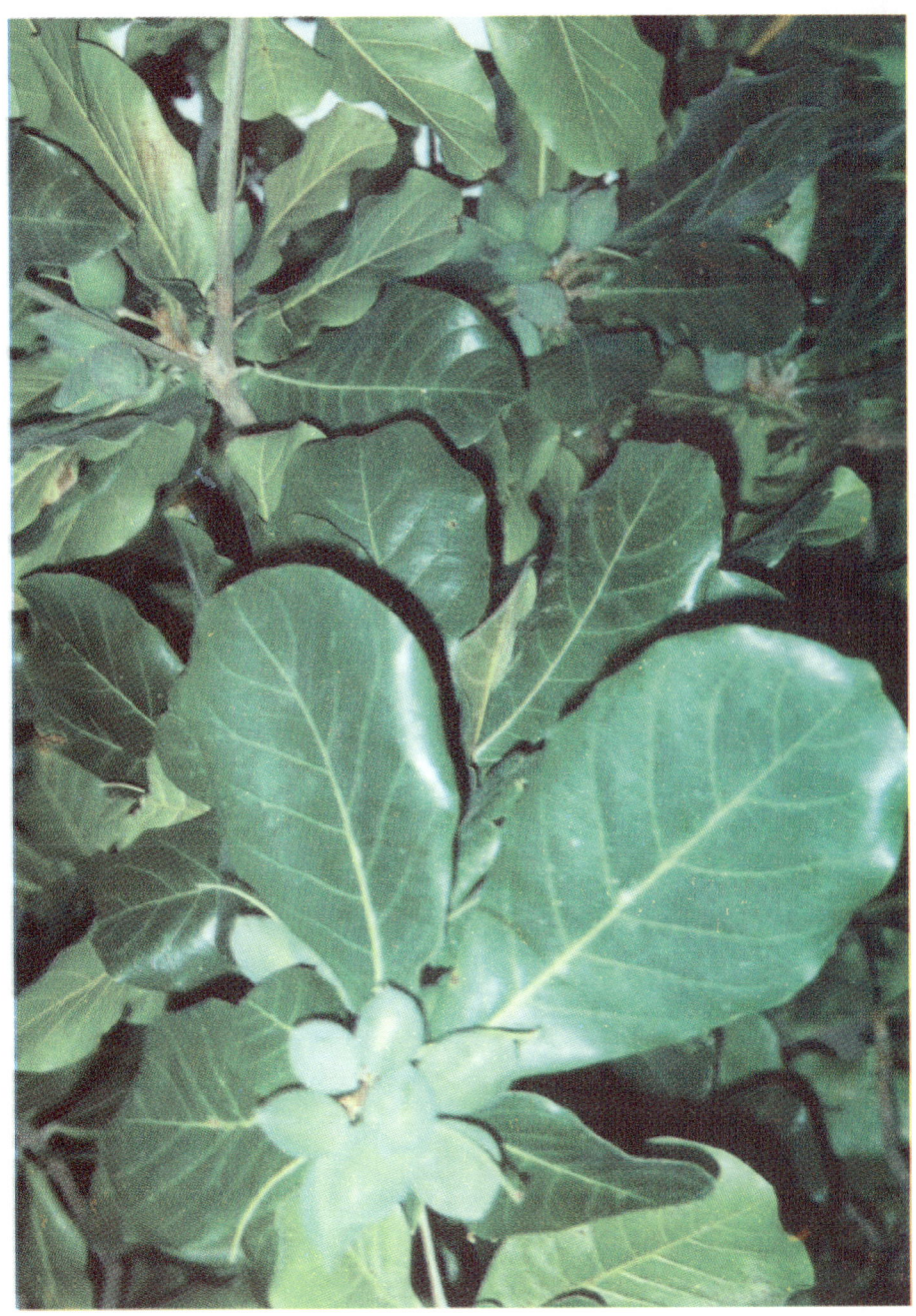

PLATE
108

Prunus amygdalis Baill.

ROSACEAE

Common Names

Eng	:	Almond
Hin	:	Badam
San	:	Badama
Ben	:	Bilatibadam
Tam	:	Vadam kottai

Parts Used

Seeds

Constituents

Fixed oil, flavones, biflavones, albuminous principle, sitosterol, octacosanol, coumarinic acid.

Uses

Demulcent, nutritive, nervine tonic, emollient, laxative.

Classification	
Kingdom	Plantae – Plants
Subkingdom	Tracheobionta – Vascular plants
Superdivision	Spermatophyta – Seed plants
Division	Magnoliophyta – Flowering plants
Class	Magnoliopsida – Dicotyledons
Subclass	Rosidae –
Order	Rosales –
Family	Rosaceae – Rose family
Genus	Prunus L. – plum

Psidium guajava L.

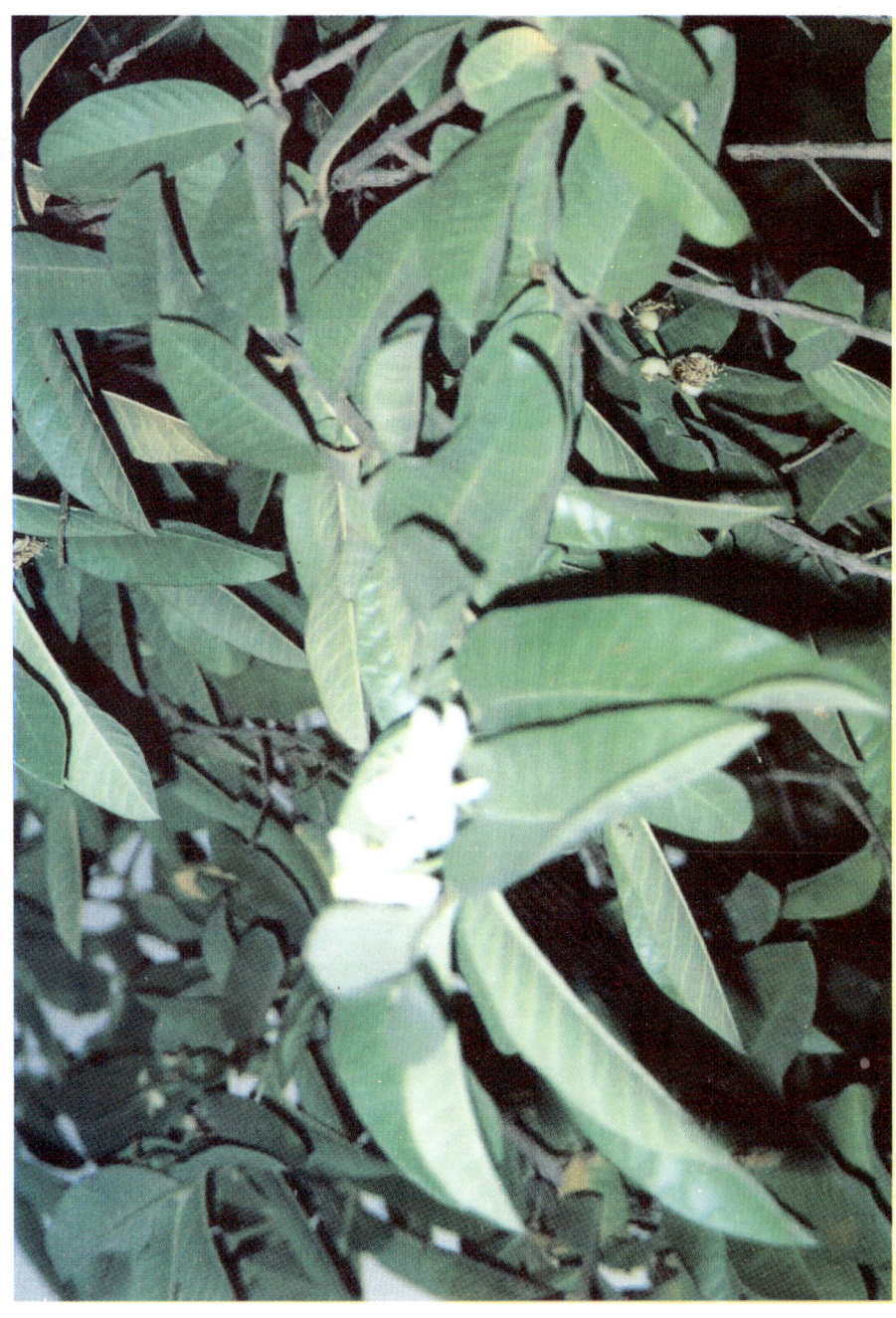

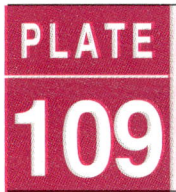

PLATE

109

Psidium guajava L.

MYRTACEAE

Common Names

Eng	:	Guava
Hin	:	Amrud
San	:	Perala
Tam	:	Koyya palam
Mal	:	Parekkai

Parts used

Fruit, leaves

Constituents

Tannins, pinene, cineol, cedrenol, globulol, terpineol, copaene, ledol, selinene, caryophyllene, the fresh flower contain ellagic acid, quercetin, oleanolic acid, the fatty acid contain protein, lauric acid, myristic acid, palmitic acid, stearic acid, oleic acid, linoleic acid

Uses

Leaves are used in the treatment of diarrhoea, for sore eyes, whooping cough, antispasmodic, antimicrobial, dysentery.

Classification	
Kingdom	Plantae – Plants
Subkingdom	Tracheobionta – Vascular plants
Superdivision	Spermatophyta – Seed plants
Division	Magnoliophyta – Flowering plants
Class	Magnoliopsida – Dicotyledons
Subclass	Rosidae –
Order	Myrtales –
Family	– Myrtle family
Genus	Psidium L. – guava

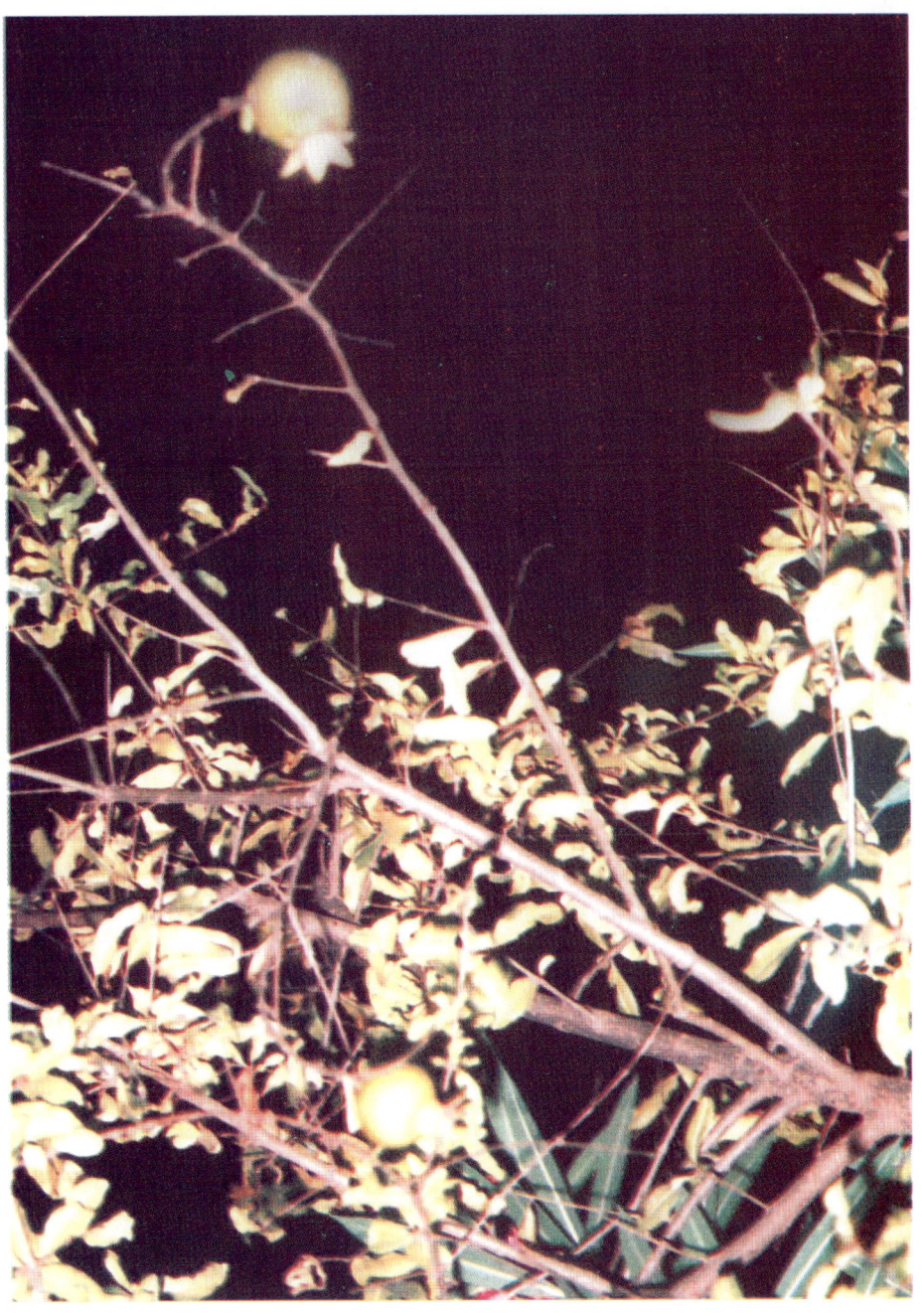

PLATE
110

Punica granatum Linn.

PUNICACEAE

Common Names

Eng	:	Pomegranate
Hin	:	Anar
San	:	Dadima palam
Tel	:	Dadima
Tam	:	Madulam
Mal	:	Matalam

Parts used

Fruit, barks and flowers

Constituents

Tannins, alkaloids- pelletierine, iso pelletierine, hyl pelletierine, pseudo pelletierine, carbohydrates.

Uses

Grains are astringent and anthelmintic, barks is used as anthelmintic, flowers and barks are astringent and stomachic.

Classification	
Kingdom	Plantae – Plants
Subkingdom	Tracheobionta – Vascular plants
Superdivision	Spermatophyta – Seed plants
Division	Magnoliophyta – Flowering plants
Class	Magnoliopsida – Dicotyledons
Subclass	Rosidae –
Order	Myrtales –
Family	Punicaceae – Pomegranate family
Genus	Punica L. – pomegranate

Rauwolfia serpentina Benth

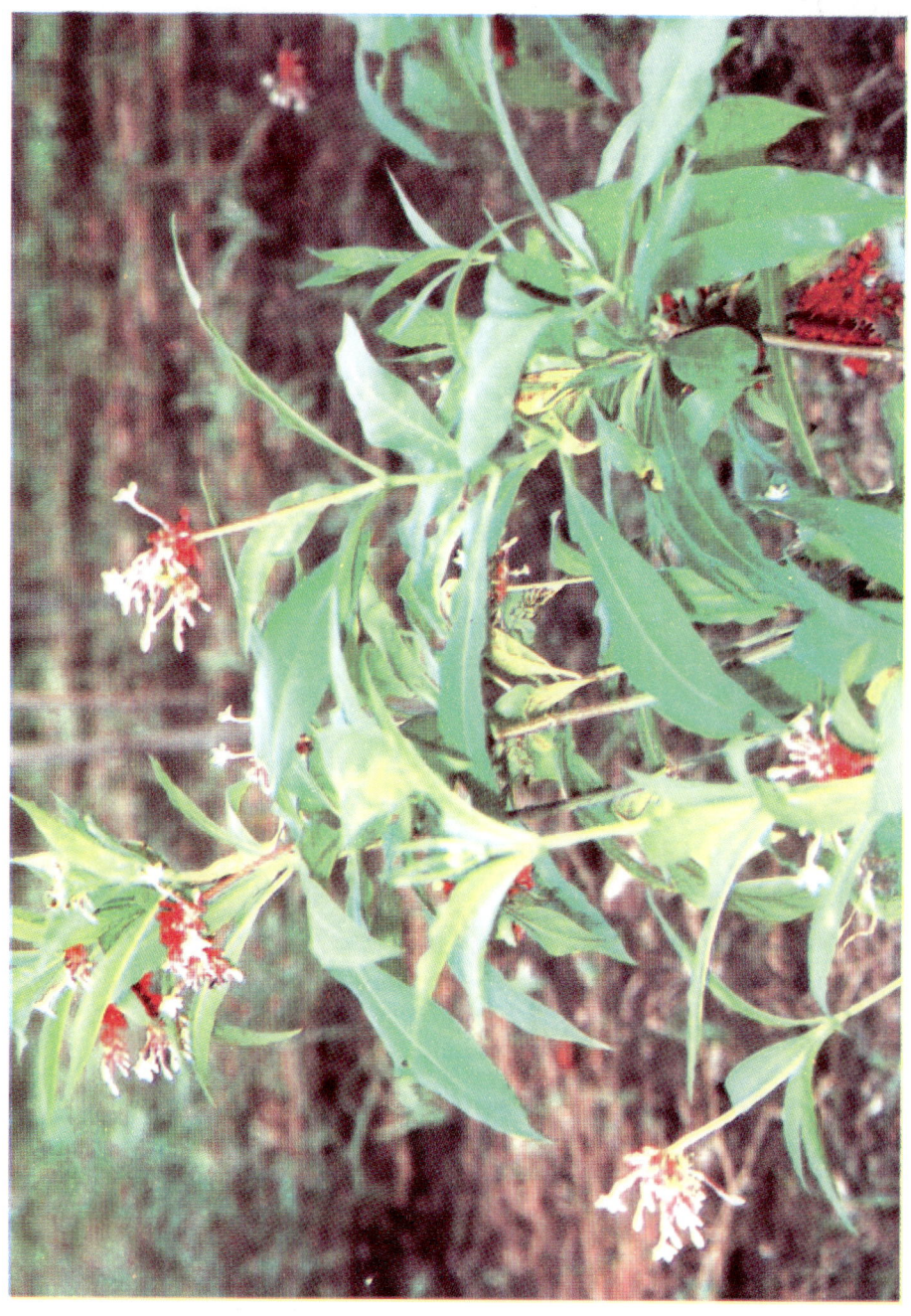

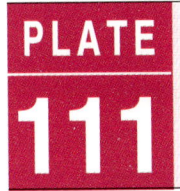

PLATE
111

Rauwolfia serpentina Benth

APOCYNACEAE

Common Names

Eng	:	Serpentine wood
Hin	:	Chota chand
Sans	:	Chandrika
Tam	:	Chivan melpodi
Mal	:	Chivan avelpori
Telu	:	Patala gandhi

Parts used

Roots & rhizomes

Constituents

Roots contain the alkaloids, ajmalimine, indobinine, yohambinine, rescinnamol, rescinnamidine, reserpine, reserpiline, rescinnamine, ajmaline, heterohyohimbine, ajmalicidine.

Uses

Anti hypertensive, reserpiline & rescinnamine reduce gaestric motility, ajmaline increase concentration of histamine, rauwolfia alkaloids are anti depresent.

Classification	
Kingdom	Plantae – Plants
Subkingdom	Tracheobionta – Vascular plants
Superdivision	Spermatophyta – Seed plants
Division	Magnoliophyta – Flowering plants
Class	Magnoliopsida – Dicotyledons
Subclass	Asteridae –
Order	Gentianales –
Family	Apocynaceae – DogBene family
Genus	Rauvolfia L. – devil's-pepper

Ricinus communis Linn

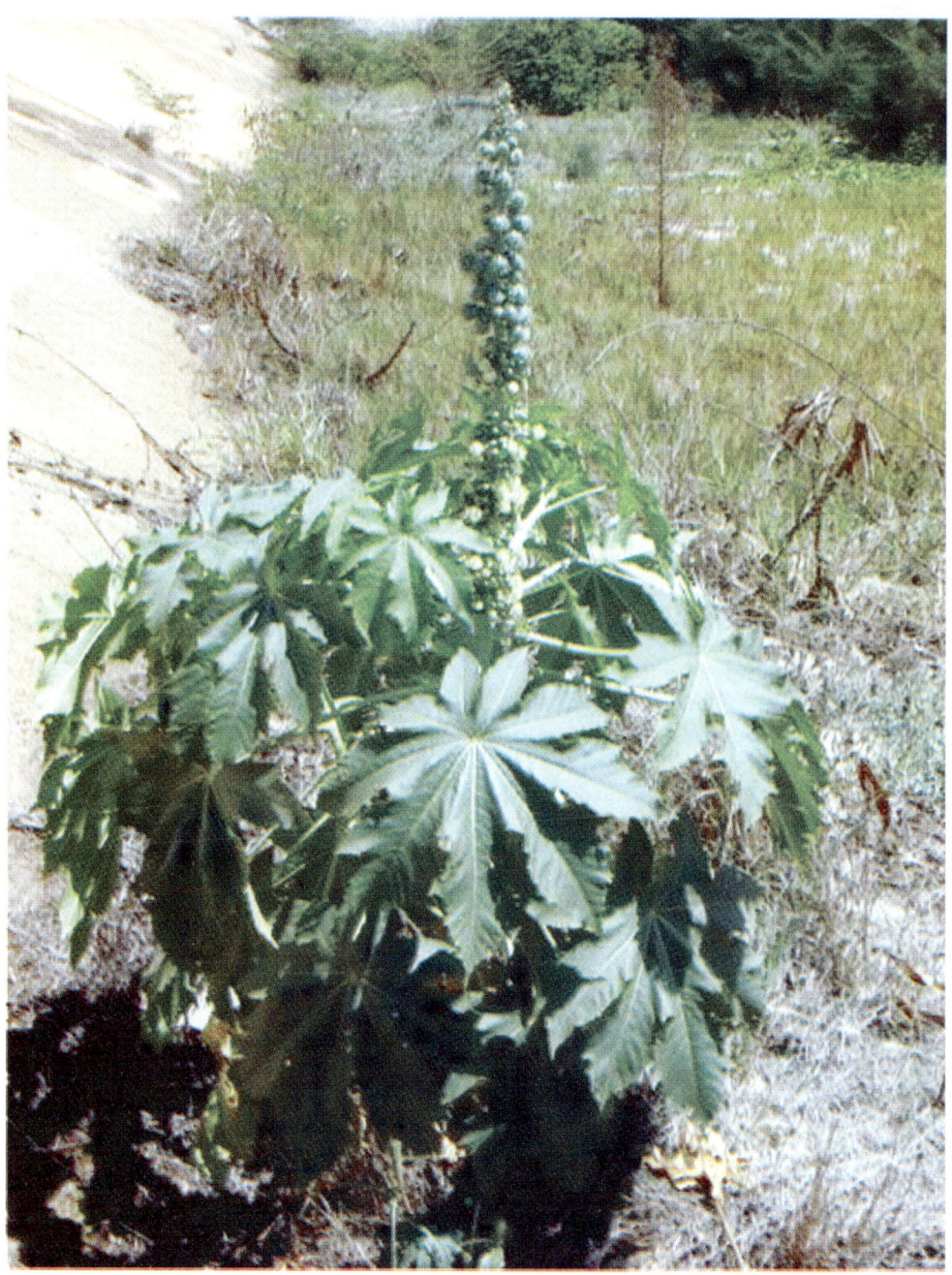

PLATE
112

Ricinus communis Linn

EUPHORBIACEAE

Common Names

Eng	:	Castor Oil
Hind	:	Erand
Sans	:	Eranda
Ben	:	Verenda
Tam	:	Amanakku
Mal	:	Chittamanakku

Parts Used

Leaves, Seeds, Oil, Root

Constituents

Fixed oil, protein, starch, mucilage, also it consist of ricinoleste or triricinolein, small quantity of palmitin, stearein

Uses

Non irritant purgative, ricinoleic acid is absorbed into the blood and tissue and is excreted with human milk, which when sucked by child causes purgative action, ricinin is a violent irritant of intestine, kidney & bladder.

Classification	
Kingdom	Plantae – Plants
Subkingdom	Tracheobionta – Vascular plants
Superdivision	Spermatophyta – Seed plants
Division	Magnoliophyta – Flowering plants
Class	Magnoliopsida – Dicotyledons
Subclass	Rosidae –
Order	Euphorbiales –
Family	Euphorbiaceae – Spurge family
Genus	Ricinus L. – ricinus

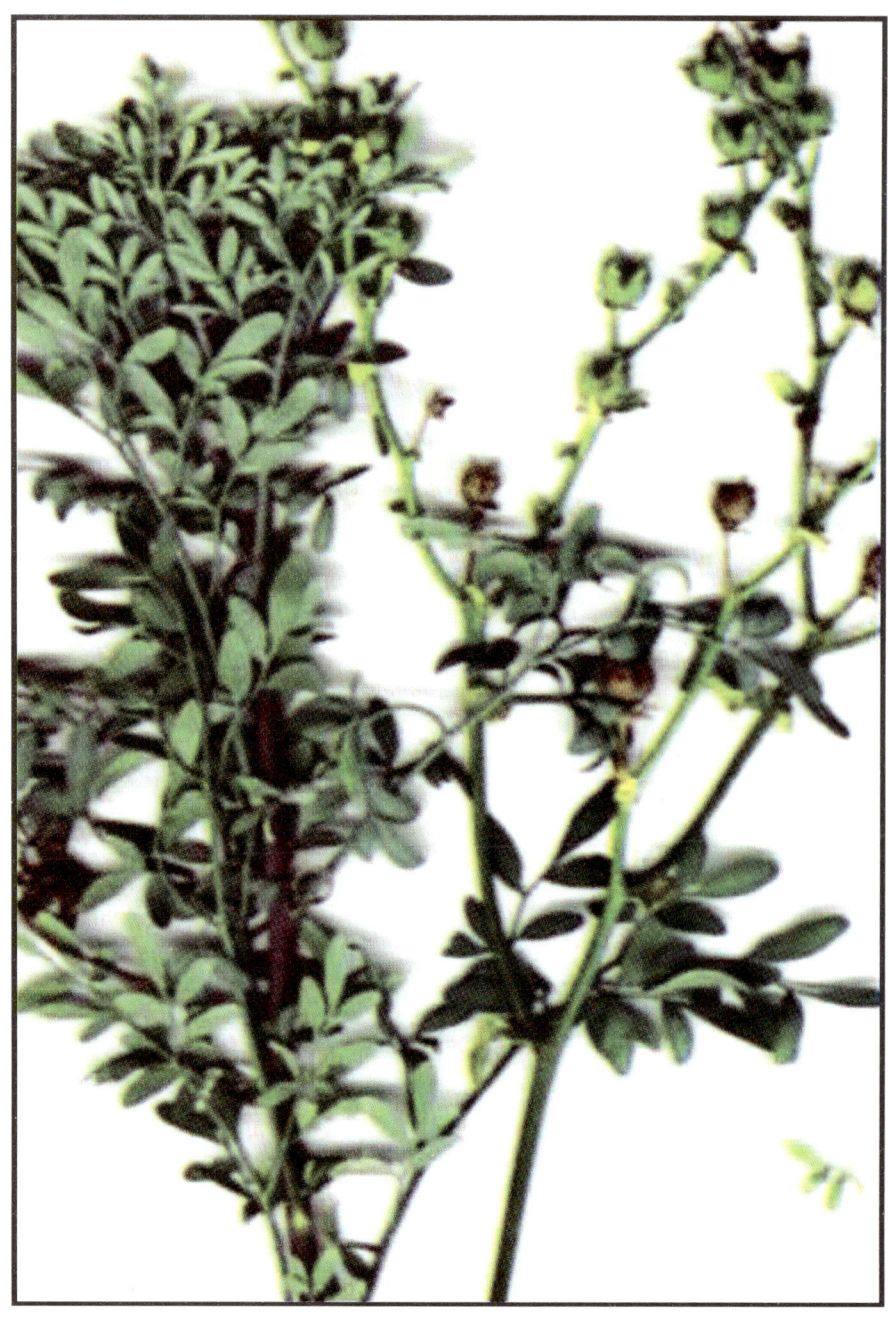

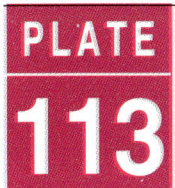

PLATE 113

Ruta graveolens Linn

RUTACEAE

Common Names

Eng	:	Common rue
Hind	:	Salap; sadab
Sans	:	Sadapala
Ben	:	Ispand
Tam	:	Arvada
Mal	:	Aruta

Parts Used

Whole Plant

Constituents

Glucoside, rutin, essential oil alkaloid, dihydrofuroacridone, gravacridiniolactate, alpha-pinene, furoquinoline alkaloid.

Uses

Antiseptic, stimulant, irritant, abortifacient, Juice of plant is antispasmodic, anthelmintic, dyspepsia, emmenegogue, aphrodisiac, rubefacient.

Classification	
Kingdom	Plantae – Plants
Subkingdom	Tracheobionta – Vascular plants
Superdivision	Spermatophyta – Seed plants
Division	Magnoliophyta – Flowering plants
Class	Magnoliopsida – Dicotyledons
Subclass	Rosidae –
Order	Sapindales –
Family	Rutaceae – Rue family
Genus	Ruta L. – rue

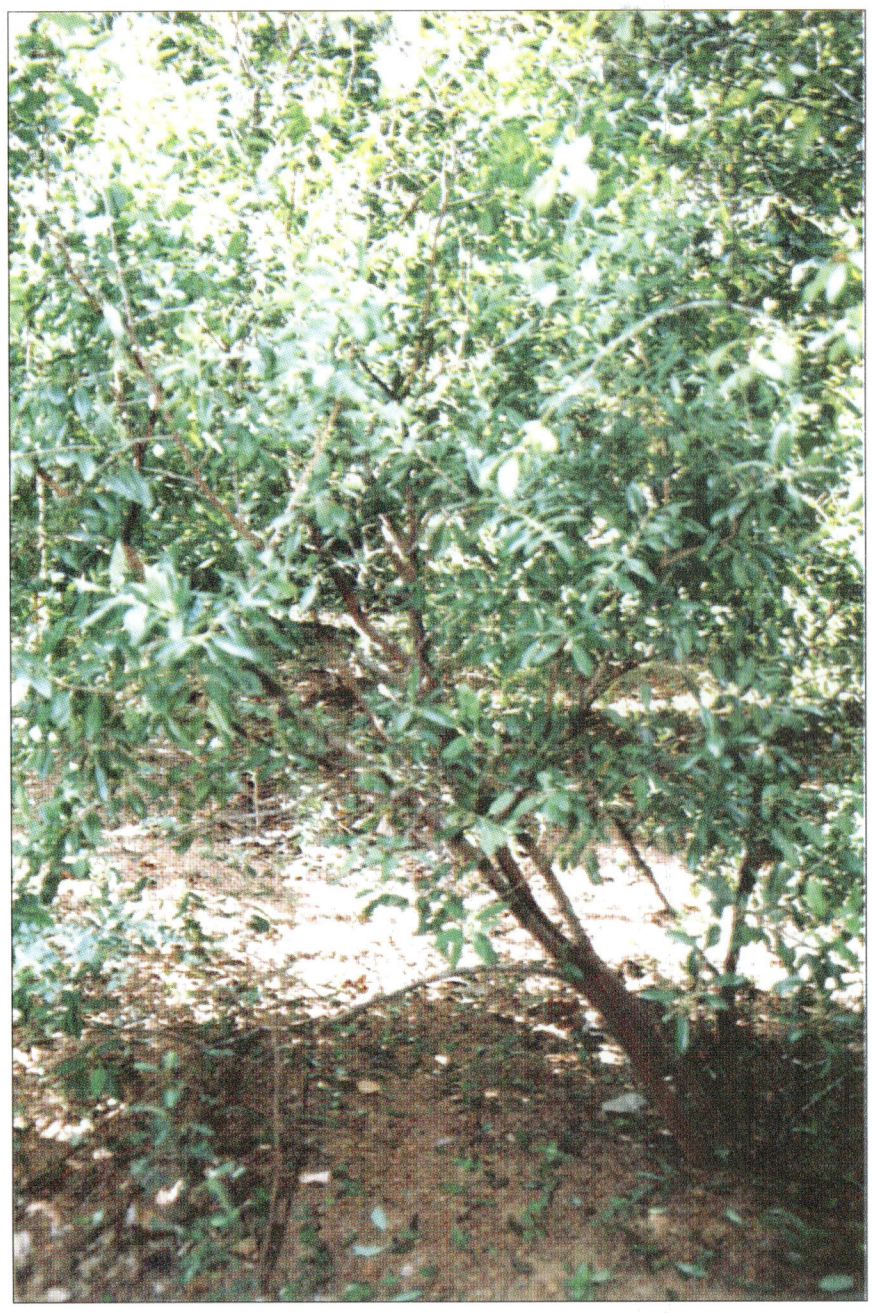

PLATE
114

Santalum album Linn

SANTALACEAE

Common Names

Eng	:	White Sandal Wood
Hind	:	safed Chandan
Sans	:	Srigandha
Ben	:	Chandan
Tam	:	Shandanak - kattai
Mal	:	Chandana maram

Parts Used

Wood

Constituents

Volatile oil, A-santalol, B-santalol, aldehyde, proteins, bisabolenols A to E, α- transbergamotenol, sesquiterpene alcohol,12, 13 - dihydroxy- α- santalol β-isomer.

Uses

Bitter, cooling, sedative, astringent, disinfectant, diuretic, stimulant, antibacterial.

Classification	
Kingdom	Plantae – Plants
Subkingdom	Tracheobionta – Vascular plants
Superdivision	Spermatophyta – Seed plants
Division	Magnoliophyta – Flowering plants
Class	Magnoliopsida – Dicotyledons
Subclass	Rosidae –
Order	Santalales –
Family	Santalaceae – Sandalwood family
Genus	Santalum L. – sandalwood

Sida cordifolia Linn

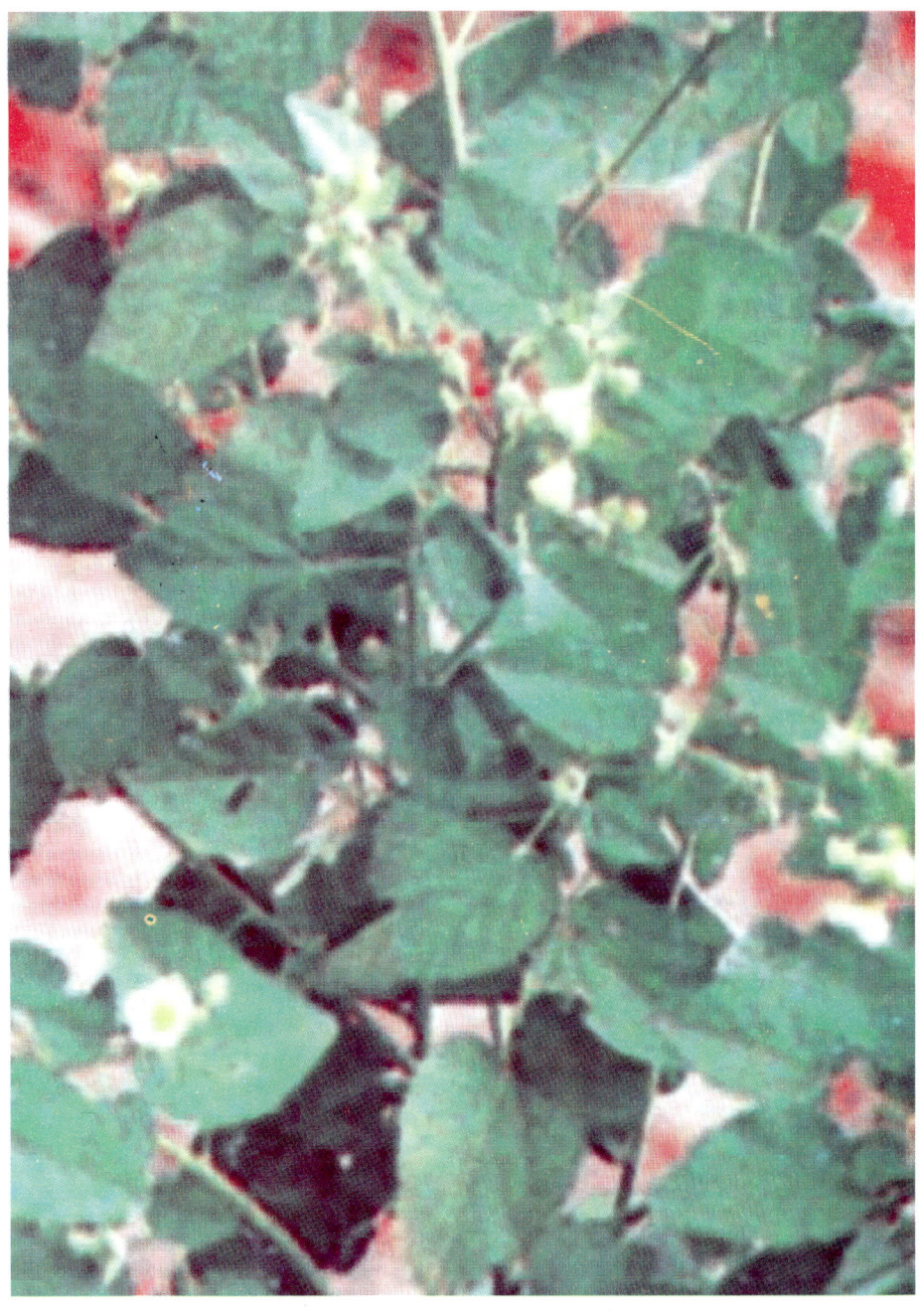

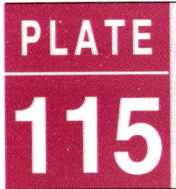

PLATE

115

Sida cordifolia Linn

MALVACEAE

Common Names

Eng	:	Llima
Hind	:	Bariar, Kungyi
Sans	:	Bala
Ben	:	Bala
Tam	:	Mayir Manikham
Mal	:	Velluram

Parts Used

Roots, leaves, seeds & stems

Constituents

Alkaloids are present in stem, root and leaves, fatty oil, phytosterol, mucins, resins, ephedrine is a main constituent.

Uses

Cooling, astringent, stomachic, tonic, aromatic, bitter, febrifuge, demulcent, diuretic, immunostimulant.

Classification	
Kingdom	Plantae – Plants
Subkingdom	Tracheobionta – Vascular plants
Superdivision	Spermatophyta – Seed plants
Division	Magnoliophyta – Flowering plants
Class	Magnoliopsida – Dicotyledons
Subclass	Dilleniidae –
Order	Malvales –
Family	Malvaceae – Mallow family
Genus	Sida L. – fanpetals

Solanum xanthocarpum Schrad

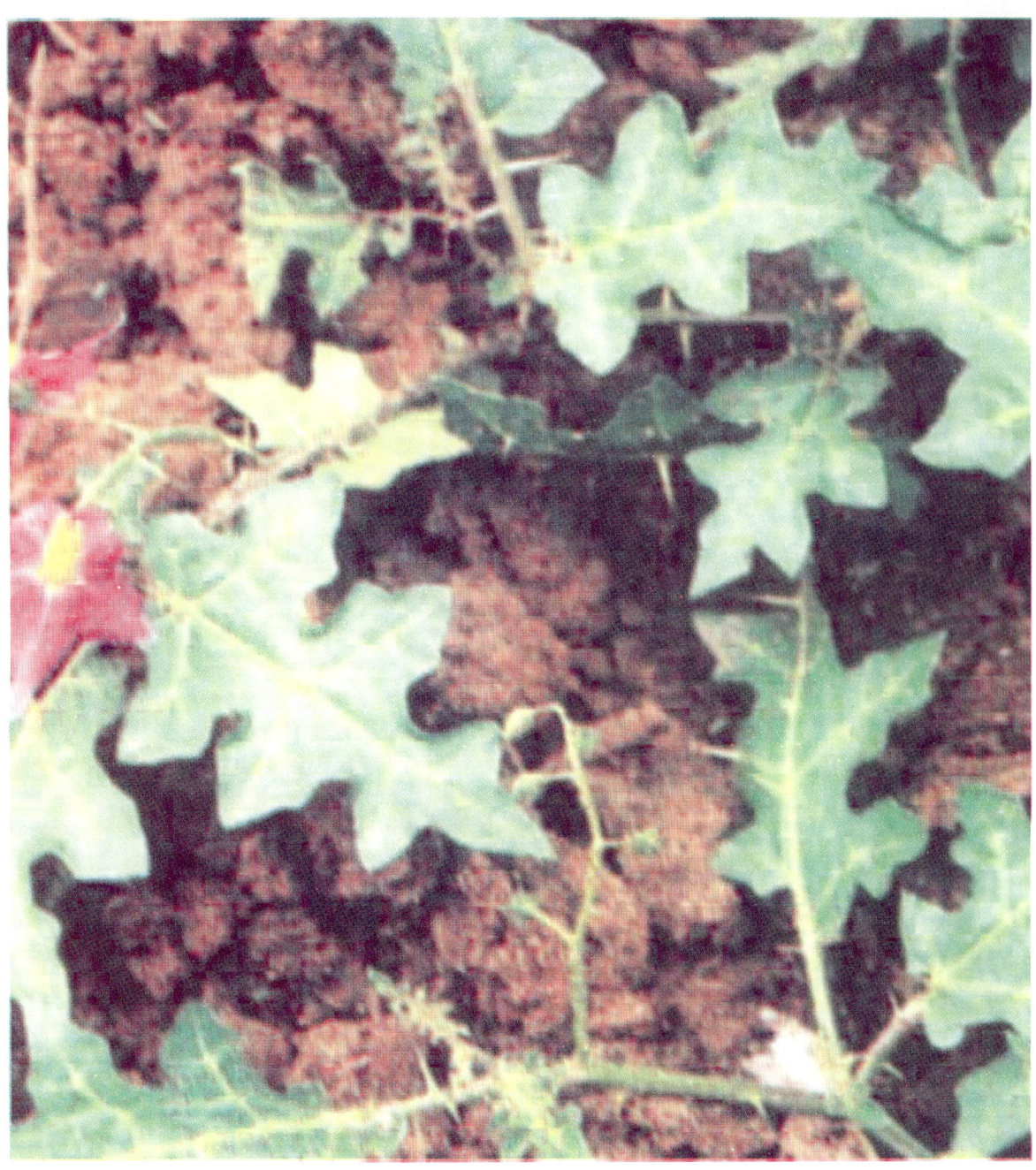

PLATE
116

Solanum xanthocarpum Schrad

SOLANACEAE

Common Names

Eng	:	Woody night shade
Hin	:	Bhutkatya
Sans	:	Kantakari
Ben	:	Kantikari
Tam	:	Kandan kattiri
Punj	:	Warumba

Parts used

Whole plant

Constituents

Glyco alkaloid termed solasodine, solasonine, solamargine, solancarpine.

Uses

Used in fever, cough, asthma, decoction of plant is used in gonorrhoea, decoction of root is used as tonic in fever and cough.

Classification	
Kingdom	Plantae – Plants
Subkingdom	Tracheobionta – Vascular plants
Superdivision	Spermatophyta – Seed plants
Division	Magnoliophyta – Flowering plants
Class	Magnoliopsida – Dicotyledons
Subclass	Asteridae –
Order	Solanales –
Family	Solanaceae – Potato family
Genus	Solanum L. – nightshade

Syzigium aromaticum (L.) Merr. & Perry

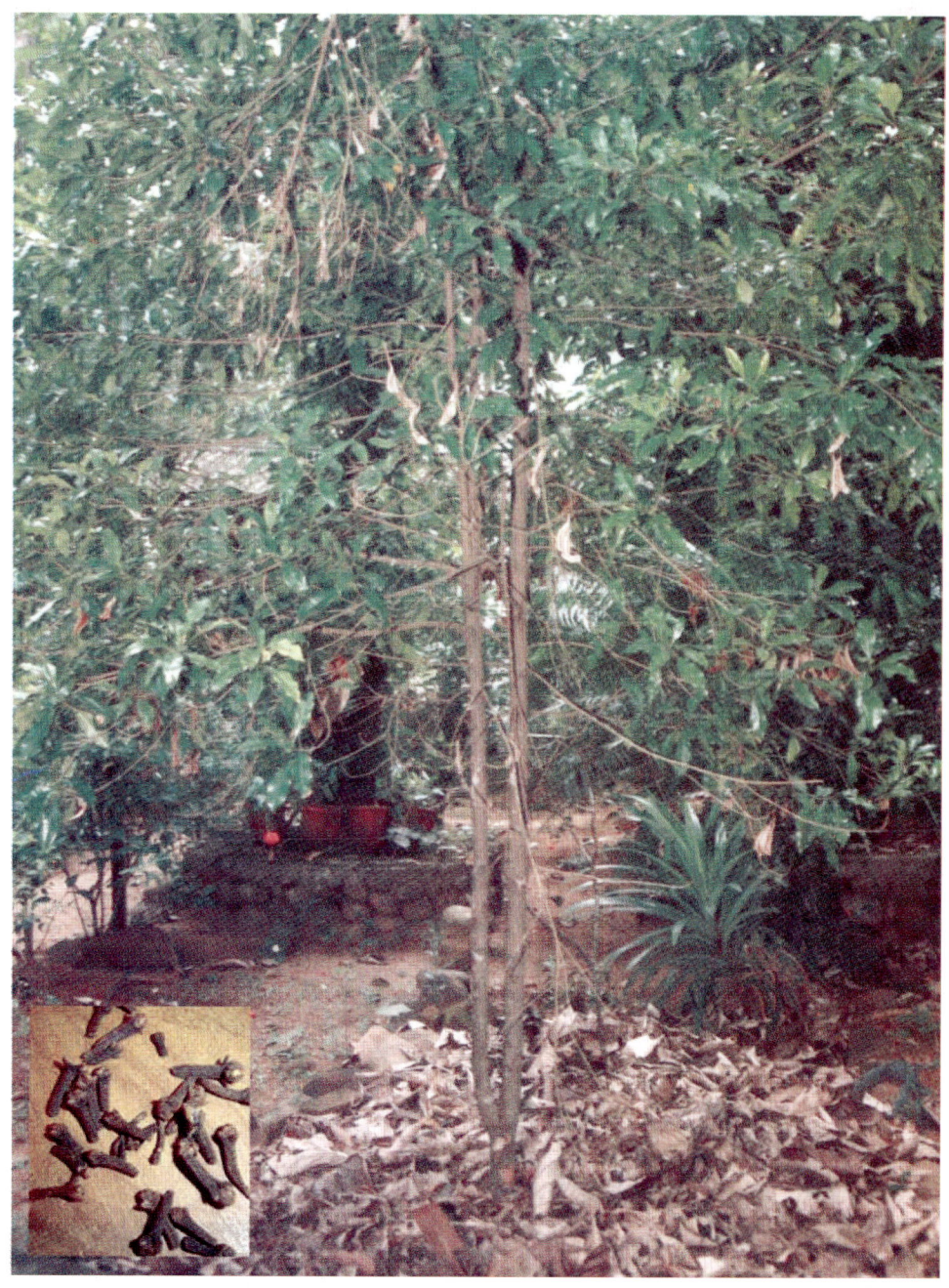

PLATE 117

Syzigium aromaticum (L.) Merr. & Perry

MYRTACEAE

Common Names

Eng	:	Clove
Hin	:	Laung
San	:	Lavangha
Tam	:	Kirambu
Ben	:	Lavang
Mal	:	Ghrambu

Parts Used

Fruits, dried flower buds, oil

Constituents

The dried leaves contain eugenol, 2- methyl- 5, 7- dihydroxy chromone 8-C-β-D- glucopyranoside, valoneic acid bis lactone, gallic acid, glycoside, ellagitannin, strictnin, gemin D, galloyeugenin, eugenin, rugosin A, D, E, casuarin, pterocarpin, galloyl peduncalagin, the clove leaf oil contain â caryophyllene, á-cubebene, farnesol.

Uses

Antioxidant, oil possesses insecticidal, antibacterial, antifungal activity, its used in dentifrices to remove stain from teeth, antihydrolytic, antiimplantation.

Classification	
Kingdom	Plantae – Plants
Subkingdom	Tracheobionta – Vascular plants
Superdivision	Spermatophyta – Seed plants
Division	Magnoliophyta – Flowering plants
Class	Magnoliopsida – Dicotyledons
Subclass	Rosidae –
Order	Myrtales –
Family	Myrtaceae – Myrtle family
Genus	Syzigium P. Br. ex Gaertn. – syzygium

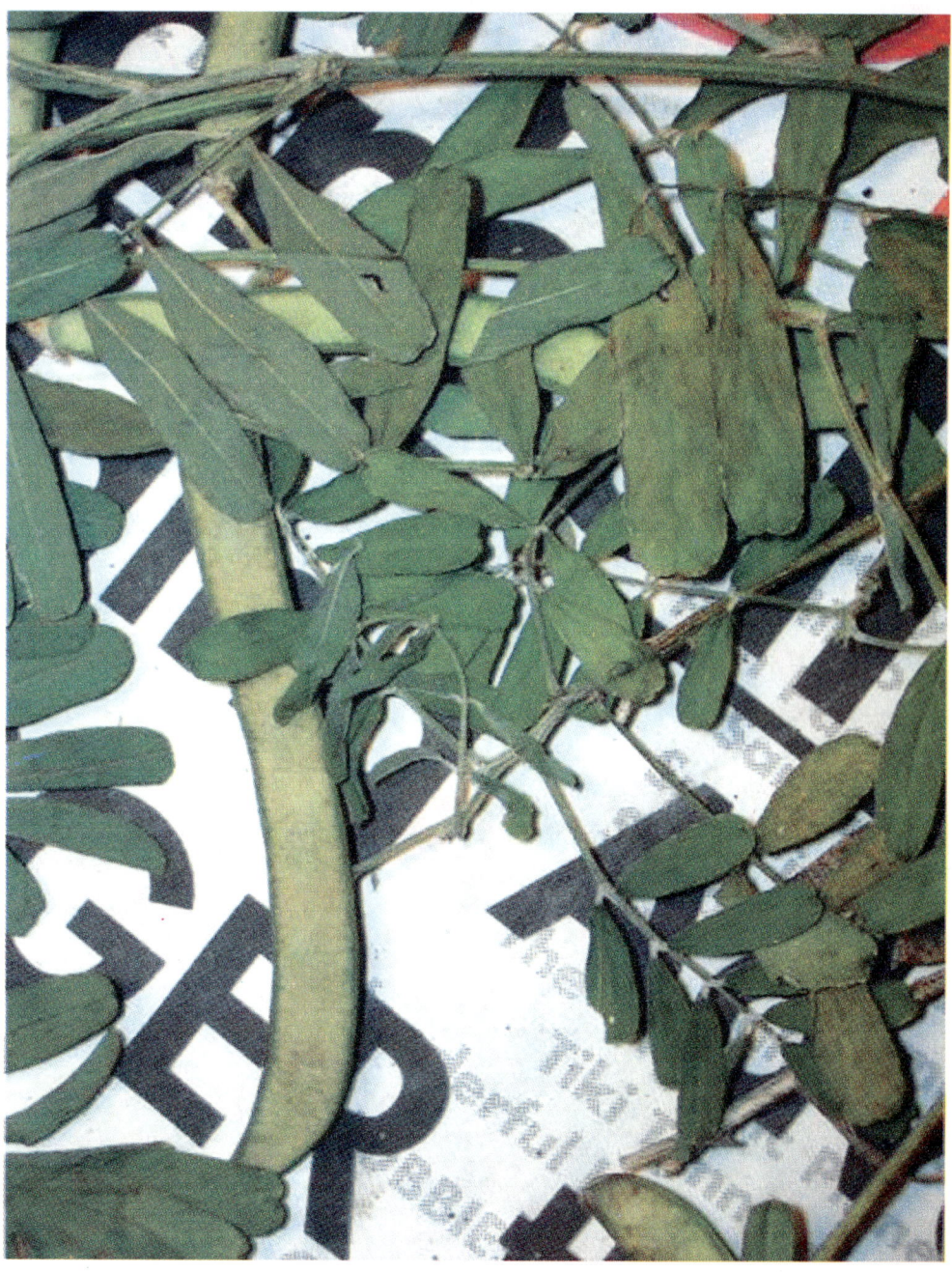

PLATE

118

Tephrosia purpurea Pers

PAPILIONACEAE

Common Names

Eng	:	Fishpoison
Hind	:	Sarphenka
Sans	:	Pulechashtree
Ben	:	Bennlgaoh
Tam	:	Kolluk-kay-welai
Mal	:	Kazhinnila

Parts Used

Leaves

Constituents

Gum, albumin, quercetin, querritrin, glycoside, pongamol, β sitosterol, ursolic acid, spinosterol- α, tetratriacontane, rotenone, tephrosin, betulinic acid, dimethylglabranin, expoxy flavones, roots contain lanceolatin B, purpuren, maackain, flemichapparin B, C.

Uses

Hypoglycaemic, leucoderma, rheumatism, hepatoprotective, febrifuge, cholagogue, tonic, laxative.

Classification	
Kingdom	Plantae – Plants
Subkingdom	Tracheobionta – Vascular plants
Superdivision	Spermatophyta – Seed plants
Division	Magnoliophyta – Flowering plants
Class	Magnoliopsida – Dicotyledons
Subclass	Rosidae –
Order	Fabales –
Family	Fabaceae – Pea family
Genus	Tephrosia Pers. – hoarypea

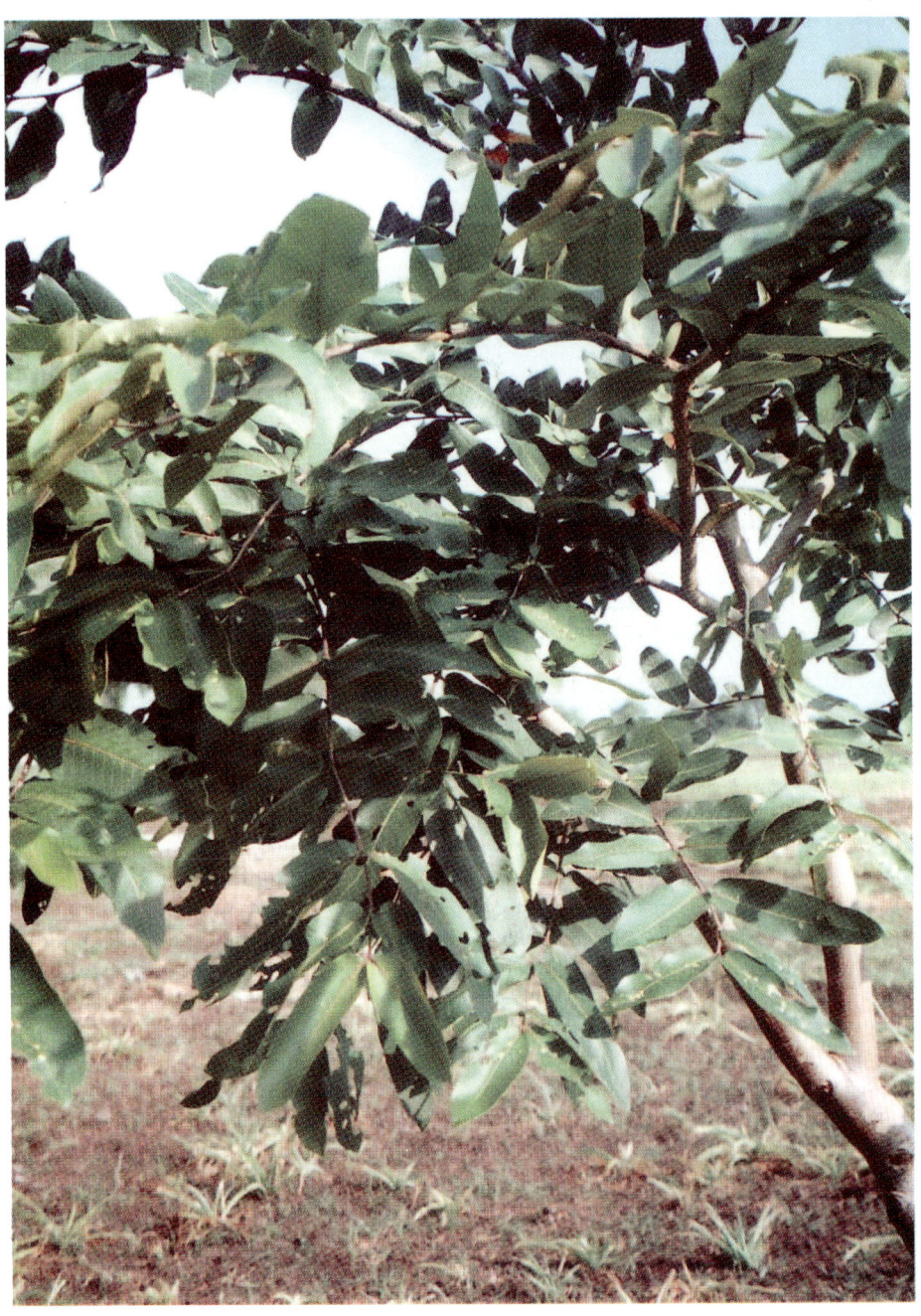

PLATE
119

Terminalia arjuna W & A

COMBRETACEAE

Common Names

Eng	:	Arjuna myrobalan
Hin	:	Arjun kahu
Sans	:	Arjuna kukubha
Ben	:	Arjun
Tam	:	Shardul
Mal	:	Vellaimaeda

Parts used

Leaves, bark

Constituents

Leaf contains carotenoids, protein, the bark contain flavour arjunolone terpenes and their glyocoside, arjungenin friedelin, arjunin, arjunctine, arjun glycoside I, II, III, arjunoside, arjunoleic acid, oleanolic acid, arjunic acid, tannins- catechol, glucotannic acid.

Use

Antifungal, anti-ischemic, cardioprotective agent in hypertension. Bark powder is diuretic, prostaglandin enhancing and has coronary risk factor modulating property, bark is hypocholesterolemic.

Classification	
Kingdom	Plantae – Plants
Subkingdom	Tracheobionta – Vascular plants
Superdivision	Spermatophyta – Seed plants
Division	Magnoliophyta – Flowering plants
Class	Magnoliopsida – Dicotyledons
Subclass	Rosidae –
Order	Myrtales –
Family	Combretaceae – Indian Almond family
Genus	Terminalia L. –

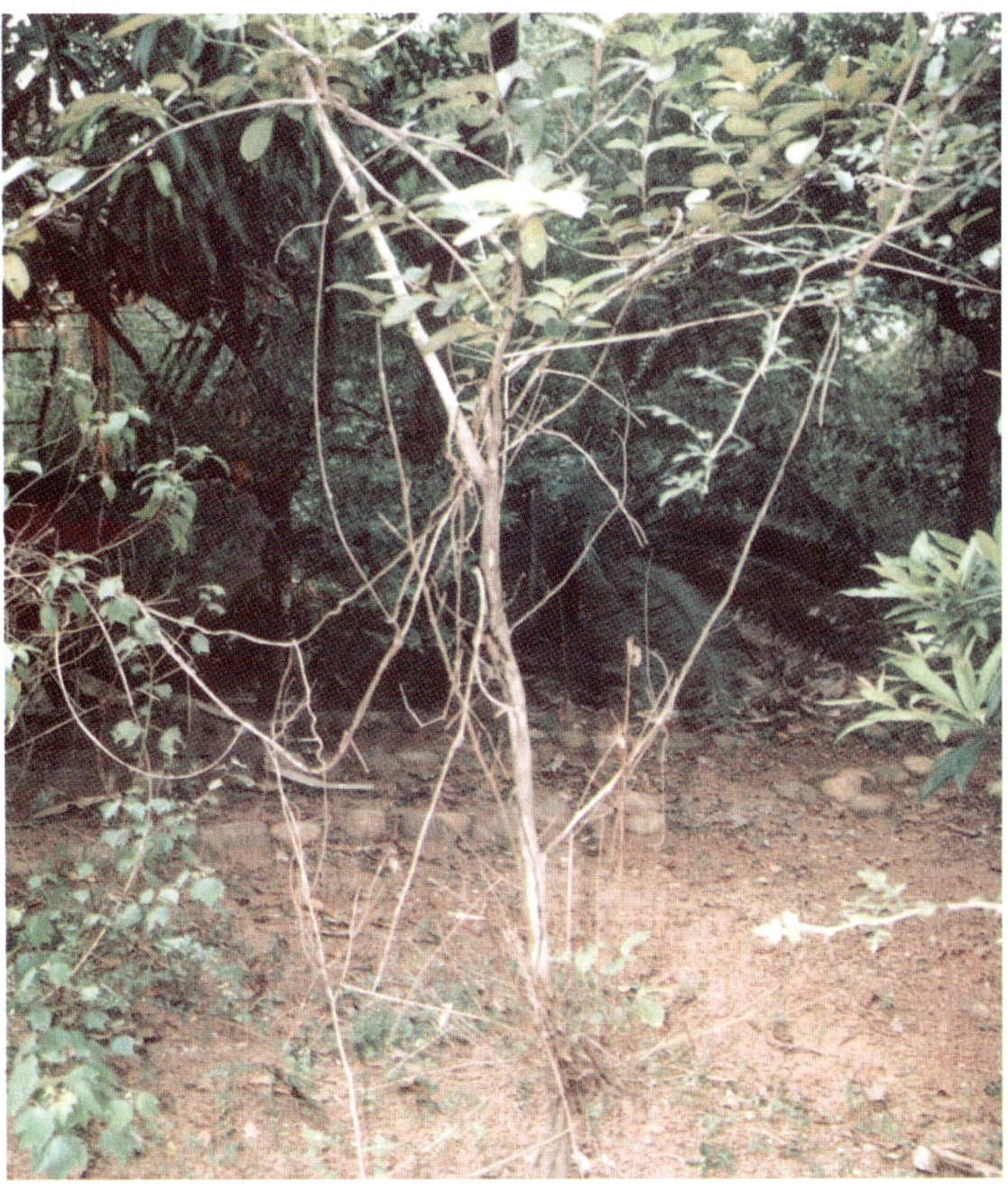

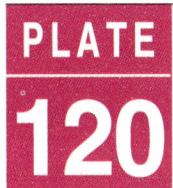

PLATE
120

Terminalia chebula Retz

COMBRETACEAE

Common Names

Eng : Myrobalan, Chebulic myrobalan
Hind : Harara, Har
Sans : Pathya, Suddha
Tam : Kadookai
Mal : Kadukkai

Parts Used

Dried Fruit

Constituents

Tannic acid, gallic acid, yellow colouring matter, chebulinic acid, stem contain triterpenoid glycoside chebuloside I, II, leaves contain terflavins B, C, D, punicalagin, punicalatin, maslinic acid, 2 α- hydroxy ursolic acid, triterpene 2 α hydroxy micromenic acid.

Uses

Fruits are highly nutritive (vitamin C), obesity, astringent, laxative, liver swelling, dropsy, ascites, antifungal, anti-inflammatory, antiarthritic, analgesic, hypoglycemic, and used in gastro intestinal disorder, anemia, purgative, alternative stomachic, fever, cough, asthma, worms.

Classification	
Kingdom	Plantae – Plants
Subkingdom	Tracheobionta – Vascular plants
Superdivision	Spermatophyta – Seed plants
Division	Magnoliophyta – Flowering plants
Class	Magnoliopsida – Dicotyledons
Subclass	Rosidae –
Order	Myrtales –
Family	Combretaceae – Indian Almond family
Genus	Terminalia L. – tropical almond

Thevetia neriifolia Juss

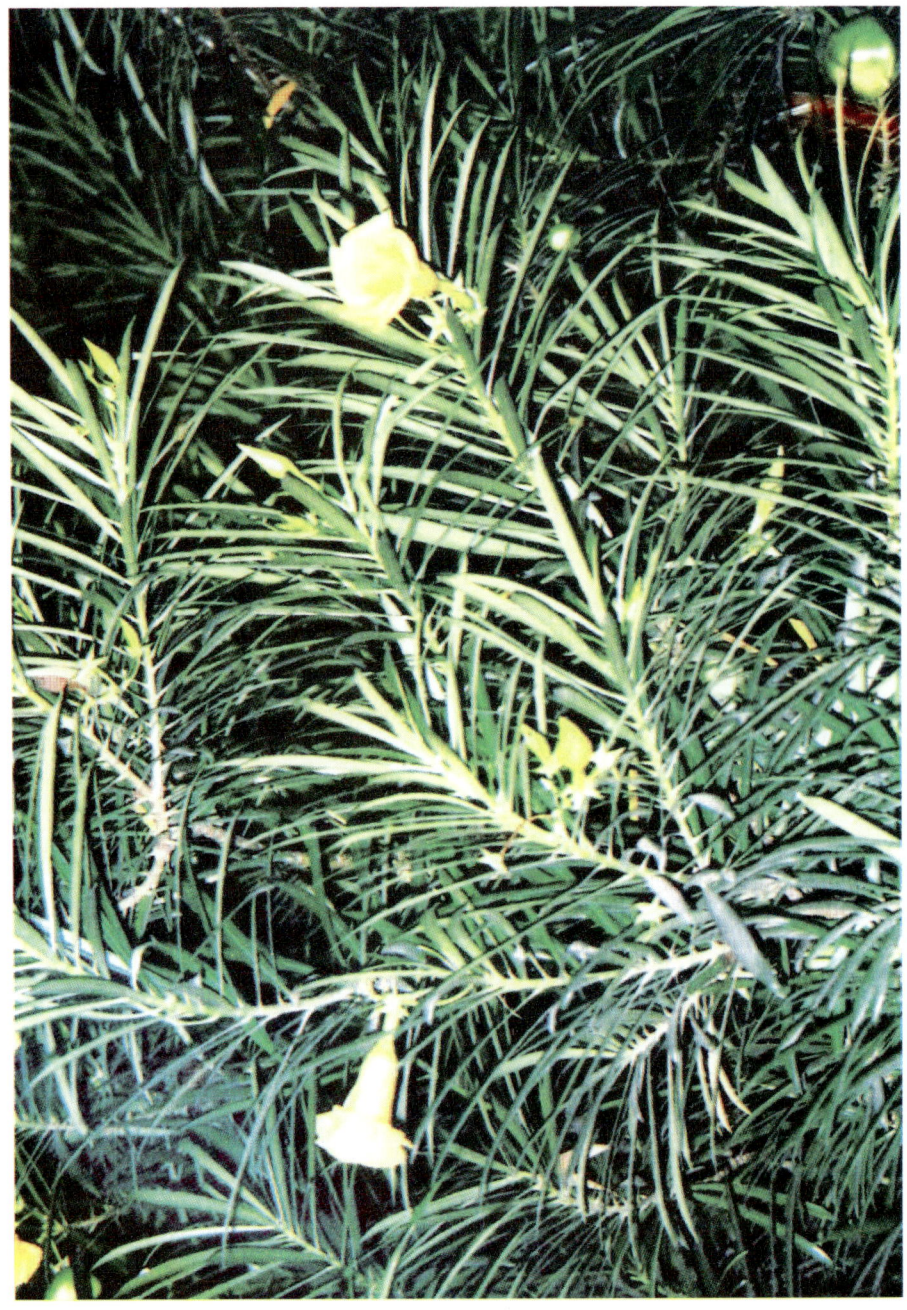

PLATE 121

Thevetia neriifolia Juss

APOCYNACEAE

Common Names

Eng	:	Yellow oleander
Hind	:	Pila kaner
Sans	:	Hapusha
Tam	:	Pachchai arali
Mal	:	Pachchai arali

Parts Used

Seeds, roots and juice.

Constituents

Cardiac glycosides- thevetine, peruvoside, sitosterol, fatty acids.

Uses

Roots of these plants are made in to a paste and applied to tumours. Seeds are used in the treatment of rheumatism, dropsy and also used as abortifacient and purgative.

Classification	
Kingdom	Plantae – Plants
Subkingdom	Tracheobionta – Vascular plants
Superdivision	Spermatophyta – Seed plants
Division	Magnoliophyta – Flowering plants
Class	Magnoliopsida – Dicotyledons
Subclass	Asteridae –
Order	Gentianales –
Family	Apocynaceae – Dogbane family
Genus	Thevetia Adans. – thevetia

Thuja occidentalis Linn

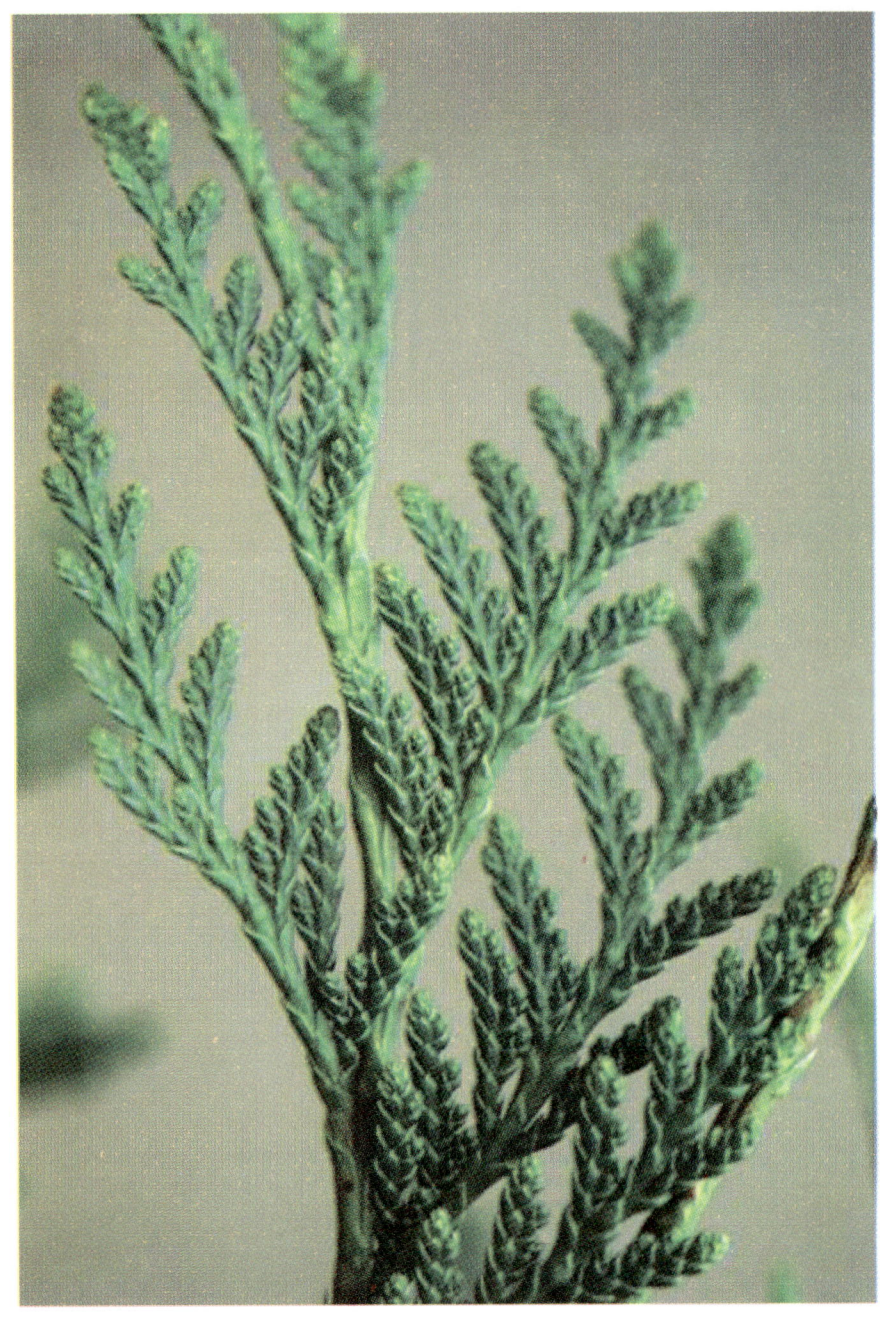

PLATE
122

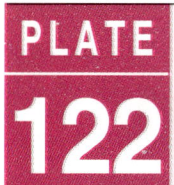

Thuja occidentalis Linn

CUPRESSACEAE

Common Names

Eng   :   Arborvitae

Parts Used

Leaves

Constituents

The major constituents are thujone, fenchole, diterpenoids including rimuene and beyerene, selarene, abietadiene, abietriene and hypoxy iso pinarene.

Uses

Used in nasal congestant and cough suppresent, aqueous extract of the drug is used as immunomodulatory.

Classification	
Kingdom	Plantae – Plants
Subkingdom	Tracheobionta – Vascular plants
Superdivision	Spermatophyta – Seed plants
Division	Coniferophyta – Conifers
Class	Pinopsida –
Order	Pinales –
Family	Cupressaceae – Cypress family
Genus	Thuja L. – red cedar

Tribulus terrestris Linn

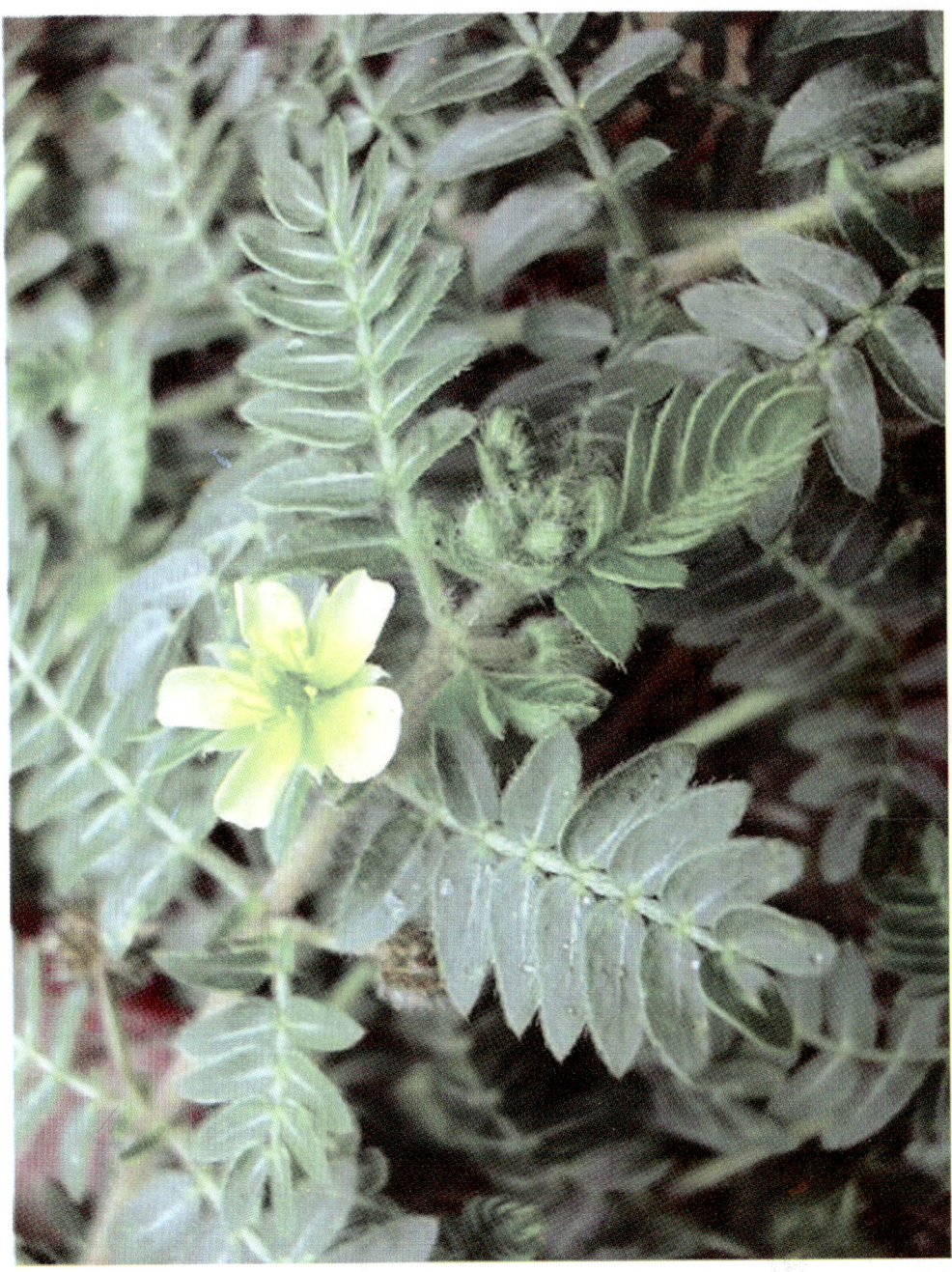

PLATE
123

Tribulus terrestris Linn

ZYGOPHYLLACEAE

Common Names

Eng	:	Small Caltrops
Hind	:	Chota gokhru
Sans	:	Ikshugandha
Ben	:	Gokhuri
Tam	:	Chrunerinche, Nerinji
Mal	:	Nerinnil, Neringil

Parts Used

Fruit & root

Constituents

Alkaloid, resin, fat, carbohydrates, β carotene, ascorbic acid, phytic acid phytate, oxalic acid, cinnamic amide derivative, terrestriamide, quercetin, diosgenic hecogenic, ruscogenic spirosta 3-, 5-diene

Uses

Amylase inhibitor, lipase activating activity, cooling, demulcent, diuretic, tonic, aphrodisiac

Classification	
Kingdom	Plantae – Plants
Subkingdom	Tracheobionta – Vascular plants
Superdivision	Spermatophyta – Seed plants
Division	Magnoliophyta – Flowering plants
Class	Magnoliopsida – Dicotyledons
Subclass	Rosidae –
Order	Sapindales –
Family	Zygophyllaceae – Creosote-bush family
Genus	Tribulus L. – punturevine

Tridax procumbens Linn

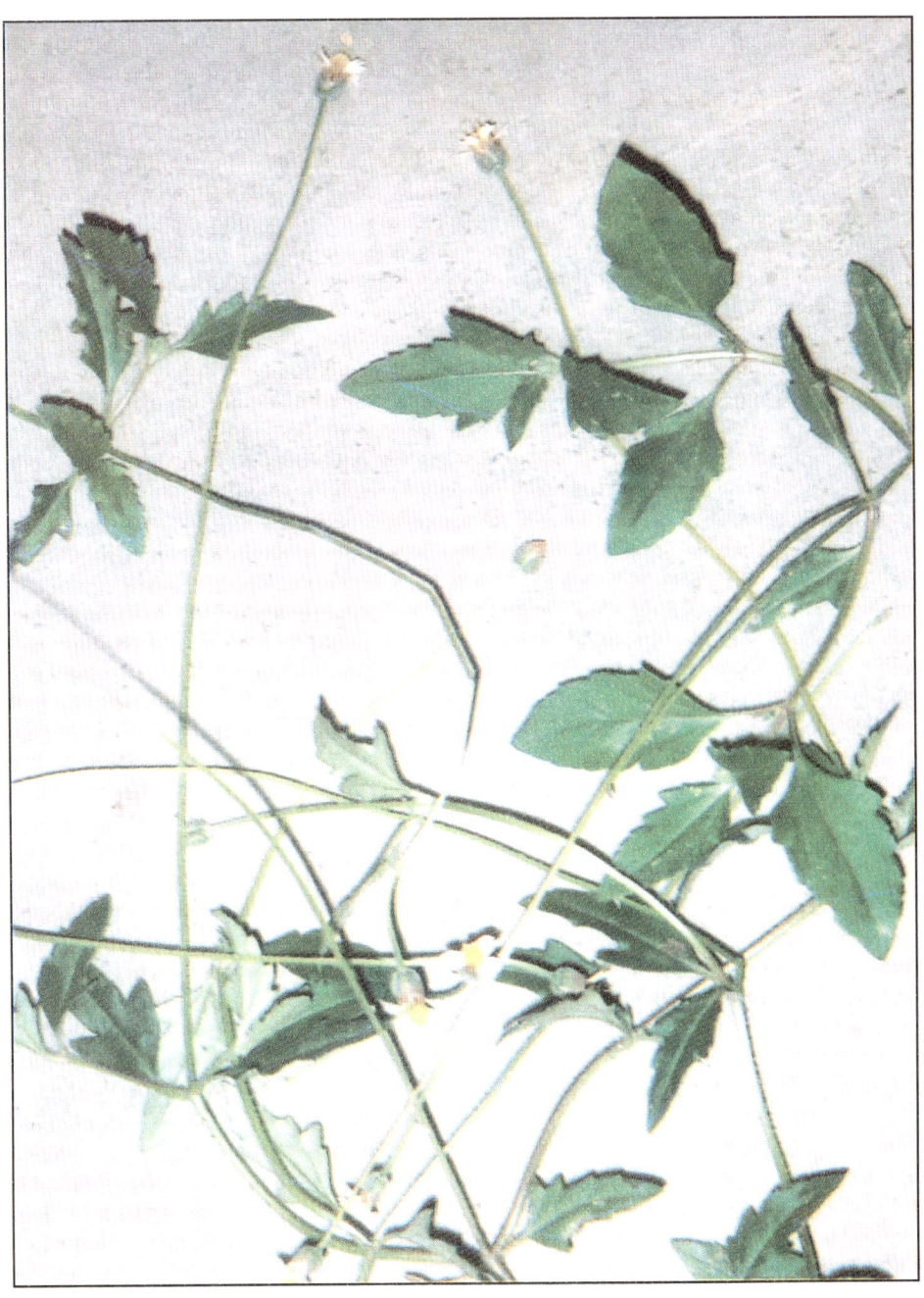

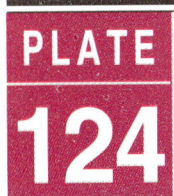

PLATE

124

Tridax procumbens Linn

COMPOSITAE

Common Names

Eng : Coat buttons
Tam : Vettukaya-thalai
Tel : Raavanaasuruditalakaai
Ka : Gabbu sanna savanthi

Parts Used

Whole plant

Constituents

Unsaponifiable fractions containing campesterol, stigmasterol, amyrin, sitosterol. Plant also contain fumaric acid, luteolin, quercitin, isoquercitin also esters.

Uses

Antidiarrhoel, antijuvenile, insect repellent, hepatoprotective.

Classification	
Kingdom	Plantae – Plants
Subkingdom	Tracheobionta – Vascular plants
Superdivision	Spermatophyta – Seed plants
Division	Magnoliophyta – Flowering plants
Class	Magnoliopsida – Dicotyledons
Subclass	Asteridae –
Order	Asterales –
Family	Asteraceae – Aster family
Genus	Tridax L. – tridax

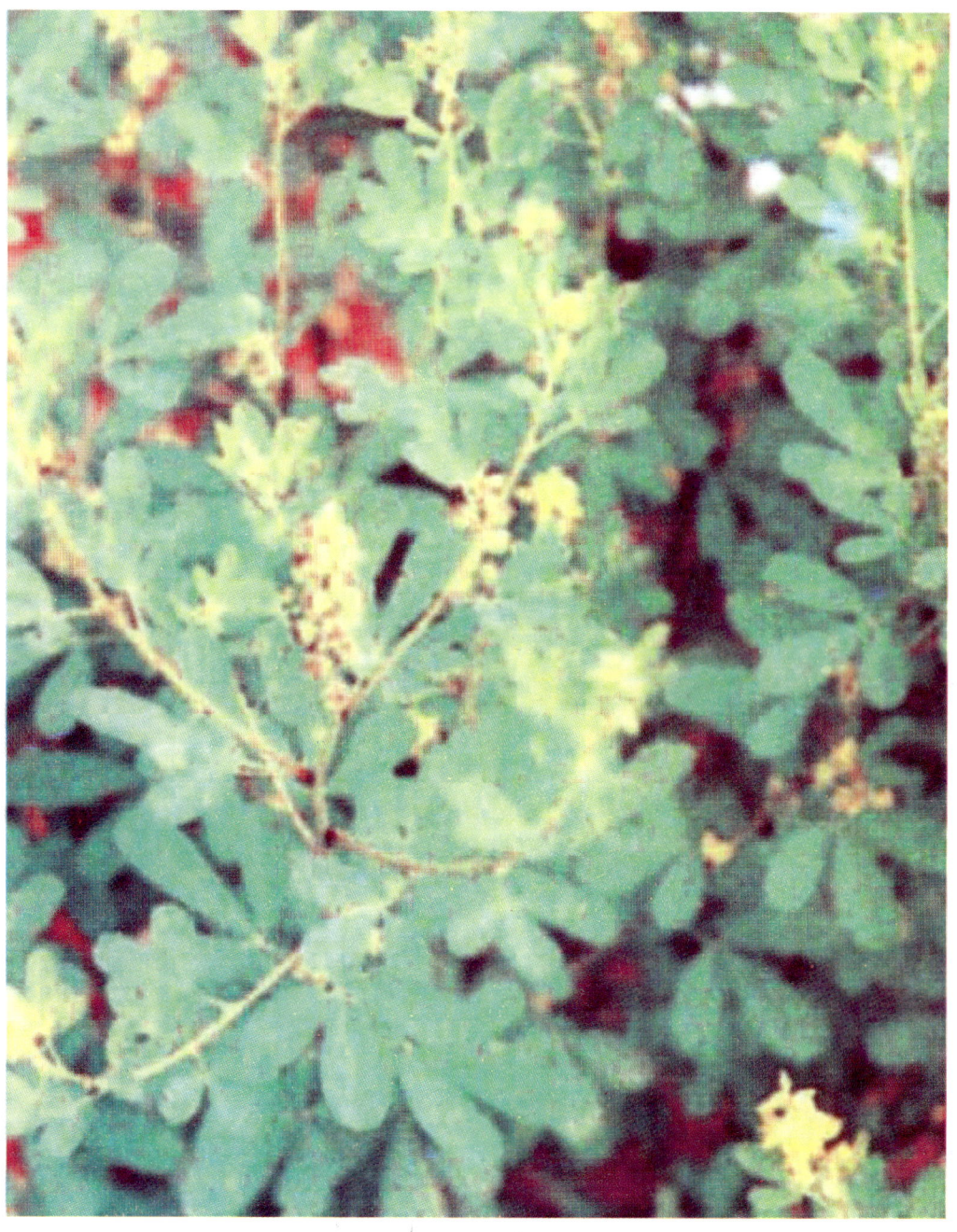

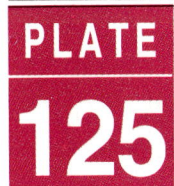

PLATE 125

Trigonella foenum graecum Linn

PAPILIONACEAE

Common Names

Eng	:	Fenugreek
Hind	:	Methi
Sans	:	Medhika
Ben	:	Methi
Tam	:	Vendayam
Mal	:	Uluva

Parts Used

Seeds, Pods, Leaves

Constituents

Globulin, albumin

Uses

Mucilaginous, demulcent, diuretic, tonic, carminative, emmenagogue, astringent, emollient, aphrodisiac.

Classification	
Kingdom	Plantae – Plants
Subkingdom	Tracheobionta – Vascular plants
Superdivision	Spermatophyta – Seed plants
Division	Magnoliophyta – Flowering plants
Class	Magnoliopsida – Dicotyledons
Subclass	Rosidae –
Order	Fabales –
Family	Fabaceae – Pea family
Genus	Trigonella L. – fenugreek

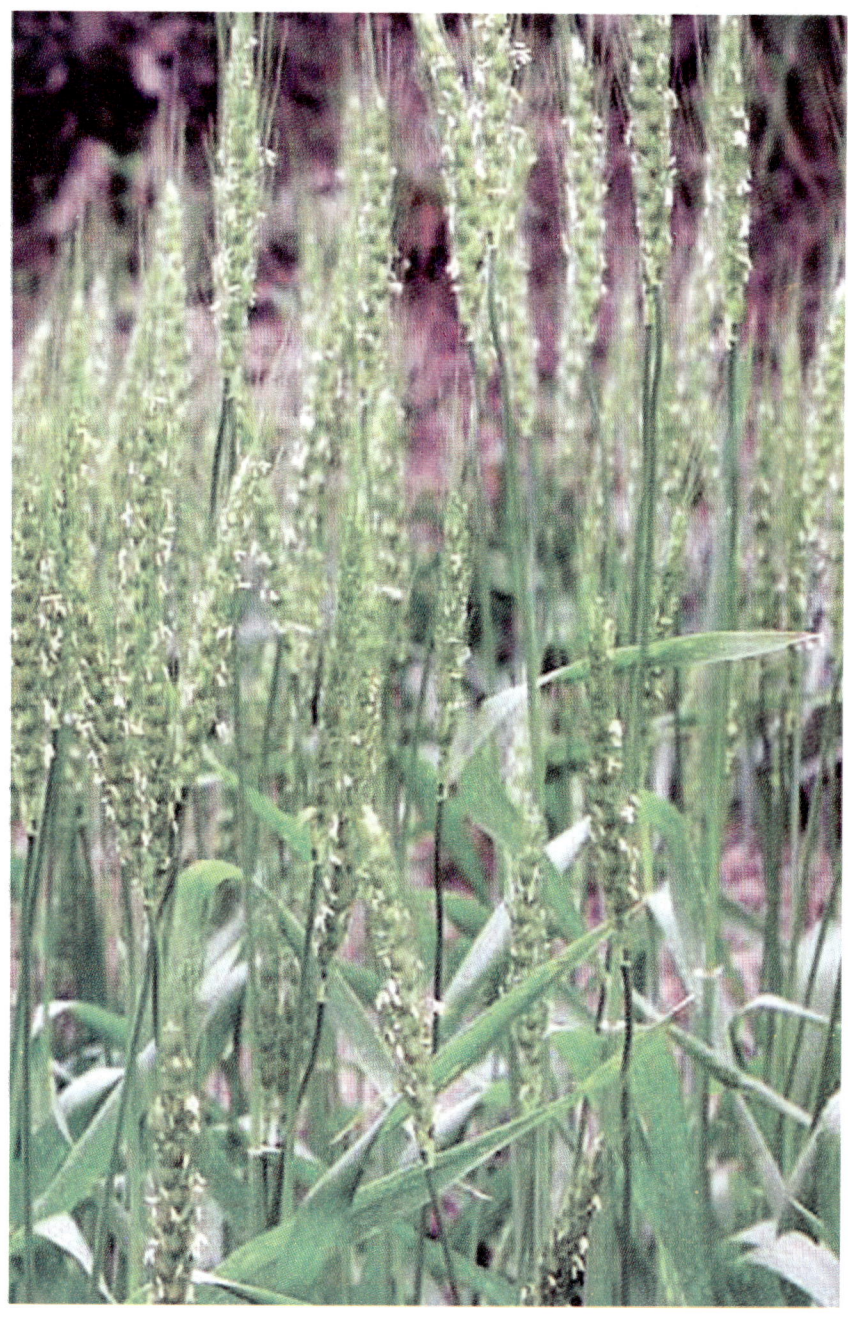

PLATE
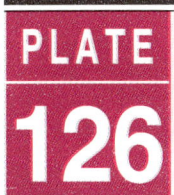
126

Triticum aestivum Linn

GRAMINAE

Common Names

Eng	:	Beardless wheat
Hin	:	Ghahun
Tam	:	Codambu
Mal	:	Godamb

Parts used

Grains

Constitunts

Fatty acid, linoleic acid, llinolenic acid, oleic acid, unsaponifiable matter, vitamin E is the main component of the unsaponifiable matter

Uses

Nutritional supplement, as a source of vitamine E, and fatty acid

Classification	
Kingdom	Plantae – Plants
Subkingdom	Tracheobionta – Vascular plants
Superdivision	Spermatophyta – Seed plants
Division	Magnoliophyta – Flowering plants
Class	Liliopsida – Monocotyledons
Subclass	Commelinidae –
Order	Cyperales –
Family	Poaceae – Grass family
Genus	Triticum L. – wheat

Verbascum thapsus Linn

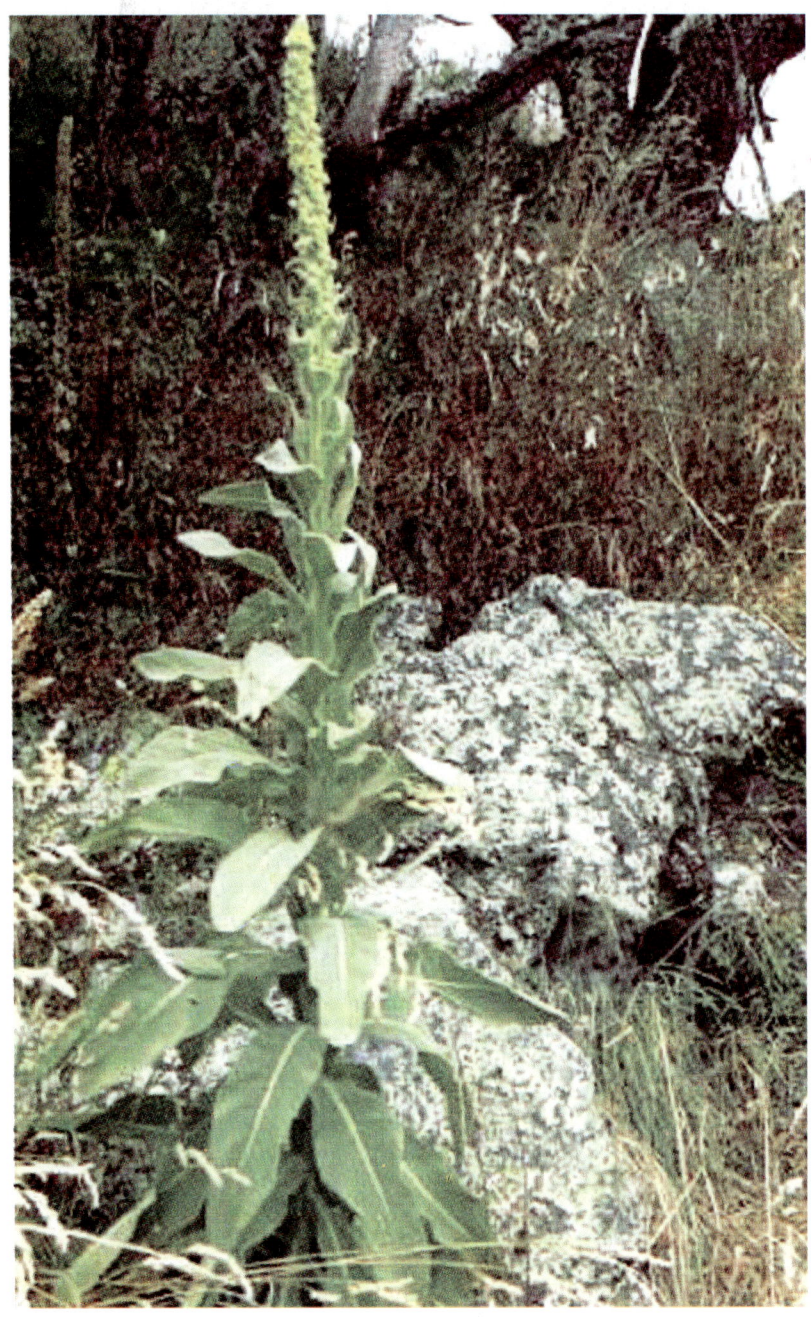

PLATE
127

Verbascum thapsus Linn

SCROPHULARIACEAE

Common Names

Eng : Common mullein
Hin : Gidar-tamaka
Pun : Valrphul
Urdu : Janglitamak

Parts used

Leaves, seeds, roots, flowers

Constituents

Flower contain volatile oil, fatty acids, leaves contain tannins, bitter principle, mucilage, saponin. Plant also contain irridoid glycosides, aucubin, sesquiterpenes, triglycosides of luteolin, verbascoside along with its aglycone. Leaves and flowers contains flavonoids.

Use

Demulcent, diuretic, antiseptic, anti asthmatic, pulmonary complaints, anti emetic, seeds are aphrodisiac, narcotic, astringent.

Classification	
Kingdom	Plantae – Plants
Subkingdom	Tracheobionta – Vascular plants
Superdivision	Spermatophyta – Seed plants
Division	Magnoliophyta – Flowering plants
Class	Magnoliopsida – Dicotyledons
Subclass	Asteridae –
Order	Scrophulariales –
Family	Scrophulariaceae – Figwort family
Genus	Verbascum L. – mullein

Vitex negundo Linn

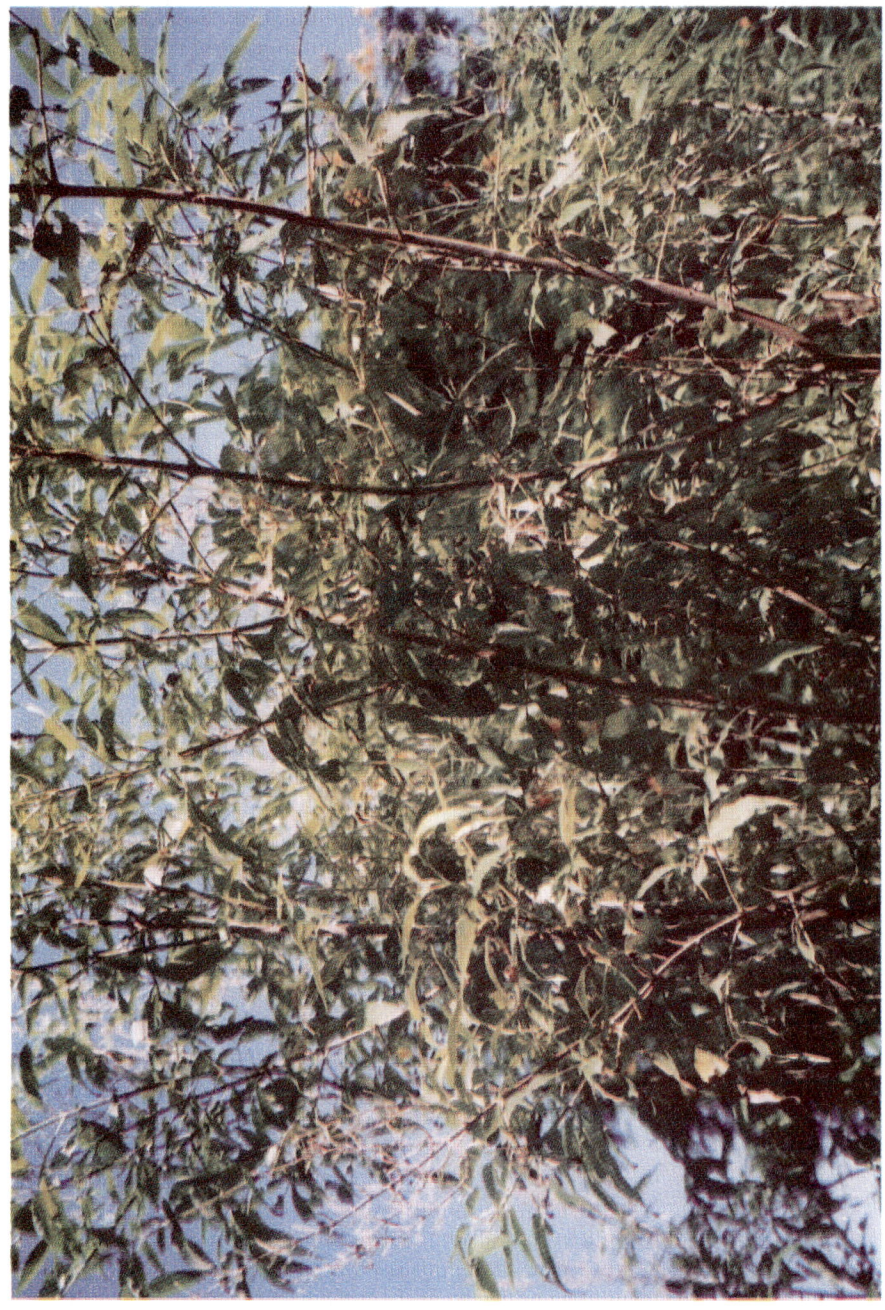

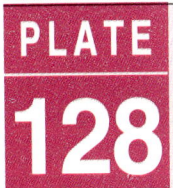

PLATE
128

Vitex negundo Linn

VERBENACEAE

Common Names

Eng	:	Indian Privet
Hind	:	Mewri,Nengai
Sans	:	Indrani Nilpushpa
Ben	:	Nirgundi,Nisinda
Tam	:	Nirkkundi Nochi
Mal	:	Indrani,Nochi,Vellanochi

Parts Used

Leaves, Bark, Root

Constituents

Glycoside, resin,essential oil, acid resin, organic acid, alkaloid, colouring matter, iridoid glycosides, isomeric flavanones, sitosterol, stigmasterol, vanillic acid, benzoic acid derivative, negundoside, nishindaside.

Uses

Antiseptic, stimulant, irritant, abortifacient, Juice of plant is antispasmodic, dyspepsia, emmenegogue, aphrodisiac, rubefacient.
Tonic, pungent, bitter acrid taste, astringent, stomachic, antehelminthic, promote growth of hair, in constipation, inflammation, leucoderma, asthma, painful teething of children, acute rheumatism, headache.

Classification	
Kingdom	Plantae – Plants
Subkingdom	Tracheobionta – Vascular plants
Superdivision	Spermatophyta – Seed plants
Division	Magnoliophyta – Flowering plants
Class	Magnoliopsida – Dicotyledons
Subclass	Asteridae –
Order	Lamiales –
Family	Verbenaceae – Verbena family
Genus	*Vitex* L. – chastetree

Withania somnifera Dunal

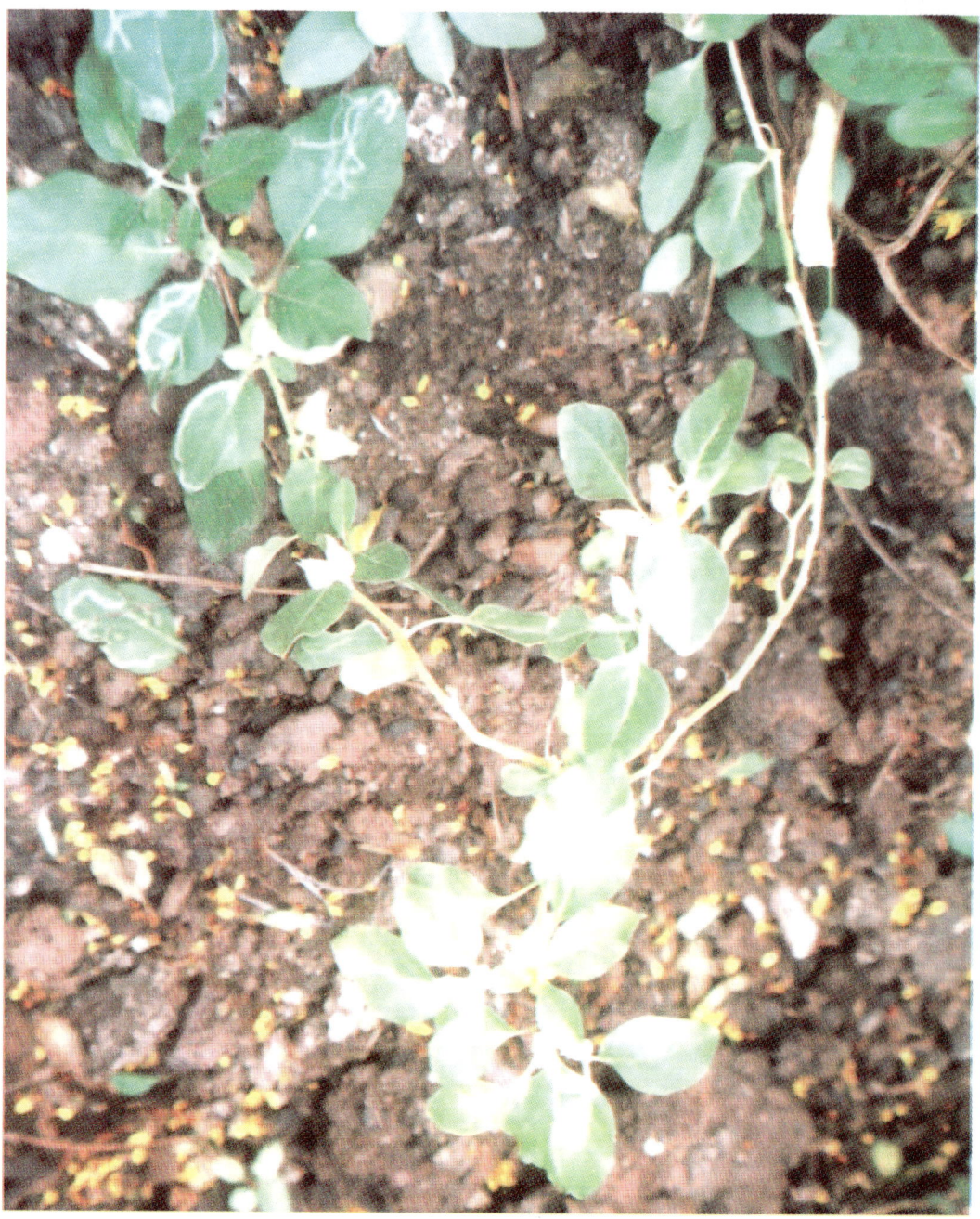

PLATE
129

Withania somnifera Dunal

SOLANACEAE

Common Names

Eng	:	Winter cherry
Hin	:	Asgandh
Sans	:	Ashvagandha
Tam	:	Achuvagandi
Mal	:	Pevette
Tel	:	Penneroo gadda

Parts used

Roots and rhizomes

Constituents

Withanolide is the main constituent, D-deoxyphysalo lactone, 5 β-oh-6x- cl-withanolide D and withanolide C, 5 dehydeoxy withanolide R, withasomniferin A, coagulin, withasomidienone, 2 glucowihanolide are also present.

Uses

Decrease the arterial diastolic blood pressure, it is classified as tranqulizer antidepressant, anti stress, anti inflammatory.

Classification	
Kingdom	Plantae – Plants
Subkingdom	Tracheobionta – Vascular plants
Superdivision	Spermatophyta – Seed plants
Division	Magnoliophyta – Flowering plants
Class	Magnoliopsida – Dicotyledons
Subclass	Asteridae –
Order	Solanales –
Family	Solanaceae – Potato family
Genus	Withania D – withania

Zea mays Linn

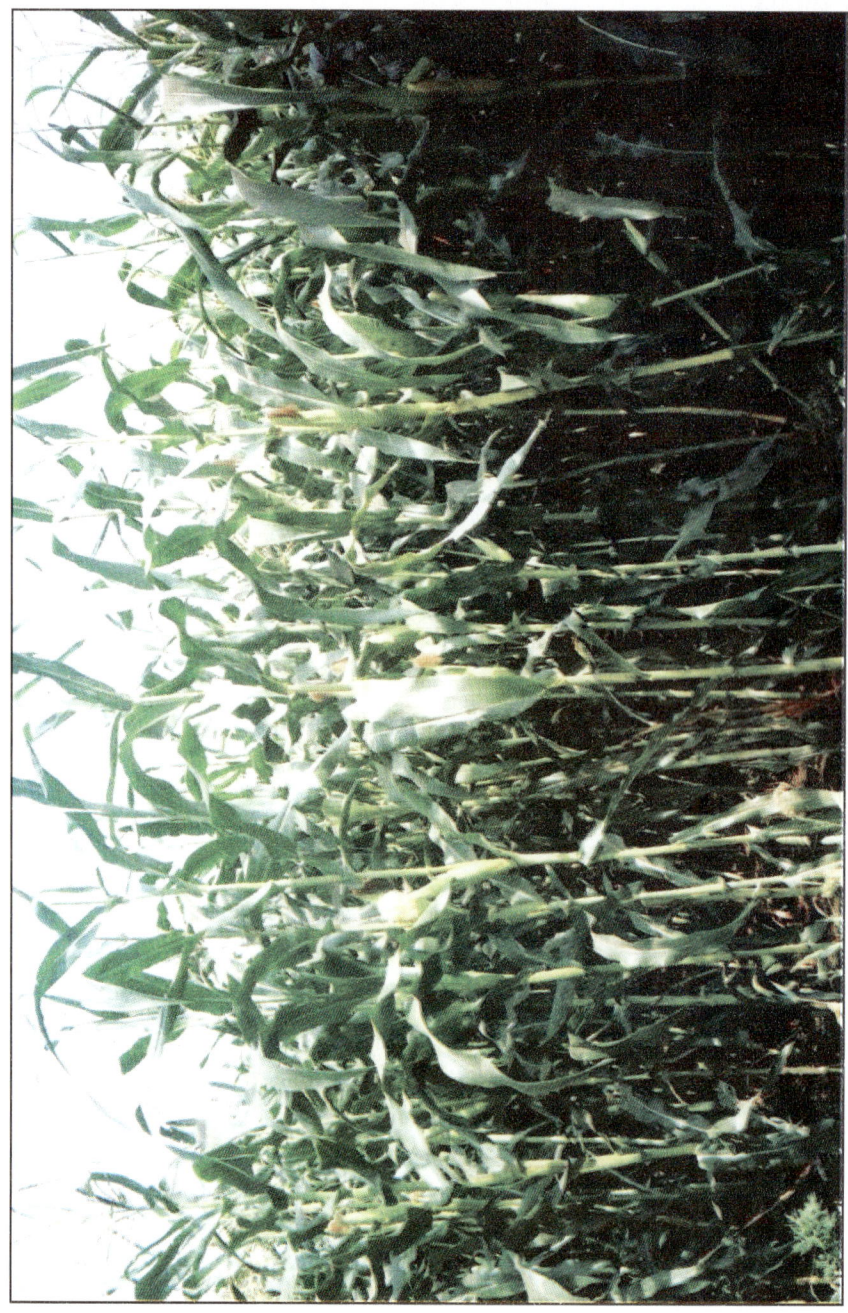

PLATE
130

Zea mays Linn

GRAMINEAE

Common Names

Eng	:	Maize, Indian corn
Hin	:	Makka, Bhutta
San	:	Yavanala
Ben	:	Bhuththe
Tam	:	Makka cholam
Mal	:	Cholam

Parts Used

Grains

Constituents

Polysaccharides, amylose, β amylose, amylopectin

Uses

Nutritive, demulcent, protective, absorbent.

Classification	
Kingdom	Plantae – Plants
Subkingdom	Tracheobionta – Vascular plants
Superdivision	Spermatophyta – Seed plants
Division	Magnoliophyta – Flowering plants
Class	Liliopsida – Monocotyledons
Subclass	Commelinidae –
Order	Cyperales –
Family	Poaceae – Grass family
Genus	Zea L. – corn

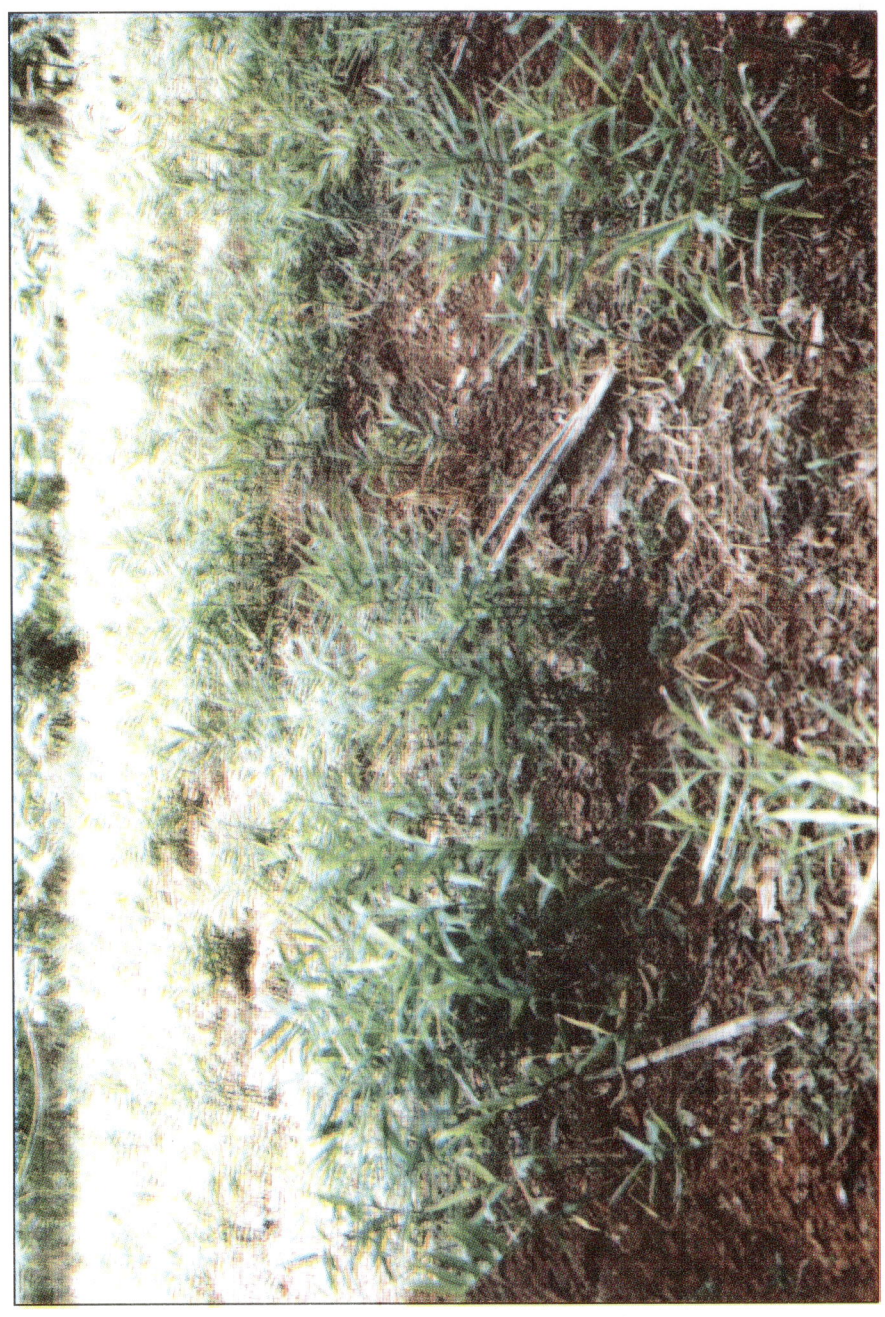

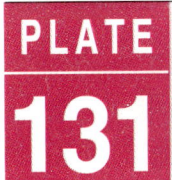

PLATE
131

Zingiber officinale Roscoe

ZINGIBERACEAE

Common Names

Eng	:	Ginger
Hind	:	Sonth
Sans	:	Srangavera
Ben	:	Sonth, Fresh-Adrak
Tam	:	Shukhu, Fresh-inji
Mal	:	Chukka, Fresh inji

Parts Used

Scraped and dried rhizome

Constituents

Aromatic volatile oil, camphene, phellandrene, zingiberene, cineol, borneol, gingerol.

Uses

Aromatic, stimulant, carminative, stomachic, digestive, local stimulant, rubefacient.

Classification	
Kingdom	Plantae – Plants
Subkingdom	Tracheobionta – Vascular plants
Superdivision	Spermatophyta – Seed plants
Division	Magnoliophyta – Flowering plants
Class	Liliopsida – Monocotyledons
Subclass	Zingiberidae –
Order	Zingiberales –
Family	Zingiberaceae – Ginger family
Genus	Zingiber P. Mill. – ginger

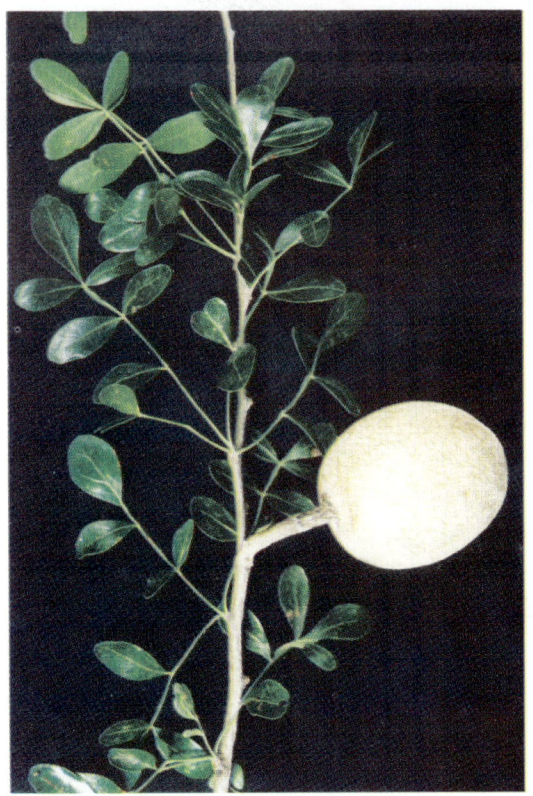

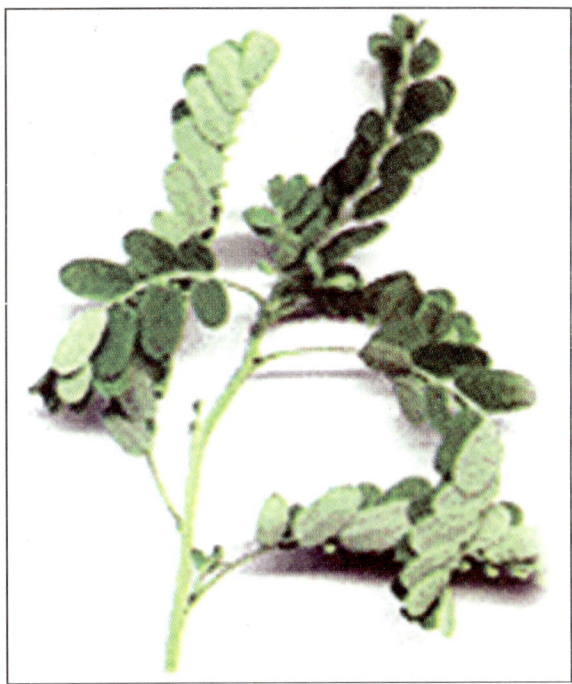

Phyllanthus niruri Linn

Feronia elephantum Corr

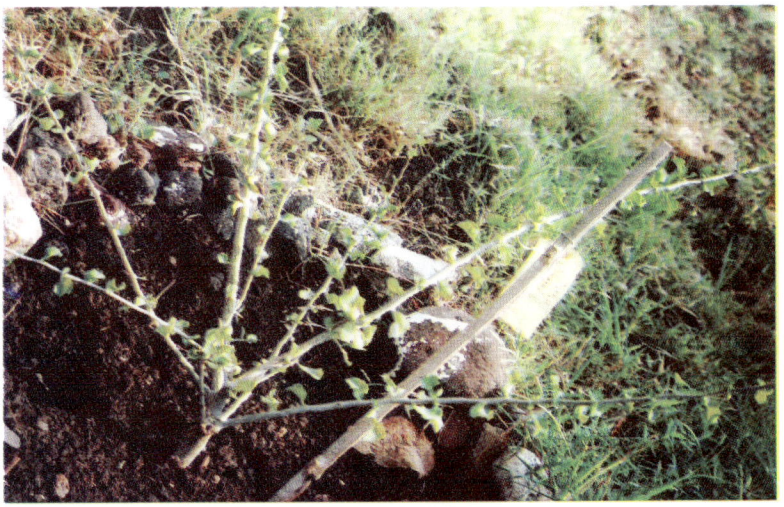

Commiphora weightii Arnott

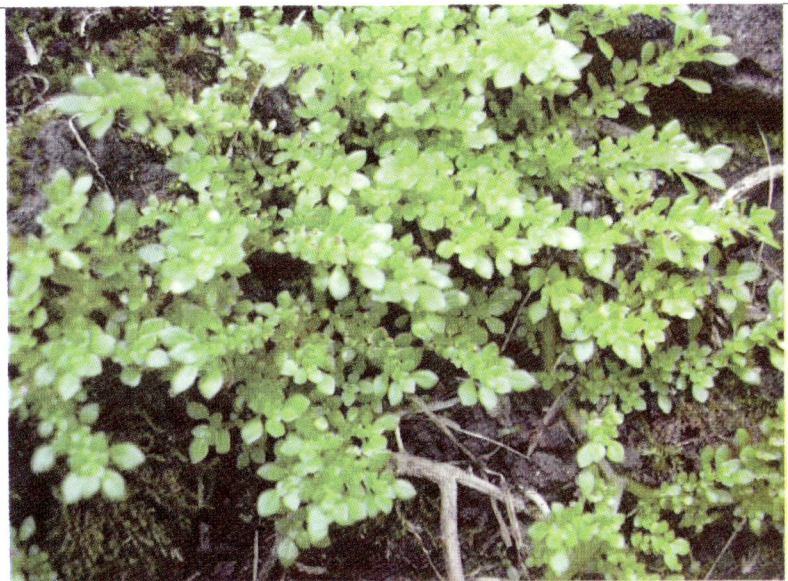

Pilea microphylla Liebm

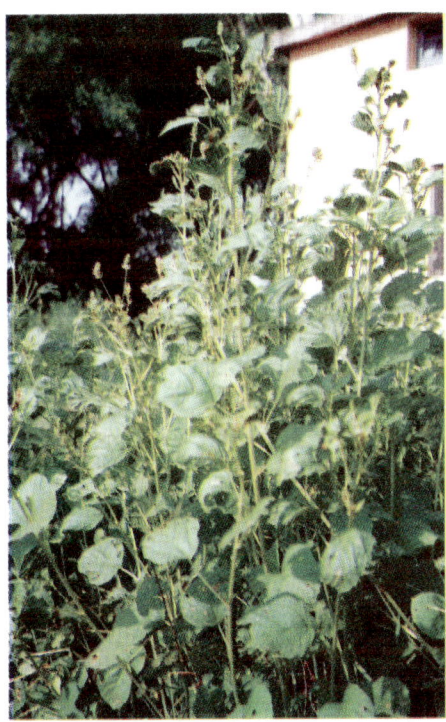

Coleus forskoli Poir

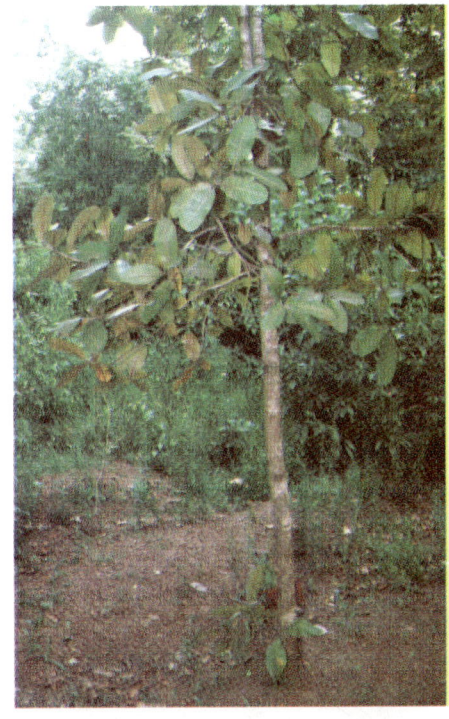

Semecarpus anacardium LinnReferences

References

- *Asima Chaterjee, Satyesh Chandra Prakashi, The treatise on Indian Medicinal Plants, Vol 6, Vol 1, National Institute of science communication, New Delhi, 2001.*

- *Bhattacharjee SK, Handbook of Medicinal Plants, 3rd Revised edition, Pointer Publishers, Jaipur, 2001*

- *Chopra RN, Chopra LC, Varma BS, Supplement to glossary of Indian Medicinal Plants 1st Edn reprint, Publications and Information Directorate, New Delhi, 1974.*

- *Gyanandra Pandey, Anticancer Herbal Drugs in India, 1st Edn, Sri Satguru Publication, Delhi, 2002.*

- *Gyanandra Pandey, Uncommon Plant drug of Ayurveda, 1st Edn, Sri Satguru Publication, Delhi, 1994.*

- *Guide to Popular Natural Product, Facts and Comparisons, 1999.*

- *Gupta KRL, Hindu Practice of Medicine, 2nd Edn, Sri Satguru Publication, Delhi, 1986.*

- *Indian Herbal Pharmacopoeia, Vol I, II, Indian Drug Mfgs Association Mumbai, Regional Research Laboratory Jammu Tawi, 1999.*

- *Indian Pharmacopoeia, Vol 1, 3rd edition, Ministry of Health and Family Welfare, Govt. of India, Controller of Publication, New Delhi, 1985.*

- *Jean Bruneton, Pharmacognosy, 2nd Edn, Lavoisier Publishing Inc, USA, 1999.*

- *Karnik CR, Pharmacology of Ayurvedic medicinal Plant, 1st Edn, Sri Satguru Publication, Delhi, 1996.*

- *Karnick CR, Pharmacopeial Standards of herbal plants Ist edition Vol I & II, Sri Satgara Publicators, Delhi, 1994.*

- *Kritikar KR, Basu BP, An ICS, Indian Medicinal Plants, 2nd Edn, Vol I-IV, Bishen Singh Mahendrapal Singh, DahraDun,2004.*

- *Kokate CK, Purohit AP, Gokhale SB, Pharmacognosy, 19th Edn, Nirali Prakashan, Delhi, 2002.*

- *Kurian JC, Plants that heals, 5th edn, Oriental watchman publishing house, Pune, 2003.*

- *Michael Mc Gufflin, Christopher Hobbs, Roy Upton Alicia Goldberg, Botanical Safety Handbook, Library of Congress Cataloging in Publication Data, 1999.*

- *Mohammed Ali, Text book of pharmacognosy, 1st Edn, CBS Publishers and Distributers, Delhi, 1994.*

- *Pal DC & Jain SK, Tribal Medicine, Ist edition, Naya Prakash, Calcutta, 1998.*

- *Rita Singh, Vedic Medicines, 1st Edn, Anmol Publications Pvt Ltd, Delhi, 1998.*

- *Sammabamurty AVSS, Subramanyam NS, Medicinal Plant in Industry, Ist edition, CBS Publishers distributors, New Delhi, 2000.*

- *Shiva MP, Alok Lehri M, Alka Shiva, Aromatic Medicinal Plants, International Book Distributors, Dehradun, 2002.*

- *Sivarajan VV and Balachandran I, Ayurvedic drugs and their plant sources, Oxford and IBH Publishing Co.Pvt. Ltd, New Delhi, 2002.*

- *Subhash R, Sunanda R and Pavanjape MH, Ayurvedic Treatment of Common diseases, Edn 1, Sri Satguru Publications, Delhi, 1999.*

- *Trease and Evans, Pharmacognosy, Edn 15, W.B.Saunders, London, 2002.*

- *The Wealth of India, Vol. 1-5, Publication and Information Directorate, Council for Scientific and Industrial Research, New Delhi, 1985.*

Index

BOTANICAL NAME	FAMILY	ENGLISH NAME	PAGE NO.
Daucus carota Linn	Umbelliferae	The carrot	111
Digitalis lanata Ehrh.	Scrophulariaceae	Grecian Fox glove	113
Digitalis purpurea Linn	Scrophulariaceae	Fox glove	115
Eclipta prostrata L	Compositae	False daisy	117
Elettaria cardamomum Maton	Zingiberaceae	Cardamom	119
Ephedra gerardiana Linn	Gnetaceae	Ephedra	121
Erythroxylum coca Lam	Erythroxylaceae	Coca leaves	123
Eucalyptus globulus Labill	Myrtaceae	Australian fever	125
Euphorbia hirta Linn	Euphorbiaceae	Australian asthma herb	127
Euphorbia neriifolia Linn	Euphorbiaceae	Common milk hedge	129
Evolvulus alsinoides Wall & Linn	Convolvulaceae	Slender dwarf morning-glory	131
Ferula assafoetida Linn	Umbelliferae	Asafoetida	133
Ficus bengalensis Linn	Urticaceae	Banyan Tree	135
Ficus glomerata Roxb	Moraceae	Cluster- fig	137
Ficus religiosa Linn	Moraceae	Sacred fig	139
Foeniculum vulgare Miller	Umbelliferae	Indian sweet fennel	141
Gaultheria procumbens L.	Ericaceae	Betula oil	143
Gentiana lutea L.	Gentianaceae	Yellow gentian	145
Ginkgo biloba L.	Ginkgoaceae	maiden hair tree	147
Glycyrrhiza glabra Linn	Papilionaceae	Sweet wood, Liquorice	149
Gossypium herbaceum Linn	Malvaceae	Cotton	151
Hibiscus rosasinensis Linn	Malvaceae	China rose, shoe flower plant	153
Holarrhena antidysenterica Wall	Apocynaceae	Kurchi, Tellicherry	155
Ipomoea batatas Poir	Convolvulaceae	Sweet potato	157
Jasminum grandiflorum Linn	Oleaceae	Spanish Jasmine	159
Jatropha curcus Linn	Euphorbiaceae	Angular leaved physic nut	161
Lantana camara Linn	Verbenaceae	Lantana, wild sage	163
Lawsonia inermis Linn	Lythraceae	Henna, Samphire	165
Mangifera indica Linn	Anacardiaceae	Mango	167
Manihot esculentum Pohl	Euphorbiaceae	Tapioca	169
Mentha arvensis Linn	Labiatae	Japanese mint	171
Mentha piperita Linn	Labiatae	Peppermint	173

BOTANICAL NAME	FAMILY	ENGLISH NAME	PAGE NO.
Mentha spicata Linn	Labiatae	Spearmint	175
Mimosa pudica Linn	Mimosaceae	Sensitive plant, humble plant	177
Momordica charantia Linn	Cucurbitaceae	Bitter gourd	179
Moringa oleifera Lam	Moringaceae	Horse radish	181
Murraya koenigii Linn	Rutaceae	Curry leaf	183
Musa paradisica Linn	Scitaminaceae	Banana	185
Nerium indicum Linn	Apocynaceae	Oleander	187
Nicotiana tabacum, Linn	Solanaceae	Tobacco	189
Ocimum basilicum Linn	Labiatae	Sweet basil	191
Ocimum sanctum Linn	Labiatae	Holy basil	193
Oryza sativa Linn	Graminae	Rice	195
Panax ginseng C. Meyer	Araliaceae	Chinese ginseng	197
Papaver somniferum Linn	Papaveraceae	Bale-wort	199
Passiflora edulis Sims	Passifloraraceae	Purple passion fruit	201
Passiflora foetida Linn	Passifloraraceae	Purple passion fruit	203
Passiflora mollisima Bailey	Passifloraraceae	Benana passion fruit	205
Passiflora quadrangularis Linn	Passifloraraceae	Giant granadilla	207
Phyllanthus emblica Linn	Euphorbiaceae	Indian Goose Berry	209
Piper longum Linn	Piperaceae	Dried catkins, long pepper	211
Piper nigrum Linn	Piperaceae	Black Pepper	213
Plantago ovata Forsk	Pantaginaceae	Ispaghula	215
Prunus amygdalis Baill.	Rosaceae	Almond	217
Psidium guajava L.	Myrtaceae	Guava	219
Punica granatum Linn.	Punicaceae	Pomegranate	221
Rauwolfia serpentina Benth	Apocynaceae	Serpentine wood	223
Ricinus communis Linn	Euphorbiaceae	Castor Oil	225
Ruta graveolens Linn	Rutaceae	Common Rue	227
Santalum album Linn	Santalaceae	White Sandal Wood	229
Sida cordifolia Linn	Malvaceae	Llima	231

333 305